Immunopathology

Sixth International Convocation on Immunology

Organizing Committee

Boris Albini
Giuseppe A. Andres
Ernst H. Beutner

Joseph H. Kite, jr.
Morris Reichlin
Felix Milgrom, Chairman

**Sixth International Convocation
on Immunology**

Niagara Falls, N.Y., June 12–15, 1978

Immunopathology

Editors
Felix Milgrom and Boris Albini,
Buffalo, N.Y.

74 figures and 62 tables, 1979

S. Karger
Basel · München · Paris
London · New York · Sydney

International Convocations on Immunology

National Library of Medicine Cataloging in Publication
  International Convocation on Immunology, 6th, Niagara Falls, N.Y., 1978
  Immunopathology/editors, Felix Milgrom and Boris Albini.—Basel; New York: Karger, 1979
  Sponsored by the Center for Immunology of the State University of New York at Buffalo
  1. Immunology—congresses 2. Pathology—congresses I. Milgrom, Felix, ed. II. Albini, Boris, ed.
  III. State University of New York at Buffalo. Center for Immunology
  W3 IN6856 6th 1978 i/QW 504.3 I5li 1978
  ISBN 3-8055-2971-6

© Copyright 1979 by S. Karger AG, 4011 Basel (Switzerland), Arnold-Böcklin-Strasse 25
Typeset by Asco Trade Typesetting Ltd., Hongkong
Printed in Switzerland by Thür AG Offsetdruck, Pratteln

ISBN 3-8055-2971-6

Contents

Immunologically Mediated Systemic Diseases

Immunopathology of Infectious Diseases

Effector Mechanisms in Immunopathology

Workshops

Acknowledgements

The Center for Immunology and the Convocation Committee gratefully acknowledge the generous contributions in support of this convocation from

Abbott Laboratories
Biological Corporation of America
Biotest-Serum Institut GmbH
Burroughs Wellcome Company
Ciba-Geigy Corporation
Corning Medical
Cutter Laboratories, Inc.
E. I. du Pont de Nemours & Company, Inc.
Hoffmann-LaRoche Inc.
Hooker Chemicals & Plastics Corporation
S. Karger AG

Lederle Laboratories
Mallinckrodt, Inc.
Merck Sharp & Dohme Research Laboratories
Ortho Diagnostics Inc.
Rochester Scientific Company, Inc.
The Squibb Institute for Medical Research
State University of New York at Buffalo
Technicon Corporation
Medical Products Division, Union Carbide Corporation
Wampole Laboratories
Warner-Lambert/Parke-Davis

Introduction

At the beginning of the immunological era, those beneficial immune mechanisms were studied which permit man and animals to recover from infectious diseases and to resist repeated infections.

Jules Bordet was the first to show that not only microorganisms and their products but also completely harmless foreign substances are antigenic and elicit immune responses. Furthermore, he demonstrated that serum of a guinea pig immunized with rabbit red blood cells would cause disease and death when injected into rabbits. This and other observations made *Ehrlich and Morgenroth* coin the term *horror autotoxicus*, 'fear of self-poisoning', to point out that a healthy man or animal would refuse formation of autoantibodies, i.e., antibodies combining with autologous antigens. *Ehrlich and Morgenroth* realized that the lack of formation of autoantibodies is a rather complex phenomenon requiring some immunologic homeostatic mechanisms. As early as 1900 they spoke about the existence of anti-autolysins which prevent the appearance of autolysins and therefore serve as guardians of the *horror autotoxicus* principle. One cannot help admiring these intuitive statements which predicted what we now call anti-idiotypic antibodies and their role in controlling autoimmunity.

Since the very beginning of the 20th century, formation of autoantibodies, both harmful and harmless, was described under natural and experimental conditions. The pathogenic role of immune responses to autologous antigens has been studied by many investigators. In this country, these studies were pioneered by *Ernest Witebsky* and *William Dameshek*. One of the editors of this volume had the unique privilege to co-chair with these two investigators a comprehensive conference on 'Autoimmunity' organized by the New York Academy of Sciences precisely 13 years ago.

Studies on immediate hypersensitivity reactions initiated in 1902 were continued quite extensively. With his description of serum sickness, *von Pirquet* initiated important studies on the pathogenic role of immune complexes.

The pathogenicity of immune mechanisms active in the course of an infectious disease was clearly described in 1890 by *Robert Koch* in his studies on tuberculosis. Thereafter, many instances of immunopathologic lesions in infectious diseases have been documented.

It is rather obvious that immunological mechanisms quite frequently bring more harm than benefit. Still, it is difficult to condemn the basically teleological immune mechanisms. The damage which they inflict may be conceived as the result of their overeagerness to help, a crime of passion. The field of immunopathology is almost as old as the science of immunology. During over ninety years, studies conducted in this field have made most significant contributions to the practice of medicine.

This book summarizes the proceedings of the *Sixth International Convocation on Immunology*. The organizing committee of this convocation undertook the ambitious goal of preparing a program that would review comprehensively the field of immunopathology. The committee considered it very appropriate that this meeting should be organized by the academic community of Buffalo where immunopathological studies, initiated by *Ernest Witebsky* in the late 1940s, have been conducted in the Department of Microbiology and The Center for Immunology for three decades. The committee succeeded to assemble at this meeting most of the leading research workers in the field. All of them are our friends and many of them had been previously associated with us. It was attempted to achieve a balance between authoritative reviews of well-established concepts and reports on recent data and new hypotheses. We hope that this book will be both informative and provocative. *F. M.*

B. A.

Self-Recognition

Immunopathology. 6th Int. Convoc. Immunol., Niagara Falls, N.Y., 1978, pp. 1–6 (Karger, Basel 1979)

Is Autoimmunity an Aberration of Physiological Mechanisms?

Pierre Grabar

Institut Pasteur, Paris

All observable pathological phenomena may be exaggerations or inhibitions of physiological mechanisms, with the exception of those cases in which exogeneous agents intervene. Applying this concept, I envisaged the formation of autoantibodies (auto-Abs) not as an aberration of a defense mechanism, but as an exaggeration of a normal physiological mechanism. In simple organisms, nutrition is realized by phagocytosis. This phenomenon exists in all animals, and I assume that it would have disappeared during evolution if it were not necessary. In higher animals, phagocytosis is facilitated by opsonization due to Abs. Thus, one may suppose that Abs participate in a mechanism derived from nutrition. The blood transports many varied and important substances, such as O_2, CO_2, lipids, metals, enzymes, hormones, vitamins, etc., such transport being effected by carriers specific for these substances.

In 1947, and particularly in 1953 at the International Microbiological Congress in Rome [16, 17], I proposed the consideration of the immunoglobulins (at that time known only as 'γ-globulins') as specific 'transporteurs' of metabolic and catabolic products. Evidently, when transporting catabolic products, they are auto-Abs and I assumed that they should be considered as a normal physiological phenomenon.

Some observations can be interpreted as showing the role of Abs as specific 'transporteurs' of metabolites, for example the appearance of Abs to milk proteins in children fed with milk [10], the presence of anti-bovine serum albumin Abs in dogs nourished with beef [18] and mice receiving bovine serum albumin *per os* [2], the reaction of normal sera with glycogen [18], etc. The formation of Abs to nutritional products occurs because these substances escaped total degradation by digestive enzymes.

As mentioned previously, the 'transporteurs' of catabolites are auto-Abs. In a large number of publications, it has been shown that auto-Abs exist normally, that they can appear and that they can be induced experimentally, particularly when Freund's adjuvant is used. In the majority of known cases of the appearance of auto-Abs, destructive or necrotic lesions of certain tissues are observed and the auto-Abs react specifically with components of these tissues [20]. If we assume that, in the particularly interesting case of the NZB mouse, the etiology of the observed anomalies is viral, it is possible to explain the appearance of several different auto-Abs as the virus may attack numerous tissues including the thymus. The experimental induction of auto-Abs against erythrocytes has been achieved in another strain of mice by the injection of their own red blood cells previously heated to 49 °C [22].

The existence of auto-Abs has been also demonstrated in normal sera, for example: (a) All human sera contain cryoagglutinins [12]. (b) Human serum contains panagglutinins which agglutinate red or white cells of the same organism which have been previously treated with neuraminidase or a protease [34]. These panagglutinins opsonize aging cells, which are then phagocytosed. *Kay* [25] has observed that aged erythrocytes have IgG on their surface. (c) Auto-Abs reacting with degradation products of different classes of immunoglobulin [33] and with fibrinogen cleavage products [32] have been detected in normal human and animal sera. (d) It has been known for a long time that the serum of adult snakes neutralizes their own venom [9]. (e) Nearly all normal sera contain Abs to myelin, which are non-pathogenic [14]. (f) Sera of healthy persons may contain Abs capable of reacting with various tissue extracts, and also with elastin [20], nuclear components [26] and even nucleic acids [9]. Sera of young SJL/J mice also contain antinuclear factors and anti-RNA Abs [7]. In general, the quantity of auto-Abs in human or animal sera increases with age. This may be due to the development of various lesions during life. More auto-Abs can certainly be found in normal sera by the use of very sensitive methods. For example, *Jormalainen and Mäkelä* [24], using the particularly sensitive method of phage labelling, found that normal sera contain Abs reacting with various haptens. Generally, the search for auto-Abs is only undertaken when pathological phenomena are observed, whereas they may also exist in the absence of such phenomena, when routine analysis is not performed. The probable existence of complexes of auto-Abs with autoantigens (auto-Ags) in normal sera may render the detection of auto-Abs more difficult. We may conclude that auto-Abs exist normally and that they can appear as a consequence of abundant tissue destruction, microbial- or viral-induced lesions, thermal injury, etc., and that they may be considered to be an exaggeration of a normal physiological mechanism, the formation of 'transporteurs' of catabolic products.

In an attempt to explain the mechanism involved, I will consider two of the important steps in Ab formation; the first of which is the recognition of the immunogenicity of the Ag and the last step which is the actual synthesis of a specific Ig, a process which is certainly dependent upon genetic information.

It is well known that rabbits, in contrast to mice, do not form Abs to pneumococcal polysaccharides when injected with purified polysaccharides, but form such Abs well when injected with pneumococci. Thus, they possess cells capable of synthesizing these Abs, and if they do not respond, there must be another reason. In addition, it is known that some children are incapable of forming certain Abs. The same also exists in certain animal species or strains. These cases could be explained as being due to a genetic absence of cells capable of synthesizing the corresponding Abs, but it seems established [5] that the genetic factors influencing the formation of Abs to certain Ags relate to the activity of T cells and not the B cells which actually synthesize the Ab molecule. Thus, in these cases genetic control intervenes in the mechanism of Ab formation at a step other than the final synthesis of the Ab molecule. The existence of genetic enzyme deficiencies are well known [13], and we may suppose that they interfere with the normal immunological mechanisms. Whatever the final step of Ab formation, however, the actual synthesis must be the same for Abs to both self and non-self Ags and cells capable of such synthesis must be present normally since the appearance of both categories of Abs can be induced experimentally.

For many years and again recently [19, 20], I have proposed that the simplest explanation of self recognition is that under normal conditions, self Ags are degraded and lose their immunogenicity. In cases where this degradation does not occur and the auto-Ags remain intact, they are immunogenic. Recently, *Mehta* [29] proposed a concept similar to my old hypothesis.

In pathological cases of auto-Ab formation, as mentioned earlier, abundant destruction of cells or tissues can generally be observed. The degradation of their constituents by autolytic enzymes is inhibited because the excess of substrates inhibits the enzymatic activity and, consequently, these constituents retain their immunogenicity. In experimentally induced auto-Ab formation, Freund's adjuvant is almost always used. As has been established, this adjuvant inhibits proteolytic enzymes [27] and thus the degradation of auto-Ags can be avoided and their immunogenicity preserved.

Enzymatic processes have been observed to play an important role in immunogenicity, for example: (a) *Ryan and Lee* [35] found a correlation between resistance to protein degradation by macrophages and immunogenicity. (b) The formation of Abs to nucleic acids can be achieved if these substances are injected in a form in which they are not degraded by nucleases, whereas, if injected in a pure form, degradation occurs and no Abs are produced [31]. (c) *Sela et al.* [36] have observed that the formation of Abs to a certain polypeptide in different strains of mice depends upon differences in the rate of metabolism of this Ag. (d) The importance of the rate of metabolic degradation of erythrocytes and of some bacterial Ags in the antibody response of high and low Ab producer strains has been studied by *Biozzi et al.* [8]. In both cases, slower degradation favors the formation of Abs.

It is well known that it is easier to induce auto-Abs when modified auto-Ags or cross-reacting Ags are used. This again seems to indicate that it is the immunogenicity which is important. Cells capable of forming auto-Abs are present, but the metabolism of the modified Ags used may be different from that of the native Ags, thus explaining the difference in response. We may conclude that the role of enzymes is very important in the first step of auto-Ab formation, that is the immunogenicity of self Ags. This concept is particularly simple, based on well-known facts, and does not need particular *ad hoc* hypothesis. It does not, however, exclude some other possible mechanisms.

In the induction of experimental tolerance, it is assumed that the Ag can exist in a tolerogenic form, but the characteristics of this form are not well established. The simplest example is probably that in which non-polymerized IgG can act as tolerogen whereas the polymerized molecule does not induce tolerance. It is thus possible that auto-Ags could also exist in a tolerogenic form, for example, as partially degraded molecules. *Ada et al.* [1] induced tolerance to an undegraded Ag by use of its degradation products and *Benjamin and Hershey* [6] with degradation products of bovine serum albumin. At the present time, it remains uncertain if, in general, Ags must act as a complete molecule or must first be degraded. For example, according to *Ault et al.* [4], non-metabolizable Ags can induce tolerance; this can be interpreted as suggesting that the Ag must be metabolizable to be immunogenic. On the other hand, we have induced Abs in the rabbit to hidden groupings of a native protein [15] which would mean that this Ag was modified following injection.

Although the exact process of activation of the immunocompetent cell is not well established, the possibility exists that a tolerogen can block this mechanism. With Mrs. *Escribano*, we have shown that the formation of Abs specific for a chemical hapten in rats by their immunization with this hapten coupled with a carrier protein can be inhibited by previous injections of the same free and non-reactive hapten [21]. Thus, a small molecule containing only one determinant group is capable of inducing a certain degree of tolerance. The same mechanism may occur with incompletely degraded self Ags.

Calne et al. [11] have shown that a prolongation of renal allograft survival in pigs can be obtained by injections of large quantities of serum or of spleen extracts. In human transplantation, previous multiple transfusions (particularly of donor serum) enhance graft survival. *Hasek et al.* [23] have induced graft tolerance in the rat by the injection of sera from donor strain rats. Experiments performed by *Feldman* and co-workers [37] have shown that serum constituents can inhibit the sensitization of self cells. Components possessing the specificity of transplantation Ags have been detected in and even isolated from the serum [30]. These substances may act as tolerogens and are probably degradation products of histocompatibility Ags.

Many different explanations of autoimmunization have been proposed. I think that the theory of forbidden clones and the intervention of somatic mutations in the mechanism of autoimmunization have been abandoned. I exclude also the proposed idea that auto-Ags must be modified and thus become in some way foreign to the organism. It is true that modified self Ags more readily induce auto-Abs, but these Abs once formed exhibit equal reactivity with the unmodified determinants of the native Ag. It has also been suggested that auto-Abs are formed following the uncovering of self Ags which normally have no contact with immunocompetent cells. However, we now know that auto-Abs are also formed against tissues in continuous contact with the blood, such as liver [3], or even Igs [33] and serum albumin

[28]. Thus this suggestion cannot be proposed as a general mechanism, although hidden self Ags are possibly more highly immunogenic.

On the contrary, it is evident that suppressor cells, their products and thymic hormones play an important role. If the soluble suppressor factors are Ag-specific, it is possible that they modulate the immunogenicity of auto-Ags and that enzymatic processes may be involved. They may, however, act at another step in the mechanism of Ab formation, but this problem will be considered in other reports.

In summary, my concept is that the self-recognition is mainly enzymatic. Under normal conditions, auto-Ags are degraded by autolytic enzymes and become non-immunogenic or possibly tolerogenic. In cases of tissue destruction provoked by exogenous agents, however, the abundance of available tissue components inhibits the activity of the enzymes present. The non-degraded self Ags are immunogenic, and induce auto-Ab formation. The actual synthesis of the specific Igs is the same for Abs to both self and non-self Ags. In both cases, the main role of these Abs is the cleaning up of the organism, and thus, they participate in the same physiological mechanism as 'transporteurs' of metabolic and catabolic products. This concept does not exclude the intervention of suppressor cells and of thymic factors, which may even participate in the mechanism described.

References

1 Ada, G. L.; André, C.; Lambert, R.; Bazin, H., and Heremans, J. F.: The tissue localization, immunogenic and tolerance-inducing properties of antigens and antigen fragments. Cold Spring Harb. Symp. *32*: 381–393 (1967).
2 André, C.; Parish, C. R.; Nossal, G. J. V., and Abbot, A.: Interference of oral immunization with the intestinal absorption of heterologous albumins. Eur. J. Immunol. *4*: 701–704 (1974).

3 Arnason, B.; Salomon, J. C. et Grabar, P.: Anticorps antifoie et anti-immunoglobulines sériques chez les souris classiques et axéniques; étude comparative par nécrose aiguë provoquée par le tetrachlorure de carbone. C. r. hebd. Séanc. Acad. Sci., Paris 259: 4882–4885 (1964).

4 Ault, K. A.; Unanue, E. R.; Katz, D. H., and Benacerraf, B.: Failure of lymphocytes to reexpress antigen receptors after brief interaction with a tolerogenic D-amino acid copolymer. Proc. natn. Acad. Sci. USA 71: 3111–3114 (1974).

5 Benacerraf, B.: The genetic mechanisms that control the immune response and antigen recognition. Annls. Immunol. Inst. Pasteur, Paris 125C: 143–164 (1974).

6 Benjamin, D. C. and Hershey, C. W.: The termination of immunological unresponsiveness to the cyanogen bromide fragments of BSA in rabbits J. Immun. 113: 1593–1598 (1974).

7 Bentwich, Z.; Bonavida, B.; Peled, A., and Haran-Ghera, N.: Evaluation of auto-antibodies and serum abnormalities in SJL/J mice (abstr.). Israel J. med. Scis. 8: 670 (1972).

8 Biozzi, G.; Stiffel, C.; Mouton, D.; Bouthillier, Y. et Decreusefond, C.: La régulation génétique de la synthèse des immunoglobulines au cours de la réponse immunologique. Annls. Immunol. Inst. Pasteur, Paris 125C: 107–142 (1974).

9 Boquet, P.: Venins des serpents (Flammarion, Paris 1948).

10 Burgin-Wolff, A. und Gerger, E.: Die Bildung von Antikörpern gegen verschiedene Kuhmilch-Proteine bei Neugeborenen, Kindern, Erwachsenen und Graviden. Experientia 19: 22–23 (1963).

11 Calne, R. Y.; Davis, D. R.; Hadjiyannakis, E.; Sells, R. A.; White, D.; Herbertson, B. M.; Millard, P. R.; Joysey, V. C.; Davies, D. A. L.; Binns, R. M., and Festenstein, H.: Immunosuppressive effects of soluble cell membrane fractions, donor blood and serum on renal allograft survival. Nature, Lond. 227: 903–906 (1970).

12 Dacie, J. V.: Occurrences in normal human sera of 'incomplete' forms of cold auto-antibodies. Nature, Lond. 166: 36 (1950).

13 Dreyfus, J. C.: Bases moléculaires des maladies enzymatiques génétiques. Biochimie 54: 559–571 (1972).

14 Edington, T. S. and Delessio, D. J.: The assessment by immunofluorescence methods of humoral anti-myelin antibodies in man. J. Immun. 105: 248–255 (1970).

15 Escribano, M. J.; Keilova, H. et Grabar, P.: Etude de la gliadine et de la gluténine après réduction ou oxydation. Biochim. biophys. Acta 127: 94–100 (1966).

16 Grabar, P.: Les globulines du sérum sanguin (Desoer, Liège 1947).

17 Grabar, P.: Mise en évidence par hémagglutination passive de réactions de divers sérums normaux avec quelques substances macromoléculaires. 6th Congr. Int. Microbiol., Rome 1953, vol. 2, pp. 303–304.

18 Grabar, P.: Réaction de divers sérums normaux avec des substances macromoléculaires naturelles ou synthétiques. Annls. Inst. Pasteur, Paris 88: 11–23 (1955).

19 Grabar, P.: Formation d'auto-anticorps et leurs activités. Annls. Inst. Pasteur, Paris 118: 393–402 (1970).

20 Grabar, P.: Hypothesis. Auto-antibodies and immunological theories. Clin. Immun. Immunopath. 4: 453–466 (1975).

21 Grabar, P. et Escribano, M. J.: Induction de tolérance immunitaire par des haptènes libres non réactifs. C. r. hebd. Séanc. Acad. Sci., Paris 282D: 1833–1836 (1976).

22 Halpern, B. et Bourdon, G.: Syndrome immunohématologique expérimental ayant des caractères de l'anémie hémolytique autoimmune. C. r. hebd. Séanc. Acad. Sci., Paris 173D: 2712–2717 (1971).

23 Hašek, M.; Chutná, I.; Holáň, V., and Sládeček, M.: Induction of transplantation tolerance using serum as antigen source. Nature, Lond. 262: 295–296 (1976).

24 Jormalainen, S. and Mäkelä, O.: Anti-hapten antibodies in normal sera. Eur. J. Immunol. 1: 471–477 (1971).

25 Kay, M. B.: Mechanism of removal of senescent cells by human macrophages in situ. Proc. natn. Acad. Sci. USA 72: 3521–3525 (1975).

26 Laffin, R. J.; Bardawil, W. A.; Pachas, W. N., and McCarthy, J. S.: Immunofluorescent studies on the occurrence of anti-nuclear factor in normal human serum. Am. J. Path. 45: 465–479 (1964).

27 Lee, J. W.; Metcalf, R. M., and Ryan, N. L.: Effect of Freund's complete adjuvant on lysosomal enzymes. Int. Archs Allergy appl. Immun. 39: 609–615 (1970).

28 Lenkei, R. and Ghetie, V.: Methods for detection of antialbumin auto-antibodies in hepatic diseases J. immunol. Meth. 16: 23–30 (1977).

29 Mehta, N. G.: The crucial role of phagocytosis and lysosomal destruction of antigens. Med. Hypothesis 2: 141–146 (1976).

30 Oh, S. K.; Pellegrino, M. A.; Ferrone, S.; Sevier, E. D., and Reisfeld, R. A.: Soluble HLA antigens in serum. Eur. J. Immunol. 5: 161–166 (1975).

31 Plescia, O. J. and Braun, W.: Methylated bovine serum albumin as a carrier for oligo- and poly-nucleotides; in Plescia and Braun Nucleic acids in immunology, pp. 5–17 (Springer, Berlin 1968).

32 Plow, E. F. and Edgington, T. S.: Immune response

to the cleavage-associated neo-antigens of fibrinogen in man. J. clin. Invest. *56:* 1509–1518 (1975).

33 Rivat, L.: Anti-immunoglobulines humaines. Revue fr. Transfus. *16:* 279–287 (1973).

34 Rosenberg, S. A.; Schwartz, S., and Baker, A.: Natural antibodies to 'cryptic' membrane antigen exposed by treatment with neuraminidase. Behring Inst. Mitt. *55:* 204–208 (1974).

35 Ryan, W. L. and Lee, J. W.: Antigen catabolism by lysosomal enzymes. Immunochemistry *7:* 251–265 (1970).

36 Sela, M.; Mozes, E., and Shaerer, G. M.: Thymus-independence of slowly metabolized immunogens. Proc. natn. Acad. Sci. USA *69:* 2696–2700 (1972).

37 Wekerle, H.; Cohen, I. R., and Feldman, M.: Lymphocyte receptors for auto-antigens; autologous serum inhibits self-recognition. Nature new Biol. *241:* 25–26 (1973).

Dr. P. Grabar, Institut Pasteur, F-75724 Paris Cedex 15 (France)

Immunopathology. 6th Int. Convoc. Immunol., Niagara Falls, N.Y., 1978, pp. 7–10 (Karger, Basel 1979)

Self-Recognition and Tolerance within the Immune System[1]

Benvenuto Pernis

Departments of Microbiology and Medicine, College of Physicians and Surgeons, Columbia University, New York, N.Y.

It is an accepted fact that the immune system normally does not produce antibodies directed against components of the same organism: it is tolerant to self-molecules; indeed, this ability to distinguish self from nonself is an essential feature of the immune system. The mechanisms through which this ability is achieved, however, are far from clear; the immune system cannot make the distinction of self from nonself on the basis of some general chemical property of the antigens (or of the self-molecules) nor can it rely on genetic restrictions even within one species, since the genes that control antibodies and those that control antigens reassort independently.

The immune system must therefore 'learn' to distinguish self from nonself on the basis of operational criteria that are not fully known to us. Some of these criteria can, however, be envisaged. One of the most widely accepted criteria, considered to be valid since the proposal by *Burnet* [1] of the clonal selection theory of antibody formation, is that a macromolecule is tolerogenic if it is present in fetal life and persists in the body in appreciable amounts throughout life. In other words, for the immune system, self is what is always there.

It is clear that this definition of self does not include the antibodies themselves since antibodies of a given specificity appear and wane in the serum during life in connection with the corresponding antigenic challenges. Antibodies should therefore be also antigens, at least for what concerns those sets of determinants (idiotypes) that differ from one antibody molecule to another. The production of a set of antibodies against an antigen should therefore be followed by a second wave of antibodies against these antibodies, and so forth. A series of events of this kind has been proposed, in general terms, in a view of the regulation of the immune system considered as a network of mutually interacting clones that extends, practically without interruptions, to include all the immunocytes present in one organism [8, 9]. The possibility of direct interactions between different antibodies produced by the same individual has far-reaching implications both for the physiology and for the pathology of the immune system and has been the subject of extensive experimental studies in recent years.

As a result of these studies [4, 5, 15], there is no doubt that an antibody response against the idiotypes of various immunoglobulins can be induced in individuals that have the same genotype as those that produced the idiotypes themselves. From studies of this

[1] Supported in part by NIH grant RO1 A1 14398.

kind the conclusion has been drawn that 'idiotypes should not be strictly considered self-antigens' [4]. These observations however, do not necessarily imply that anti-idiotype antibodies are regularly produced by the same individual that produces the idiotype, and that idiotype-anti-idiotype complexes are normally formed in the body in appreciable amounts. In this connection, the following data should be considered:

(a) Most experiments have been performed by immunizing an individual different from the one that had produced the idiotype.

(b) When the same individual is immunized, anti-idiotype antibodies are produced at a different time with respect to the production of the idiotype [13, 14].

(c) The immunization procedure with the idiotype included in Freund's adjuvant certainly can induce reactions that are different from those that may follow the appearance in the body of newly synthesized, soluble immunoglobulins.

(d) In some experiments [4], the assay procedure may have detected cold or low affinity anti-idiotype antibodies unable to produce significant amounts of immune complexes *in vivo*.

(e) Most of the experiments based on the immunization with syngeneic idiotypes have been performed (in the mouse) using as antigens myeloma proteins belonging to one class only (usually IgA). It is conceivable that in natural conditions of idiotype production different classes of immunoglobulins will carry the idiotype and that some of these (not IgA) might be very efficient in suppressing the production of the corresponding anti-idiotype. It is noteworthy [15] that with IgG myeloma proteins, even Freund's adjuvant is not sufficient to induce syngeneic anti-idiotypes and that it has been necessary to use hapten-coupled molecules [7] in hapten-primed animals. Therefore, we should focus our attention on the results of those investigators [3, 10, 11] who observed production of anti-idiotype as the direct and simple consequence of the appearance of the idiotype in the organism. These observations are all very interesting, but they do not show that the formation of idiotype-anti-idiotype complexes *in vivo* is part of the normal course of an immune response. In particular the data of *Cosenza* [3] indicate that the number of anti-idiotype-producing cells (up to a maximum of 2,000 cells per spleen) was minimal in comparison with the number of cells producing the idiotype (more than 10^5 per spleen) so that any idiotype-anti-idiotype complex that might have been produced would have been far in the antigen excess zone (idiotype excess).

Indeed, it appears to me that the immune system operates in a way to prevent the production of appreciable amounts of idiotype-anti-idiotype complexes; it is in fact to be expected that these complexes of immunoglobulins would be highly pathogenic *in vivo*. In order to achieve this, the simultaneous synthesis of idiotypes and anti-idiotypes is not allowed, at least not at levels equivalent to those of a measurable antibody response.

The basic element of this regulation would be a process of *clonal exclusion* whereby the products of B lymphocyte clones would be active in a symmetrical process of suppression where the product of one clone would suppress the cells that carry interacting receptors irrespective of which is the antigen and which is the antibody. In other words, the anti-idiotype would suppress the idiotype and the idiotype would suppress the anti-idiotype, whichever comes first.

Experimental observations support this view. In fact, the suppression of the idiotype by anti-idiotype antibody is well documented [12]. The reverse phenomenon, that is, the suppression of anti-idiotype production by previous administration of soluble idiotype, clearly has been shown by *Iverson and*

Dresser [7]. It appears indeed that immunoglobulins in sufficient concentration and in soluble form can very well suppress the clones with which they interact.

The principle of clonal exclusion, in all probability, only applies to those clones that produce significant amounts of immunoglobulins, that is to those which have a corresponding plasma-cell compartment. As long as clones are composed only of lymphocytes, potential interactions at the level of the membrane receptors may be without any pathological consequence. It is probably impossible to conceive an immune system without interacting clones if the diversity is such that in a mouse 10^6-10^7 different clones are simultaneously present.

It follows from what I am saying that, in a given moment, the diversity of the plasma cell compartment of an immune system (and therefore that of the serum immunoglobulins) would be much more limited than that of the lymphocyte compartment. This limitation would be the consequence of regulatory processes that, at a given time, allow the maturation to plasma cells of only those lymphocyte clones that will produce antibodies that do not conflict in idiotype-antiidiotype interaction with the products of those other clones that already have members in the plasma cell compartment and are actively secreting immunoglobulin molecules. This view considers the existence of a regulatory gate, at the level of the maturation to plasma cells, that selects from a vast repertoire of lymphocyte clones those that produce 'non-conflicting' immunoglobulins.

In support of this one might quote the results of the experiments of *Cazenave* [2] who has observed that the extreme diversity of the idiotypes that various rabbits produce upon immunization with one antigen (several animals made antibodies differing in idiotypes when immunized with ribonuclease) can be sharply reduced by appropriate manipulation of the immune system. In fact, various animals immunized with anti-idiotype antibodies that were producing antianti-idiotypes made cross-reacting idiotypes when challenged with the original antigen (RNase). Similar observations were reported by *Urbain et al.* [17].

The simpler interpretation of these findings is that all rabbits can produce a wide variety of idiotypes when challenged with RNase, but that in fact only a very small proportion of this potential is expressed at the level of immunoglobulin-secreting clones, and that precisely those clones are selected for maturation to plasma cells that do not find conflicting anti-idiotype-producing clones. The treatment inducing the production of anti-anti-idiotypes clearly results in the elimination of the anti-idiotype itself. Therefore, the original idiotype is favored following the challenge by the extraneous antigen. The number of nonmanipulated rabbits that have to be immunized with RNase before finding any two that produce cross-reacting idiotypes, possibly may give an estimate of the ratio of the diversity of the lymphocyte compartment versus that of the plasma cell compartment, the latter being several hundred times smaller than the former. Of course, this is valid only if one considers the immune system at *one given moment*, whereas throughout the life of the individual a much larger proportion of the lymphocyte repertoire may find an occasion of maturation to plasma cells, always following the rule of avoiding interactions with those clones which *at that time* are being involved in active immunoglobulin secretion.

The cellular and molecular basis of this postulated process of selection may form the object of future studies; it appears likely that idiotype-specific helper or suppressor T lymphocytes are involved, but direct interactions between B clones may also achieve the same result. In fact, athymic (nude) mice do not show any evidence of abnormal deposits of immunoglobulin complexes in their kidneys.

In any event, it appears to me that the immunoglobulin molecules themselves merit attention with respect to the processes that I have discussed. It appears that immunoglobulins that are very good antigens when aggregated or administered with adjuvants, have a potent tolerogenic activity if presented in soluble form. The latter property may be connected with some given structural feature of the immunoglobulins and may render this family of molecules different from other proteins as immunogens. This way of viewing immunoglobulins as immunogens is the exact opposite of that expressed by *Cosenza et al.* [4] that I have quoted beforehand.

Independently from theoretical considerations, it is probably worthwhile to study both the idiotype-suppressing ability of anti-idiotype antibodies belonging to different classes of immunoglobulins, and, the ability of idiotypes borne by immunoglobulins of different classes to inhibit the production of the corresponding anti-idiotypes. It may well be that the variety of molecular classes that can be produced by a given B clone is important in the regulation of the immune system. Such studies are currently under way in our laboratory.

References

1 Burnet, F. M.: The clonal selection theory of acquired immunity (Cambridge University Press, Cambridge 1959).
2 Cazenave, P. A.: Idiotypic-anti-idiotypic regulation of antibody synthesis in rabbits. Proc. natn. Acad. Sci. USA *74:* 5122–5125 (1977).
3 Cosenza, H.: Detection of anti-idiotype reactive cells in the response to phosphorylcholine. Eur. J. Immunol. *6:* 114–116 (1976).
4 Cosenza, H.; Augustin, A., and Julius, M. H.: Induction and characterization of 'autologous' anti-idiotypic antibodies. Eur. J. Immunol. *7:* 273–278 (1977).
5 Eichmann, K.: Expression and function of idiotypes on lymphocytes. Adv. Immunol. *26:* 195–254 (1978).
6 Iverson, G. M.: Ability of CBA mice to produce anti-idiotypic sera to 5563 myeloma protein. Nature, Lond. *227:* 273–274 (1970).
7 Iverson, G. M. and Dresser, D. W.: Immunological paralysis induced by an idiotypic antigen. Nature, Lond. *227:* 274–276 (1970).
8 Jerne, N. K.: Towards a network theory of the immune system. Annls Immunol. Inst. Pasteur, Paris *125:* 373–389 (1974).
9 Jerne, N. K.: The immune system: a web of V-domains. Harvey Lect. *70:* 93–110 (1976).
10 Kluskens, L. and Köhler, H.: Regulation of immune response by autologous antibody against receptor. Proc. natn. Acad. Sci. USA *71:* 5083–5087 (1974).
11 McKearn, T. J.; Stuart, F. P., and Fitch, F. W.: Anti-idiotypic antibody in rat transplantation immunity. J. Immun. *113:* 1876–1882 (1974).
12 Nisonoff, A. and Bangasser, S. A.: Immunological suppression of idiotypic specificities. Transplantn Rev. *27:* 100–134 (1975).
13 Rodkey, L. S.: Studies of idiotypic antibodies. J. exp. Med. *139:* 712–720 (1974).
14 Rodkey, L. S.: Studies of idiotypic antibodies: reaction of isologous and autologous anti-idiotypic antibodies with the same antibody preparations. J. Immun. *117:* 986–989 (1976).
15 Sakato, N. and Eisen, H. N.: Antibodies to idiotypes of isologous immunoglobulins. J. exp. Med. *141:* 1411–1426 (1975).
16 Sakato, N.; Janaway, C. A., and Eisen, H. N.: Immune responses of BALB/c mice to the idiotype of T15 and other myeloma proteins of BALB/c origin: implications for an immune network and antibody multi-specificity. Cold Spring Harb. Symp. quant. Biol. *41:* 719–724 (1977).
17 Urbain, J.; Wikler, M.; Franssen, J. D., and Collignon, C.: Idiotypic regulation of the immune system by the induction of antibodies against anti-idiotypic antibodies. Proc. natn. Acad. Sci. USA *74:* 5126–5130 (1977).

Dr. Benvenuto Pernis, Departments of Microbiology and Medicine, College of Physicians and Surgeons, Columbia University, New York, NY 10032 (USA)

Immunopathology. 6th Int. Convoc. Immunol., Niagara Falls, N.Y., 1978, pp. 11–15 (Karger, Basel 1979)

Autoreactive T Lymphocytes?

M. Feldman, S. Segal, M. Fogel and E. Gorelik

Department of Cell Biology, Weizmann Institute of Science, Rehovot

The question of whether lymphocytes possessing receptors for self antigens normally exist in the resting state of the immune system has been argued since the discovery of self tolerance. The concept of clonal deletion formulated by *Burnet* [1]—distinct from regulation of self-reactive lymphocytes via blocking factors or suppressor cells, as the basis for self-nonself discrimination—still constitutes one of the basic problems of immunology. Conceivably, these alternative mechanisms of self tolerance are not mutually exclusive. The lack of reactivity to some self antigens may be based on blocking or suppressor mechanisms, whereas clonal deletion may determine self tolerance to other antigens. In this regard, antigens which are distributed throughout the organism in relatively high concentration, such as the circulating serum proteins or the cell-surface histocompatibility antigens which exist on every cell, are of special interest. Obviously, the question of whether lymphocytes do exist which possess receptors for such self antigens, as distinct from organ-specific or differentiation antigens, should be raised with regard to each of the major classes of lymphocytes, i.e. the T and the B cells.

B Lymphocytes Reacting against Autologous Serum Proteins Appear following Polyclonal Activation

To test whether B cells recognizing autologous antigens exist in the normal organisms, *Möller* and his associates [7, 10] studied whether polyclonal activation of B lymphocytes would result in antibody production to self antigen. In a recent study, they activated spleen cells by LPS, then demonstrated that such cells produced antibodies with specificity for autologous serum coupled to SRBC [11]. Since highly purified serum albumin inhibited the plaque-forming cell (PFC) response to serum-coupled SRBC, it appears that the PFC responded to autologous serum albumin [11]. The antibodies produced by the PFC were of the IgM type, i.e. antibodies which could be produced without the cooperation of T lymphocytes. The absence of IgG antibodies seemed to indicate that, at least in this system, T cells recognizing autologous serum albumin were not manifested. Thus, self-reactive B lymphocytes do exist in the normal resting state. These do not seem to manifest a state of tolerance to thymus-dependent antigens such as serum albumin.

The tolerance to such antigens seems, therefore, to be determined at the T cell level. From experiments carried out so far, T cells with receptors to immunogens of autologous serum albumin have not been detected.

Are there T Lymphocytes with Receptors to Self Cell-Surface Antigens?

To study whether T lymphocytes with receptors to autologous cell-surface histocompatibility antigens exist, experiments were performed in our laboratory using the cell culture system for *in vitro* sensitization of T lymphocytes [5]. Rat lymphocytes of thymus, spleen, or lymph node origin were seeded for sensitization on monolayers of syngeneic embryonic fibroblasts or syngeneic adult thymus reticulum. Following 5 days of sensitization, cytotoxic T cells manifesting specific activity against syngeneic target cells developed [2, 3, 5]. Thus, autosensitization against autologous cell-surface antigens seemed to have been obtained. To demonstrate that indeed T lymphocytes possessing receptors to self antigens exist in the resting state, their depletion was attempted by using syngeneic monolayers of rat cells as cellular immunoadsorbents. Lymphocytes which adhered to the syngeneic monolayers could be autosensitized in culture, whereas those which did not adhere were depleted of the capacity to be autosensitized, although they retained the capacity to react against allogeneic cells [3]. Experiments made by *Ilfeld et al.* [8] seemed to indicate that the self antigens which signalled autosensitization in these experiments are determinants coded by the MHC.

Autosensitization in all these studies was carried out in culture media containing xenogeneic serum (horse or fetal calf). Sensitization against autologous or syngeneic cells in the presence of syngeneic rather than xenogeneic serum did not result in the generation

Table I. Effect of xenogeneic serum (FCS) on the specificity of *in vitro* sensitization of C57BL/6J spleen cells against syngeneic fibroblasts and tumor cells

Sensitizing cells	Target cells	% cytotoxicity[1] at lymphocyte-to-target cell ratios of:			
		50:1	25:1	10:1	1:1
3LL	3LL	−64.0	−51.0	−33.0	−22.0
C57BLf	C57BLf	−11.3	−10.2	−9.2	—
C57BLf	3LL	−40.2	−35.2	−23.1	−24.7
3LL	C57BLf	−9.8	—	−7.2	—
C3Hf	3LL	−17.6	−20.9	—	−14.5

Normal C57BL/6J spleen cells were sensitized for 5 days on monolayers of either normal syngeneic fibroblasts (f) or 3LL tumor cells, in the presence of 15% FCS, and tested at various ratios for their cytotoxic activity against both types of target cells.

[1] In this and the next tables, negative values represent reduced uptake of isotope in test wells (as the result of cytolytic activity, as compared to control wells). Positive values represent increased uptake of isotope in test wells as compared to control wells.

of anti-self effector T lymphocytes. This was interpreted as indicating that autologous serum contains specific factors (possibly soluble antigens) which block the T cell receptors for self cell-surface antigen [3, 15].

More recent studies carried out in our laboratory with mouse cells led us to reexamine the conclusions regarding the existence of T cells reactive against self cell-surface antigens of the MHC [6]. We have been studying the *in vitro* immunogenic properties of the 3LL Lewis lung carcinoma, a tumor which appeared spontaneously in a C57BL mouse and was maintained by serial subcutaneous transplantation in syngeneic recipients. We found that syngeneic lymphocytes could be sensitized in culture against cell-surface antigens of the 3LL cells. The resulting cytotoxic T lymphocytes (CTL) were cross tested with CTL generated in response to mouse fibroblasts, to assess the

Table II. Sensitization of C57BL/6J spleen cells on 3LL monolayers in the presence of syngeneic mouse serum results in specific antitumor cytotoxic lymphocytes[1]

Exp. No.	Spleen cell donor	Sensitizing cells	Serum used during sensitization	Serum used during effector phase	% cytotoxicity on 3LL target cells
1	Normal	3LL	FCS	FCS	−30
		3LL	FCS	SMS	+13
		3LL	SMS	SMS	−44.4
		3LL	SMS	FCS	−48
2	Normal	3LL	FCS	FCS	−41.2
		3LL	FCS	SMS	−18.9
		3LL	SMS	SMS	−63.4

[1] See footnote to table I.

specificity of the effector lymphocytes generated in culture. Such tests indicated (table I) that not only CTL generated on monolayers of the syngeneic 3LL cells lysed 3LL cells, but also CTL generated on syngeneic fibroblasts lysed 3LL targets, although to a somewhat lesser extent. Since the 3LL cells are more susceptible to T cell cytotoxicity than fibroblasts, the cross reactivity obtained in these experiments could be attributable to cell-surface self immunogens (i.e. self H-2 or fetal antigens) shared by the normal fibroblasts and the tumor cells. Alternatively, it could be argued that since the syngeneic sensitization was carried out in culture medium containing fetal calf serum (FCS), the FCS determinants, possibly coupled to the MHC antigens, constituted the actual immunogens as 'altered self' [4, 12]. If the anti-3LL cytotoxic lymphocytes produced in the presence of FCS were sensitized to FCS determinants adsorbed onto the 3LL cell surfaces, then such cytotoxic lymphocytes should lyse 3LL targets only in the presence of FCS, but not when the target 3LL cells were tested in syngeneic mouse serum (SMS). Table II indicates that this, in fact, was the result. On the other hand, if anti-3LL cytotoxic lymphocytes generated in the presence of SMS (1 %) were sensitized against genuine

Table III. Specificity of in vitro sensitization of C57BL/6J spleen cells on monolayers of syngeneic 3LL carcinoma cells[1]

Sensitizing cells	Target cells	% cytotoxicity at lymphocyte-to-target cell ratios of:		
		25:1	12:1	4:1
3LL	3LL	−36.1	−41.7	−51.3
3LL	C57BLf	+13.7	+12.8	+3.1
C57BLf	C57BLf	−8.4	−6.6	−3.3
C57BLf	3LL	+5.0	+7.9	+8.1

[1] See footnote to table I.

membrane antigens of the 3LL cells, they should lyse target cells irrespective of the serum in which they were tested. Indeed, anti-3LL CTL generated in cultures containing SMS lysed 3LL targets incubated in either SMS or FCS (table II).

Hence, tumor cells could sensitize syngeneic lymphocytes in the presence of syngeneic serum. Could the CTL thus generated in SMS lyse syngeneic normal fibroblasts? To study this, we sensitized C57BL lymphocytes against 3LL tumor cells in SMS, then cross-tested the lytic activity against 3LL and against C57BL fibroblasts (table III). We found that sensitization against 3LL in the absence of FCS resulted in effector lymphocytes which lysed 3LL targets but not C57BL fibroblasts (table III). Thus, lymphocytes possessing receptors for the tumor antigens could be detected in this system, yet there were no indications for reactivity against antigens of the normal fibroblasts.

These experiments indicated that 'autosensitization' in cell culture in the presence of FCS generated cytotoxic T lymphocytes directed against FCS determinants coupled to self cell-surface antigens. The FCS determinants appeared to have altered the self antigens in a manner probably similar to the alteration caused by hapten determinants [12] or viruses [4]. Since all previous experiments suggesting T cell autosensitization *in vitro* using rat cells were carried out in the presence of xenogeneic serum (horse), the resulting effector T lymphocytes might have been directed not against the actual normal self antigens but rather against horse serum altered self determinants. T lymphoytes seem, therefore, to possess receptors against MHC antigens coupled to horse or to fetal calf serum [9]. Yet, so far we have no indication that the normal organism possesses T cells which can recognize, i.e. specifically bind to, unmodified antologous cell-surface MHC antigens.

Conclusions

We wish to state that B lymphocytes recognizing self antigens, even those circulating in high concentration (such as serum albumin), do exist. On the other hand, T cells capable of recognizing, in the resting state, the non-organ-specific self histocompatibility antigens via cell receptors for antigen have not been demonstrated. Such cells may not exist in the normal organism, or should they exist, the affinity of their receptors for unaltered

self must be extremely low. This is in agreement with the observation that polyclonal activation of T cells elicited reactivity against alloantigens but not against self H-2 [10]. The lack of self-reactive cells need not constitute the basis for T cell tolerance of other more localized self antigens such as differentiation antigens. Lymphocytes possessing antigen receptors for differentiation antigens such as the myelin basic protein may exist in the organism. Their reactivity to self antigens under normal conditions may be blocked either via the soluble antigen which can compete for the cell receptors with the immunogenic form of macrophage-bound antigen [13], or via suppressor cells.

References

1 Burnet, F. M.: The clonal selection theory of acquired immunity (Vanderbilt University Press, Nashville 1959).
2 Cohen, I. R.; Globerson, A., and Feldman, M.: Rejection of tumor allografts by mouse spleen cells sensitized *in vitro*. J. exp. Med. *133:* 834–845 (1971).
3 Cohen, I. R. and Wekerle, H.: Autosensitization of lymphocytes against thymus reticulum cells. Science *176:* 1324–1325 (1972).
4 Doherty, P. C. and Zinkernagel, R. M.: T-cell-mediated immunopathology in viral infections. Transplantn Rev. *19:* 89–120 (1974).
5 Feldman, M.; Cohen, I. R., and Wekerle, H.: T cell mediated immunity *in vitro*: an analysis of antigen recognition and target cell lysis. Transplantn Rev. *12:* 57–90 (1972).
6 Fogel, M.; Segal, S.; Gorelik, E., and Feldman, M.: Specific cytotoxic lymphocytes against syngeneic tumors are generated in culture in the presence of syngeneic, but not xenogeneic, serum. Int. J. Cancer *22:* 329–334 (1978).
7 Hammarström, L.; Smith, E.; Primi, D., and Möller, G.: Induction of antibodies to red blood cells by polyclonal B-cell activators. Nature, Lond. *263:* 60–61 (1976).
8 Ilfeld, D.; Carnaud, C., and Klein, E.: Cytotoxicity of autosensitized lymphocytes restricted to the H-2K end of identical targets. Immunogenetics *2:* 231–240 (1975).

9 Peck, A. B.; Wigzell, H.; Janeway, C., jr., and Anderson, L. C.: Environmental and genetic control of T cell activation *in vitro*: a study using isolated alloantigen-activated T cell clones. Immunol. Rev. *35*: 146–180 (1977).

10 Primi, D.; Hammarström, L.; Smith, E. C. I., and Möller, G.: Characterization of self-reactive B-cells by polyclonal B-cell activators. J. exp. Med. *145*: 21–30 (1977).

11 Primi, D.; Smith, E. C. I.; Hammarström, L., and Möller, G.: Polyclonal B-cell activators induce immunological response to autologous serum proteins. Cell. Immunol. *34*: 367–375 (1977).

12 Shearer, G. M.: Cell-mediated cytotoxicity to trinitrophenyl-modified syngeneic lymphocytes. Eur. J. Immunol. *4*: 527–533 (1974).

13 Steinman, L.; Cohen, I. R.; Teitelbaum, D., and Arnon, R.: Regulation of autosensitization to encephalitogenic myelin basic protein by macrophage-associated and soluble antigen. Nature, Lond. *265*: 173–175 (1977).

Dr. M. Feldman, Department of Cell Biology, The Weizmann Institute of Science, 76100 Rehovot (Israel)

Immunopathology. 6th Int. Convoc. Immunol., Niagara Falls, N.Y., 1978, pp. 16–20 (Karger, Basel 1979)

Self-Recognition and the Thymus[1]

Jeannine Charreire, Claude Carnaud and Jean-François Bachs[1]

INSERM U 25, Hôpital Necker, Paris

Several sets of data suggest that clones of B and T lymphocytes recognizing 'self antigens' are present during ontogeny and persist in adult life. Such clones remain normally silent in spite of their continuous exposure to 'self' antigenic environment. Yet, they can be activated under certain conditions which fall into two main categories: the first category is connected with the antigenic stimulus *'per se'*. For instance, syngeneic tissue antigens modified by the presence of a virus [6], a chemical (hapten) [14], strong alloantigens [20], or mitogens [10] can trigger these self-recognizing clones. These will differentiate into either autoantibody-secreting plasmocytes or T killer cells specific for syngeneic targets. To the second category belong the various situations of immunological imbalance leading to autoimmune manifestations. Such situations are found in adult [3, 4] or newborn thymectomized (Tx) animals [15], in aging subjects [7, 9], in normal individuals whose suppressor cells have been removed *in vivo* by cyclophosphamide treatment [12] or by *in vitro* incubation [unpublished data], and in spontaneous autoimmune syndromes

like that of NZB mice [17]. A common denominator can be found between the first and second category of activating factors: the regulatory role of the thymus. Indeed, the different immunological imbalances quoted share the property of an associated partial or total cessation of thymic function. As for the relationship between thymus and antigenic recognition, it needs only to be recalled that this organ has been postulated to be the site of generation of T cell receptor diversity [11], of inactivation of potentially autoreactive clones [2] and, more recently, of positive selection of clones reacting with both H-2 self and H-2 plus any potential modification [21].

In this context, it would be interesting to obtain direct evidence for manifestations of autoreactivity at the level of thymocytes which represent a homogeneous population of immature T cells. For that purpose, we have used, in parallel, two approaches: the first, attempting to characterize autoantigen-binding cells by identification of lymphocytes forming rosettes with syngeneic erythrocytes; the second, consisting of studying the development of an autoreactive immune response —the syngeneic graft-versus-host (GVH) reaction.

[1] Presented by Dr. *J.-F. Bach.*

Autologous Rosette-Forming Cells (A-RFC)

A low proportion of normal lymphoid cells bind autologous (or syngeneic) erythrocytes (A-RFC). Such A-RFC are prevalent in the thymus (table I). Their number is augmented after adult thymectomy and returns to normal values after injection of various thymic preparations, i.e. thymosin fraction V, thymic humoral factor, *facteur thymique sérique* (FTS) [4], or thymopoietin [19]. Recent studies using Thy-1 and Ly markers indicate that A-RFC are composed of both Ly 123$^+$ and Ly 23$^+$ cells [submitted for publication].

Thymic A-RFC appear as early as the 17th day of gestation in mice. Their number increases progressively to reach a peak at day 2 after birth. A sudden decline then occurs [*Charreire and Pyke*, in preparation], and the A-RFC incidence goes down to adult level at 1 week of age. Thymic A-RFC level increases dramatically during the regeneration phase following newborn thymus grafting, returning to normal values when the wave of proliferation is terminated.

The nature of the A-RFC is not definitively determined. Thy-1 and Ly studies indicate that they belong to the T cell lineage. Morphological studies confirm their lymphoid nature and exclude macrophages (as also shown by absence of colloidal carbon uptake). B cell involvement is excluded by A-RFC passage through Ig anti-Ig columns of Degalan beads. As for their classification into T cell subsets, the effects of adult thymectomy and of thymic factors indicate that A-RFC include both immature Ly 123$^+$ T cells and more mature Ly 23$^+$ cells.

The specificity for 'self' of the A-RFC phenomenon is shown by the larger number of A-RFC found when thymocytes are mixed with syngeneic erythrocytes than with erythrocytes from congenic resistant strains of mice or from other species. Competition experiments based upon blocking of A-RFC receptors with syngeneic or allogeneic erythrocyte membranes led to similar conclusions. It is probable, however, that the H-2 specificity of A-RFC is partly masked by the presence on H-2 erythrocytes of public incompatible specificities shared by erythrocytes of the various mouse strains studied. On the other hand, non-specific factors described in several rosette systems [19] might also account for partial cross-reactivity between erythrocytes of different haplotypes.

Table I. Frequency of autologous rosette-forming cells in newborn and grafted thymuses (mean ± SE)

Population	Number of experiments	Number of A-RFC per 1,000 lymphocytes at WC/RBC ratios of		
		1 : 4	1 : 16	1 : 64
Newborn thymocytes (D + 1)	4	2.2 ± 0.2	32.4 ± 9.0	71.5 ± 19
Grafted thymocytes (D + 9)[1]	6	6.5 ± 1.7	11.0 ± 2.7	69.4 ± 11.1
Adult thymocytes	18	1.0 ± 0.3	3.1 ± 0.5	17.2 ± 3.7

[1] Newborn thymuses (D + 1) are grafted under the kidney capsule. Nine days later, the grafted lobes are removed and tested for A-RFC incidence.

Syngeneic Cytotoxicity

In lymphoid organs from normal mice, we have observed the presence of cells spontaneously cytotoxic for syngeneic erythrocytes. The cytotoxicity may be demonstrated after an 18-hour incubation at 37 °C by the release of radioactive chromium or hemoglobin. A role for macrophages in the cytotoxicity is unlikely as the lymphoid cell preparation retains killing ability after nylon wool filtration. Among lymphoid cells, T cells are probably involved, since thymocytes represent the most efficient source of cytotoxic cells and since the cytotoxic phenomenon is inhibited after depletion by anti-Thy-1 or by anti-Ly 2 sera (but not by anti-Ly 3 serum). As already described for A-RFC, syngeneic cytotoxicity increases after adult thymectomy and is inhibited by FTS.

Much remains to be learned on the mechanisms of such a syngeneic model of cytotoxicity. In particular, the optimal lysis observed at low effector/target cell ratio should be explained. One possibility could be that only a minority of erythrocytes can serve as target. Thus, the chances of interaction between an effector cell and the right target would be very much dependent upon the amount of erythrocytes introduced into the assay. An alternative hypothesis could be a target competition between erythrocytes and effector cells themselves. Only by lowering the number of the effector cells would it be possible to demonstrate a cytotoxic effect on the labeled erythrocytes. The physiological and, more particularly, the immunological relevance of this syngeneic cytotoxicity is unknown. In any case, it should be distinguished from the plaques formed with bromelain-treated syngeneic erythrocytes which, at variance with the phenomenon described above, need complement and only appear after 48 h of preculture of effector cells. It could play a role in the elimination of certain subpopulations of red cells, in particular aged erythrocytes.

Syngeneic GVH Reaction

Normal allogeneic spleen cells injected in the foot pads of mice induce a significant increase in the weight of the corresponding popliteal lymph node. On the other hand, syngeneic control cells do not induce any increase in popliteal lymph node weight.

Table II. Reactivity of newborn versus adult thymocytes in syngeneic popliteal lymph node assay

Experiment	Thymocyte origin[1]	Number of injected cells	Average weight of popliteal LN mg $\pm$ SE	Index[2]
1	Adult	1×10^7	1.70 ± 0.17	1.59
	Newborn	1×10^7	2.70 ± 0.21	
2	Adult	10×10^6	1.01 ± 0.06	1.43
	Newborn	10×10^6	1.45 ± 0.13	
3	Adult	5×10^6	1.64 ± 0.13	1.33
	Newborn	5×10^6	2.18 ± 0.23	
4	Adult	5×10^6	1.15 ± 0.11	1.62
	Newborn	5×10^6	1.87 ± 0.10	

[1] Each experimental group includes 8–10 lymph nodes. Reaction is measured on day 8.

[2] $\text{Index} = \dfrac{\text{Average weight of LN exposed to newborn thymocytes}}{\text{Average weight of LN exposed to adult thymocytes}}.$

Table III. Autoreactivity of thymocytes recovered from a regenerating newborn thymus graft measured in syngeneic popliteal lymh node assay[1]

Experiment	Thymocyte origin	Average weight of popliteal LN mg ± SE	Index
1	Normal thymocytes	1.01 ± 0.06	
	Grafted thymocytes	1.81 ± 0.23	1.79
2	Normal thymocytes	1.06 ± 0.08	
	Grafted thymocytes	1.45 ± 0.15	1.87

[1] For details, see footnote to table II.

However, when the spleen cell donor is ATx, a significant adenomegaly of the local popliteal node is found in syngeneic combinations. This effect of adult thymectomy can be shown as early as 4 weeks after the operation and reaches its maximum at 3 months. It is also possible to show the presence of autoreactive cells among thymocytes, provided these thymocytes come from newborn animals. Indeed, no reactivity is seen with adult thymocytes which behave like adult spleen cells (table II). Thymocytes recovered from a thymus undergoing self-regeneration after grafting show a significant autoreactivity in the lymph node assay if compared to normal thymocytes (table III). Finally, it appears that GVH autoreactivity is observed in all situations where high A-RFC values are found. This is not surprising since we have reported that A-RFC depleted spleen cells from ATx mice on a Ficoll-Hypaque mixture are associated with a loss of the capacity to induce a syngeneic GVH [3].

Discussion

Our data show that, in contrast to normal adult thymocytes, newborn thymocytes, proliferating thymocytes after thymus grafting, and spleen cells from ATx mice show manifestations of autoreactivity as assessed by: autologous rosette formation and syngeneic GVH. A causal relationship to A-RFC incidence is suggested both by high A-RFC levels found in these organs and by depletion experiments.

These data are reminiscent of findings obtained in other experimental models which also mimick autoreactivity, such as: *in vitro* sensitization on thymus epithelial or on fibroblast cultures [5]; mixed lymphocyte reaction against autologous spleen cells [1], autologous T cell-depleted peripheral human blood cells [13], or lymphoblastoid cell lines [16]. Two possibilities could account for the prevalence of autoreactive cells in newborn and regenerating thymus, as well as in spleens of mice submitted to adult thymectomy. First, that only immature T cells express autoreactivity as suggested by several authors in various models [4, 15]. Second, that autoreactive cells are particularly sensitive to suppressor T cells. The latter would explain the effects of adult thymectomy and cyclophosphamide [12] and be in keeping with the autoimmune syndrome of NZB mice also associated with deficiency of suppressor T cells. In that respect, thymic factors known to stimulate suppressor T cells simultaneously inhibit autologous rosette formation [4] and autosensitization [18]. The preventive effect of thymocytes [21] or of FTS [unpublished results] on hemolytic anemia and Sjögren's syndrome in NZB mice could thus be explained.

The relationship between autoreactive T

cells discussed in this paper and those involved in cell-mediated autoimmunity, or in helper function for autoantibody synthesis, remains to be determined. The specificity of the former ones for putative autoantigens and, in particular for syngeneic MHC-coded specificities, is not definitively proven, although suggested by several pieces of evidence. Finally, the relationship of these autoreactive cells with the T cells undergoing the education process of H-2 self recognition inside the thymus should be investigated.

References

1 Boehmer, H. von and Byrd, W. J.: Responsiveness of thymus cells to syngeneic and allogeneic lymphoid cells. Nature new Biol. 235: 50–52 (1972).

2 Burnet, F. M.: The clonal selection theory of acquired immunity (Cambridge University Press, Cambridge 1959).

3 Carnaud, C.; Charreire, J., and Bach, J. F.: Adult thymectomy promotes the manifestation of autoreactive lymphocytes. Cell. Immunol., 28: 274–283 (1977).

4 Charreire, J. and Bach, J. F.: Binding of autologous erythrocytes to immature T cells. Proc. natn. Acad. Sci. USA 72: 3201–3205 (1975).

5 Cohen, I. R. and Wekerle, H.: Autosensitization of lymphocytes against thymus reticulum cells. Science 176: 1324–1325 (1972).

6 Doherty, P. C.; Blanden, R. V., and Zinkernagel, R. M.: Specificity of virus immune effector T cells for H-2 K and H-2 D compatible interactions: implications for H diversity. Transplantn Rev. 29: 89–124 (1976).

7 Fournier, C. and Charreire, J.: Increase in autologous erythrocyte binding by T cells with aging in man. Clin. exp. Immunol. 29: 468–473 (1977).

8 Gershwin, M. E. and Steinberg, A. D.: Suppression of hemolytic anemia in New Zealand mice. Clin. Immunol. Immunopath. 4: 38–45 (1975).

9 Gozes, Y. and Trainin, N.: Enhancement of Lewis lung carcinoma in syngeneic host by spleen cells of C57BL/6 old mice. Eur. J. Immunol. 7: 159–164 (1977).

10 Hammarström, L.; Smith, E.; Primi, D., and Möller, G.: Induction of antibody response to autologous red blood cells in bovine spleen cells by polyclonal B cell activators. Nature, Lond. 263: 60–63 (1976).

11 Jerne, N. K.: The somatic generation of immune recognition. Eur. J. Immunol. 1: 1–9 (1971).

12 L'Age-Stehr, J. and Diamanstein, T.: Induction of autoreactive T lymphocytes and their suppressor cells by cyclophosphamide. Nature, Lond. 271: 663–665 (1978).

13 Opelz, G.; Kiuchi, M.; Takasugi, M., and Terasaki, P. I.: Autologous stimulation of human lymphocyte subpopulations. J. exp. Med. 142: 1327–1333 (1975).

14 Shaerer, G. M.; Rehn, T. G., and Schmitt-Verhulst, A. M.: Role of the murine major histocompatibility complex in the specificity of in vitro T cell mediated lympholysis against chemically modified autologous lymphocytes. Transplantn Rev. 29: 222–246 (1976).

15 Small, M. and Trainin, N.: Control of autoreactivity by a humoral factor of the thymus (THF). Cell. Immunol. 20: 1–11 (1975).

16 Svedmyr, E.; Wigzell, H., and Jondal, M.: Sensitization of human lymphocytes against autologous or allogeneic lymphoblastoid cell lines: characteristics of the reactive cells. Scand. J. Immunol. 3: 499–508 (1974).

17 Talal, N.: Autoimmunity and lymphoid malignancy: manifestations of immunoregulatory desequilibrium; in Talal, Autoimmunity, genetic, immunologic, virologic and clinical aspects, pp. 183–206 (Academic Press, New York 1977).

18 Trainin, N.; Carnaud, C., and Ilfeld, D.: Inhibition of in vitro autosensitization by a thymic humoral factor. Nature new Biol. 245: 253–255 (1973).

19 Verhaegen, H.; De Cock, W., and De Cree, J.: The effect of azathioprine and Levamisole on rosette forming cells of LC subjects and cancer patients. Clin. exp. Immunol. 29: 311–315 (1977).

20 Zarling, J. M. and Bach, F. H.: Sensitization of lymphocytes against pooled allogeneic cells. I. Generation of cytotoxicy against autologous human lymphoblastoid cell lines. J. exp. Med. 147: 1334–1340 (1978).

21 Zinkernagel, R. M.; Callahan, G. N.; Althage, A.; Cooper, S.; Klein, P. A., and Klein, J.: On the thymus in the differentiation of 'H-2 self-recognition' by T cells: evidence for dual recognition? J. exp. Med. 147: 882–896 (1978).

Dr. J.-F. Bach, INSERM U 25, Hôpital Necker, 161, rue de Sèvres, F-75015 Paris (France)

Immunopathology. 6th Int. Convoc. Immunol., Niagara Falls, N.Y., 1978, pp. 21–25 (Karger, Basel 1979)

Self-Recognition in Senescence[1]

Takashi Makinodan

Geriatric Research, Education and Clinical Center (GRECC), V.A. Wadsworth Hospital Center, and The Department of Medicine, UCLA, Los Angeles, Calif.

Introduction

Because aging is characterized by the inability to maintain homeostasis, various systems with regulatory functions are now being examined experimentally; one is the immune system. The immune system is appealing, because its homeostatic effectiveness is dependent upon its ability to distinguish nonself from self. In this paper, I wish to address myself to the issue of how aging influences immunologic vigor and self recognition.

Age-Related Changes in Immune Functions

The decline in normal immune functions with age appears to be characteristic of higher mammals, inasmuch as it has been observed in all species examined including mice, rats, guinea pigs, rabbits, dogs and humans [9, 15]. The onset and rate of decline, however, vary with the type of immune response and the species.

The first hint that normal immune functions could be declining with age came from findings of morphologists who showed in laboratory animals and humans that the thymic lymphatic mass decreased with age as a result primarily of atrophy of the cortex, beginning at the time of sexual maturity [7]. Histologically, the cortex of an involuted thymus is sparsely populated with lymphocytes which are replaced by macrophages, plasma cells and mast cells. Interestingly, *Hirokawa* [7] noted that the one tissue in the involuting thymus that manifested atrophic changes is the epithelial tissue, the producer of factors responsible for the transformation of precursor T cells into T cells. In contrast to the thymus, splenic, lymph node and bone marrow masses do not change appreciably with age. Histologically, however, these tissues also manifest changes reflective of a shift in the proportion of cell types; e.g. decrease in the size of germinal centers in lymphoid tissues and an increase in the number of plasma cells and phagocytes [2, 4].

The decline in normal immune functions is due to changes in both the cellular environment and the cells of the immune system. At present, we do not know the nature of the responsible factor(s) in the cellular environment. We suspect that two types of factors are involved; i.e. deleterious substances of molecular and viral nature, and essential substances of nutritional and hormonal nature.

[1] This is Publication No. 022 from V. A. Wadsworth GRECC, supported in part by the Department of Energy (EY 76-S-03-0034) and the V. A. Merit Review Grant (MRIS No. 5444).

Three types of cellular changes can cause immunologic aging: (a) an absolute decrease in the number of competent cells; (b) a decrease in the functional efficiency of immune cells as a result of qualitative changes intrinsic to the cells, and (c) a decrease in the functional efficiency of immune cells as a result of increase in the proportion of suppressor cells. Our study of *individual* old mice indicates that the number of immune cells in them is comparable to that of young mice, and their reduced T cell-dependent antibody response can be explained by the presence of excessive numbers of suppressor cells in about 65% of the cases, by a selective reduction in the number of at least one type of cell that exists in excess in young mice in about 25% of the cases, and by a decrease in the functional efficiency of cells in about 10% of the cases [13]. Complementary studies by others [5, 18, 22] revealed that not only is the number of antigen-responsive precursor cell units reduced in old mice, but also that the number of functional progeny cells generated by each antigen-stimulated precursor cell unit is reduced. The functional cells which emerge, however, appear to be as efficient as those in young mice. These results are consistent with the view that the decline in normal immune functions with age is due primarily to the failure of antigen-responsive precursor cells to interact with each other efficiently upon antigenic stimulation, and to the failure of these precursor cells to undergo proliferation and transformation efficiently once they are stimulated. The underlying cause for these failures appears to be due primarily to age-related alteration in cells and factors that can influence the rate of differentiation and the magnitude of clonal expansion.

All four major cell types—stem (S) cells, macrophages, T cells and B cells—are being analyzed in relation to age. The results to date indicate that they all manifest varying degrees of functional alteration [9, 15].

Stem Cells. The total number of S cells in mice generally remains relatively constant throughout the life span. Functionally, they can self-replicate *in situ* throughout the natural life span and, furthermore, they do not seem to lose their lymphohematopoietic differentiation ability. However, their clonal expansion rate declines with age, as does their rate in generating B cells and their rate in repairing ionizing radiation-induced DNA damage. These results show that the potential of stem cells to differentiate and proliferate is not compromised appreciably by old age but their capacity to do so efficiently is, as a result of inhibitory factors which emerge late in life.

Macrophages. Macrophages are not adversely affected by age in their *in vitro* handling of antigens, as judged by their: (a) capacity to cooperate with T and B cells during induction of antibody response; (b) content of lysosomal enzymes; (c) rates of engulfment and degradation of opsonized sheep red blood cells (RBC). On the other hand, macrophages are not as efficient *in situ*, when judged by blood clearance of colloidal carbon, the removal of foreign tumor cells and localization of antigens in lymphoid follicles during an immune response [9, 14]. These results indicate that decline with age in the functional activities of macrophages *in situ* is reflective of changes in their humoral regulatory factors, rather than of changes intrinsic to them.

T Cells. The total number of T cells does not decrease appreciably with age, but the proportion of subsets of T cells does appear to change. This is reflected by: (a) a decrease in various antigen- and mitogenstimulated T cell responses [9, 15]; (b) a decrease in the amount of cell surface theta antigen [1]; (c) decrease in the proportion of more mature lymph node T cells involved as amplifiers in mixed lymphocyte reactions [3]; (d) a decrease in the relative number of concanavalin-inducible circulating suppressor T cells [6]; (e) a decrease in the number of antigen-inducible spleen T helper cells [11], and (f) an increase in the number of antigen-inducible splenic T suppressor cells [19]. It would appear that the proportion of suppressor T cells may be increasing with age at the expense of helper T cells.

B Cells. The total number of B cells also does not change appreciably with age. However, their immunologic and proliferative capacities also decline, subsequent to that of T cells [15]. What has been most revealing is that associated with the decline, the proportion of suppressor B cells increases [20].

What emerges from these studies on stem cells, macrophages, T cells and B cells is that as individuals age, their immune functions wane as a result primarily of changes in the homeostatic mechanism that controls immune responses.

Influence of Age on Self-Recognition

Maintenance of immunologic tolerance to self also seems to break down as the ability of the immune system to recognize and respond efficiently to foreign antigens declines with age. This is reflected in the age-related increase in the number of individuals with autoimmune manifestation and diseases linked to autoimmunity [9].

Various approaches have been undertaken to understand the complex triangular association of aging, the loss of immunologic vigor and the breakdown in the maintenance of tolerance to self. One approach is focused on the role of regulatory T cells on antibody response to syngeneic cells. Using this approach, *Koskimies and Mäkelä* [10] found that T cell-deficient mice produced 2–3 times more antibody-forming cells in response to hapten-modified syngeneic RBC. *Naor et al.* [17] then demonstrated in aging mice that the decrease in antibody response to hapten-modified xenogeneic RBC is associated with an increase in antibody response to hapten-modified syngeneic RBC. These studies suggest that a major defect in the loss of self recognition in aging mice is associated with the loss of cells which normally would suppress antibody response to haptens closely associated to self antigens and to self antigens themselves.

Another approach takes into account the role of viruses, since it is known that viruses are intimately associated with a number of autoimmune diseases [9]. *Kay* [8], who began such a model study recently, was able to evaluate for the first time the long-term consequences (0.5–1 year) of parainfluenza viral infection in 8 different aging strains of mice and their hybrids. She found that the magnitude of age-related thymic involution is pronounced, the capacity of T cells to respond to mitogenic stimulation is reduced to background levels, and the frequency of individuals with anti-RBC autoantibodies is increased with age among strains of mice which normally do not express such autoantibodies. It would appear that the T cells may be the target of the parainfluenza infection. Another approach, described by *Weigle and Parks* [21], determines the effect of age on susceptibility, maintenance and termination of immunologic tolerance to self by examining the immunologic status of subsets of T and B cells. Their preliminary study on autoimmune-prone, short-lived NZB mice indicates that the defect resides in the B cells rather than in suppressor T cells.

Perhaps the genetic approach has been one of the most rewarding. It has revealed that: (a) H-2 genes display a considerable influence upon T and B cells of aging mice in their responsiveness to mitogens; (b) H-2 and HLA genes play a major role in autoimmunity and susceptibility to diseases, and (c) variations in life span and age-related diseases within a strain of mice congenic at the H-2 region are as great as those between strains [16]. Results of this nature indicate that the major histocompatibility complex (MHC) influences life expectancy and disease susceptibility of aging individuals, perhaps by modulating lymphocytes in their recognizance of self from nonself on an immunologic basis. This would mean that MHC could then be instrumental in age-related decline in homeostasis leading to self-destructive processes. Support of this view comes from recent epidemiological studies revealing that certain asymptomatic autoimmune parameters can be used as predictors of diseases and of life expectancy among the elderly [12].

Summary

An attempt has been made to describe briefly the complex triangular association of aging, age-related decline in immunologic vigor and age-related breakdown in maintenance of immunologic tolerance to self. It has been emphasized that the loss of immunologic vigor reflects the inability of the aging immune system to recognize and respond efficiently to foreign antigens. This is due primarily to the increase in the suppressor cells. Paradoxically, the increase in suppressor cells which can impinge upon immune cells responsive to foreign antigens is associated with a decrease in suppressor cells which can impinge upon immune cells responsive to self and altered-self antigens. Studies focused on the mechanisms responsible for age-related changes in normal and abnormal immune functions reveal that at the level of the cells, the changes can occur both in T and B cells, but at the molecular level the changes must reflect those occurring in the major histocompatibility gene complex.

References

1 Brennan, P. C. and Jaroslow, B. N.: Age-associated decline in theta antigen on spleen thymus-derived lymphocytes of B6CF$_1$ mice. Cell. Immunol. *15:* 51–56 (1975).

2 Chino, F.; Makinodan, T.; Lever, W. H., and Peterson, W. J.: The immune system of mice reared in clean and dirty conventional laboratory farms. I. Life expectancy and pathology of mice with long life spans. J. Geront. *26:* 497–507 (1971).

3 Gerbase-Delima, M.; Meredith, P., and Walford, R.: Age-related changes, including synergy and suppression, in the mixed lymphocyte reaction in long-lived mice. Fed. Proc. Fed. Am. Socs exp. Biol. *34:* 159–161 (1975).

4 Good, R. A. and Yunis, E.: Association of autoimmunity, immunodeficiency and aging in man, rabbits and mice. Fed. Proc. Fed. Am. Socs exp. Biol. *33:* 2040–2050 (1974).

5 Goodman, S. A. and Makinodan, T.: Effect of age on cell-mediated immunity in long-lived mice. Clin. exp. Immunol. *19:* 533–542 (1975).

6 Hallgren, H. M. and Yunis, E. J.: Suppressor lymphocytes in young and aged humans. J. Immun. *118:* 2004–2008 (1977).

7 Hirokawa, K.: The thymus and aging; in Makinodan and Yunis Immunology and aging; 1st ed., pp. 51–70 (Plenum Publishing, New York 1977).

8 Kay, M. M. B.: Long-term subclinical effects of parainfluenza (Sendai) infection on immune cells of aging mice. Proc. Soc. exp. Biol. Med. *158:* 326–331 (1978).

9 Kay, M. M. B. and Makinodan, T.: Immunobiology of aging: evaluation of current status. Clin. Immunol. Immunopath. *6:* 394–413 (1976).

10 Koskimies, S. and Mäkelä, O.: T-cell-deficient mice produce more antihapten antibodies against syngeneic than against allogeneic erythrocytes conjugates. J. exp. Med. *144:* 467–476 (1976).

11 Krogsrud, R. L. and Perkins, E. H.: Age-related changes in T cell function. J. Immun. *118:* 1607–1611 (1977).

12 Mackay, I. R.; Whittingham, S. F., and Mathews, J. D.: The immunoepidemiology of aging; in Makinodan and Yunis Immunology and aging; 1st ed., pp. 35–49 (Plenum Publishing, New York 1977).

13 Makinodan, T.; Albright, J. W.; Good, P. I.; Peter, C. F., and Heidrick, M. L.: Reduced humoral immune activity in long-lived old mice: an approach to elucidating its mechanism. Immunology *31:* 903–911 (1976).

14 Makinodan, T.; Perkins, E. H., and Chen, M. G.: Immunologic activity of the aged. Adv. Gerontol. Res. *3:* 171–198 (1971).

15 Makinodan, T. and Yunis, E. (eds): Immunology and aging; 1st ed. (Plenum Publishing, New York 1977).

16 Meredith, P. J. and Walford, R. L.: Autoimmunity, histocompatibility, and aging. Mech. Aging Dev. *9:* 61–77 (1979).

17 Naor, D.; Bonavida, B., and Walford, R. L.: Autoimmunity and aging: the age-related response of mice

of a long-lived strain to trinitrophenylated syngeneic mouse red blood cells. J. Immun. *117:* 2204–2208 (1976).

18 Price, G. B. and Makinodan, T.: Immunologic deficiencies in senescence. II. Characterization of extrinsic deficiencies. J. Immun. *108:* 413–417 (1972).

19 Segre, D. and Segre, M.: Humoral immunity in aged mice. II. Increased suppressor T cell activity in immunologically deficient old mice. J. Immun. *116:* 735–738 (1976).

20 Singhal, S. K.; Roder, J. C., and Duwe, A. K.: Suppressor cells in immunosenescence. Fed. Proc. Fed. Am. Socs exp. Biol. *37:* 1245–1252 (1978).

21 Weigle, W. O. and Parks, D. E.: Effect of aging on immune and tolerant states. Fed. Proc. Fed. Am. Socs exp. Biol. *37:* 1253–1257 (1978).

22 Zharhary, D.; Segev, Y., and Gershon, H.: The affinity and spectrum of cross reactivity of antibody production in senescent mice: the IgM response. Mech. Aging Dev. *6:* 385–392 (1977).

Dr. T. Makinodan, V. A. Wadsworth Hospital Center, Wilshire and Sawtelle Blvds., Los Angeles, CA 90073 (USA)

Induction of Autoimmunity

Immunopathology. 6th Int. Convoc. Immunol., Niagara Falls, N.Y., 1978, pp. 26–30 (Karger, Basel 1979)

Genetic Regulation of Immune Responses

William E. Paul

Laboratory of Immunology, National Institute of Allergy and Infectious Diseases, National Institutes of Health, Bethesda, Md.

Genetic approaches to the study of biologic phenomena provide powerful tools with which to examine complex systems because they allow the investigation of individual steps of the system in a highly controlled way. This has proved particularly true in the study of the immune response in which the examination of genetically deficient patients and animals has offered enormous insights into the mechanisms involved in specific immunity. An outstanding example of the power of genetic tools in the delineation of the immune system has come from the study of the specific immune response (*Ir*) genes of the major histocompatibility complex (MHC).

A large number of distinct examples of action of specific *Ir* genes have now been described. In general, the responses controlled by these genes have two characteristics; they are thymus-dependent responses and they are directed at molecules which are either structurally or antigenically simple. The limitation of function of *Ir* gene systems to thymus-dependent immune responses was initially interpreted as evidence that the genes expressed their function within thymus-dependent (T) lymphocytes. Indeed, one favored possibility was that the *Ir* genes were the structural genes for the specific antigen-binding receptors of T lymphocytes. Over the last several years, this possibility has become

less likely, largely as a result of studies of the role of *I*-region gene products in the regulation of cellular interactions. Indeed, T lymphocyte responses appear to depend largely on collaboration with other cell types [5]. Thus, the activation of proliferative responses by specific T lymphocytes and of responses leading to the secretion of lymphokines depends on an interaction between the T lymphocyte and an antigen-presenting cell, which appears to be a member of the macrophage-monocyte series of cells [13]. The characteristics of the antigen-presenting cell are that it is a radiation-resistant, Ia$^+$, Ig$^-$, Thy-1$^-$ adherent cell [9]. The efficient activation of primed T lymphocytes requires that the donor of the antigen-presenting cell and the donor of the responding T cell possess common allelic forms of the I-A subregion of the MHC (table I) [8, 12]. In F$_1$ animals, T lymphocytes nominally specific for a given antigen, such as the 2,4-dinitrophenyl (DNP)-derivative of ovalbumin (OVA), may be shown to actually consist of two subpopulations of cells, one which can be stimulated by DNP-OVA associated with antigen-presenting cells bearing Ia molecules derived from one parent but which fail to respond to the same antigen presented by cells possessing Ia molecules derived from the alternative parent and a second popula-

Table I. Stimulation of antigen-specific proliferative responses of primed T lymphocytes requires I-A similarity between donor of antigen-presenting cell and donor-responding cell[1]

Donor of antigen-presenting cell	Regions held in common								Response
	K	A	B	J	E	C	S	D	
A.TL (skkkkkd)[2]	+	+	+	+	+	+	+	+	+
B10.A (4R) (kkbbbbbb)	−	+	−	−	−	−	−	−	+
B10.A (5R) (bbbkkddd)	−	−	−	+	+	−	−	+	−

[1] T lymphocytes were obtained from peritoneal exudates of A.TL mice which had been previously immunized with 2,4-dinitrophenyl-ovalbumin (DNP-OVA). These cells were cultured in microtiter wells with mitomycin-C-treated spleen cells, from nonimmunized mice, which had been incubated in vitro with DNP-OVA and then extensively washed. Proliferative responses were measured by the uptake of tritiated thymidine after 5 days of culture. Adapted from Yano et al. [12].
[2] The genetic formulas for alleles at the MHC loci K, A, B, J, E, C, S and D are shown in parentheses.

Table II. Need for antigen-presenting cell to derive from a donor possessing a responder form of a specific Ir gene[1]

Responding strain $(B10 \times B10.S)F_1$

donor of antigen-presenting cell		response
strain	responder status	
$(B10 \times B10.S)F_1$	responder	+
B10	responder	+
B10.S	nonresponder	−
B10 + B10.S	responder + nonresponder	+

$(B10 \times B10.S)F_1$ mice were immunized with poly-(Glu, Ala, Tyr) [GAT] and T lymphocyte-enriched peritoneal exudate prepared 2–3 weeks later. These cells were challenged in vitro with mitomycin-treated, GAT-pulsed spleen cells from nonimmune F_1, B10, and B10.S donors and with a mixture of B10 and B10.S cells. The proliferative response was measured by the uptake of ^{3}H-thymidine after 5 days of culture. Adapted from Yano et al. [13].

tion with reciprocal specificity characteristics. This implies that the responding T lymphocyte can recognize two characteristics of the antigen-presenting cell—the conventional antigen (e.g. DNP-OVA) which It bears and the Ia type of the cell [6].

One of the most important features of Ir gene product function has come from the extension of this concept to Ir gene-controlled systems. Thus, F_1 hybrids prepared by crossing responders and nonresponders are in general responders. If such animals are immunized with an antigen, the response to which is known to be under genetic control, T lymphocytes from these animals can be activated in vitro by antigen-presenting cells obtained from the responder parent but antigen-presenting cells from the nonresponder

parent fail to activate such responses [10, 13] (table II). This result indicates that Ir genes must be expressed in the antigen-presenting cell [see 9] but it does not clarify the actual nature of the defect that leads to unresponsiveness. Two general explanations for the defect may be considered. One can be described as the absence of the clone of T cells which can recognize antigen presented by cells of the nonresponder parent; the other is the failure of the nonresponder antigen-presenting cell to perform some critical operation which is required for the subsequent activation of the responding T cell clone. The latter assumes that there is an actual chemical or physical representation of Ir gene product function on the antigen-presenting cell. For example, it has been suggested that

Ia antigens on the surface of the antigen-presenting cell have the capacity to recognize certain structural features of the antigen and to interact with it in such a way as to create a stimulatory molecule. The defect in the nonresponder would consist of a failure of the antigen-presenting cell from the nonresponder to carry out the critical interaction step. To determine whether this is, in fact, the nature of *Ir* gene product function, it will be necessary to compare antigen handling by responder and nonresponder antigen-presenting cells.

The alternative possibility is that 'antigen-processing' events occur normally on the surface of antigen-presenting cells from the nonresponder parent. Indeed, it is possible that no important molecular interactions occur on this cell. Rather, the defect in the nonresponder may involve the absence from the animal of any T cells which could recognize the antigen in question on the surface of the nonresponder antigen-presenting cell. This 'absent clone' theory implies that the *Ir* gene product is expressed in the antigen-presenting cell but that its function is simply the passive one of being recognized by some type of self-recognition structure. Furthermore, this theory suggests that the generation of T cell clones which can simultaneously recognize given self-I-region antigens and given conventional antigens is not a random process. The failure to generate a specific *set* of recognition structures would be the true functional *Ir* gene defect event though the actual genetic site to which the *Ir* genes map may be quite distinct from the site in which the genes controlling the recognition structures are located.

Both of these theories emphasize that it is in the process of cellular interactions in which the function of Ir gene products and Ia antigens are to be found. I have developed the argument leading to this view by discussing limitations on the interactions of antigen-presenting cells and T lymphocytes; precisely the same constraints exist in the interactions of T lymphocytes with B lymphocytes in the stimulation of thymus-dependent antibody responses [4].

Although *Ir* gene control is studied using simple antigens for which genetic control can easily be shown, it seems certain that the phenomena revealed by these studies regulate responses to all thymus-dependent antigens. This emphasizes the intimate participation of *MHC* gene function in all aspects of the immune system.

Closely related to the phenomenon of regulation of cellular interactions by I-region gene products is the role of MHC gene products in the specific cell-mediated lysis of virus-infected and chemically modified target cells. It is now widely appreciated that MHC gene products play critical roles in the cell-mediated cytotoxic response which develops in animals immunized with various viruses [14]. For example, mice immunized with lymphocytic choriomeningitis, vaccinia, ectromelia, influenza or vesicular stomatitis virus develop specific killer cells which are capable of lysing target cells infected with the virus used for immunization but not cells infected with other viruses. However, the capacity of cytotoxic T cells from immunized donors to destroy virus-infected target cells is markedly affected by the histocompatibility type of the target cell.

Only virus-infected cells of the same *H-2K* or *H-2D* type as the killer T cells are suitable targets for lysis. Furthermore, if one immunizes an F_1 mouse with virus, one can show that the cells which kill virus-infected target cells derived from one parent are distinct from the killer cells which lyse virus-infected target cells from the other parent. This implies that the killer T cell recognizes both MHC gene products of the target cells and viral antigens expressed by these cells. In this respect, there is great similarity between the collaboration of antigen-presenting cells and primed T lymphocytes (and of T lymphocytes and B lymphocytes) and the interaction of 'virus-specific' killer T lymphocytes and infected target cells. The principal difference in the two systems is that the T cell involved in collaborative interactions is specific for antigen and *I*-region gene products while the cytotoxic T cell is specific for antigen and *K* and/or *D* region gene products. A further analogy now exists in that specific genetic control of the ability to kill target cells bearing viruses, minor histocompatibility and chemical modifications has recently been shown [11]. In such cases, the *Ir* genes involved often map to *K* and/or *D* rather than *I*. In addition to extending the generality of specific regulation of immune responses by MHC gene products, these findings may help to clarify the mechanisms underlying the role of MHC gene products in determination of disease susceptibility.

It has been shown that a large number of human diseases occur with greater frequency in individuals of a given histocompatibility type than in individuals who are not of this type. Perhaps the best known example of this is ankylosing spondylitis, in which individuals who are HLA-B27$^+$ are approximately ninety times more likely to develop the disease than are individuals who are HLA-B27$^-$ [1]. Other diseases in which increased frequency is associated with given HLA antigens are gluten-sensitive enteropathy, Reiters' syndrome, multiple sclerosis, myasthenia gravis, rheumatoid arthritis and juvenile diabetes mellitus. In addition, it has now been shown that the incidence of juvenile diabetes mellitus is markedly diminished in individuals who possess certain HLA-D antigens [2], suggesting that MHC genes may convey resistance as well as susceptibility to disease.

The question which I wish to address is how the MHC regulation of specific immune responses might relate to MHC determination of susceptibility or resistance to individual diseases. Perhaps the most obvious and straightforward mechanism is that individuals of given distinct HLA types might lack or possess specific *Ir* genes which were critical to the development of immune responses against antigenic determinants associated with agents important in the pathogenesis of the disease. For example, it has been proposed that juvenile diabetes mellitus may result from an autoimmune process occurring as a result of a viral infection affecting the islets of Langerhans [3]. One could easily postulate that the lack of a given *Ir* gene which normally controlled responsiveness to the inciting virus might render an individual more likely to develop infection and thus to subsequently develop the disease. Alternatively, the possession of an *Ir* gene which promoted the immune response important in the subsequent 'autoimmune' reaction would also place the individual at a greater risk of developing disease. Of course, one could also achieve associations by considering the significance of the possession of *Ir* genes which protected against infection or the lack of genes which caused heightened autoimmunity.

The fact that some diseases are associated with given HLA-D antigens while others are associated with certain HLA-B antigens is consistent with developing knowledge that certain *Ir* genes are found within the I region, the human equivalent of which is HLA-D, while other *Ir* genes have now been mapped to the *D* or *K* regions, of which HLA-B is an analog.

Of course, one should not imply that specific *Ir* genes constitute the only means through which MHC gene products might lead to disease susceptibility. Other possibilities include tolerance induction through the possible resemblance of the antigens of a pathogenic agent to certain histocompatibility antigens or increased susceptibility to a given disease because the product of an allele at a MHC locus acted as a 'receptor' for certain viruses or other intracellular parasites. Nonetheless, our increasing recognition of the central role MHC gene products play in the regulation of T lymphocyte responses, including lymphokine production, T-dependent antibody synthesis, and specific cell-mediated cytotoxicity make it most likely that the very same gene products will play key roles in the processes involved in MHC control of susceptibility or resistance to disease.

References

1 Bluestone, R.: Immunogenetics and ankylosing spondylitis. Clins rheum. Dis. *3:* 255–264 (1977).

2 Gamble, D. R.; Taylor, K. W., and Cumming, H.: Coxsackie virus and diabetes mellitus. Br. med. J. *iv:* 260–264 (1973).

3 Ilonen, J.; Herva, E.; Tiilikainen, A.; Åkerblom, H. K.; Koivukangas, T., and Kouvalainen, K.: HLA-Dw2 as a marker of resistance against juvenile diabetes mellitus. Tissue Antigens *11:* 144–146 (1978).

4 Katz, D. H. and Benacerraf, B.: The function and interrelationships of T-cell receptors, Ir genes and other histocompatibility gene products. Transplantn Rev. *22:* 175–195 (1975).

5 Paul, W. E. and Benacerraf, B.: Functional specificity of thymus-dependent lymphocytes. Science *195:* 1293–1300 (1977).

6 Paul, W. E.; Shevach, E. M.; Pickeral, S.; Thomas, D. W., and Rosenthal, A. S.: Independent populations of primed F_1 guinea pig T lymphocytes respond to antigen-pulsed parental peritoneal exudate cells. J. exp. Med. *145:* 618–630 (1977).

7 Rosenthal, A. S.; Lipsky, P. E., and Shevach, E. M.: Macrophage-lymphocyte interaction and antigen recognition. Fed. Proc. Fed. Am. Socs exp. Biol. *34:* 1743–1748 (1975).

8 Rosenthal, A. S. and Shevach, E. M.: Function of macrophages in antigen recognition by T lymphocytes. I. Requirement for histocompatible macrophages and lymphocytes. J. exp. Med. *138:* 1194–1212 (1973).

9 Schwartz, R. H.; Yano, A., and Paul, W. E.: Interaction between antigen-presenting cells and primed T lymphocytes: an assessment of Ir gene expression in the antigen-presenting cell. Immunol. Rev. *40:* 153–180 (1978).

10 Shevach, E. M. and Rosenthal, A. S.: The function of macrophages in antigen-recognition by guinea pig T lymphocytes. II. Role of the macrophage in the regulation of genetic control of the immune response. J. exp. Med. *138:* 1213–1229 (1973).

11 Simpson, E. and Gordon, R.D.: Responsiveness to HY antigen; Ir gene complementation and target cell specificity. Immunol. Rev. *35:* 59–75 (1977).

12 Yano, A.; Schwartz, R. H., and Paul, W. E.: Antigen presentation in the murine T lymphocyte proliferative response. I. Requirement for genetic identity at the murine major histocompatibility complex. J. exp. Med. *146:* 828–843 (1977).

13 Yano, A.; Schwartz, R. H., and Paul, W. E.: Antigen presentation in the murine T-lymphocyte proliferative response. II. *Ir-GAT* controlled T lymphocyte responses require antigen-presenting cells from a high responder donor. Eur. J. Immunol. (in press).

14 Zinkernagel, R. M. and Doherty, P. C.: H-2 compatibility requirement for T cell mediated lysis of targets infected with lymphocyte choriomeningitis virus. Different cytotoxic T-cell specificities are associated with structure coded in *H-2K* or *H-2D*. J. exp. Med. *141:* 1427–1436 (1975).

Dr. W. E. Paul, Laboratory of Immunology, National Institute of Allergy and Infectious Diseases, National Institutes of Health, Bethesda, MD 20014 (USA)

Immunopathology. 6th Int. Convoc. Immunol., Niagara Falls, N.Y., 1978, pp. 31–35 (Karger, Basel 1979)

Autoreactivity Specific for Murine Antigens Controlled by the H-2D Region[1]

G. Cudkowicz, K. Nakano and I. Nakamura

Departments of Pathology and Microbiology, School of Medicine, State University of New York at Buffalo, Buffalo, N.Y.

Introduction

Responder spleen cells of B6D2F$_1$ hybrid mice (H-$2^{b/d}$) cultured *in vitro* with irradiated parental B6 spleen cells (H-$2^{b/b}$) generate cytotoxic T lymphocytes (CTL) specific for target cells sharing genes of the H-2^b haplotype with parental stimulators [6, 10, 11]. The F$_1$ anti-parent cell-mediated lympholysis (CML) response was developed as an *in vitro* correlate of natural resistance of lethally irradiated mice to the growth of transplanted bone marrow cells of parental or allogeneic donors [2, 3]. Anti-parent cytotoxicity can be induced in spleen cell cultures of several other hybrid strains, not only against H-2^b but also against H-2^d or H-2^k homozygous cells [4, 9, 11, 12]. Sensitive targets for such F$_1$ anti-parent CTL are mitogen-stimulated splenic lymphoblasts, thioglycollate-induced peritoneal exudate cells (PEC), or lymphoma cells.

Two major topics related to the *in vitro* development of F$_1$ anti-parent CML will be addressed in this paper: (1) the identification of the H-2 region coding for, or regulating the expression of, target determinants in H-2^b-homozygous cells; and (2) the recognition of such determinants by F$_1$ effector cells on H-2^b-heterozygous targets, a manifestation of autoreactivity. Lastly, correlations and inconsistencies between the *in vitro* and *in vivo* models of F$_1$ anti-parent cell-mediated reactions will be discussed so as to speculate on the nature of parental determinants and the mechanisms of recognition. Cytotoxic effectors were generated in 5-day B6D2F$_1$ anti-B6 mixed spleen cell cultures and then tested on cells labeled with radioactive chromium. Specific target lysis was measured in 4-hour chromium release assays; PEC were used as targets in direct cytolysis

[1] Supported by NIH Research Grants AM-13969 and CA-12844, and by NIH Contract N01-CM-53766 from the NCI.

and as cold inhibitors in competitive inhibition of specific lysis [6, 12].

Intra-*H-2* Mapping of Target Determinants

PEC from several H-2^b mouse strains were lysed to about the same extent by B6D2F$_1$ anti-B6 effectors in direct cytotoxic assays (table I, group 1). It must be noted that there was polymorphism at a multiplicity of loci other than H-2 in many of the unrelated PEC donor strains employed. The specificity of effector cells was demonstrated by the lack of significant lysis of H-2^a, H-2^d, H-2^k, and H-2^s targets (group 2). The genetic backgrounds of mice donating these PEC were matched with those of H-2^b mice so as to control for possible effects of non-H-2 associated genes. The only apparent exceptions to effector specificity for H-2^b targets were the PEC of H-2^j mice (group 3), but it is known that the H-2^j and H-2^b haplotypes share alleles of the D region specifying serologically defined antigens. PEC from mice with recombinant H-2^b haplotypes were susceptible to lysis whenever the *b* allele was present in the D region (group 4). Positivity for H-$2D^b$ was the necessary and sufficient condition for target cell lysis, irrespective of the alleles present at other H-2 regions. Critical targets in the experiments on which

Table I. Reactivity of peritoneal exudate target cells from different mouse strains with B6D2F$_1$ anti-B6 cytotoxic T lymphocytes

Group No.	Mouse strains	K I SGD ABJEC	Qa-1	Qa-2	Tla	Direct lysis of target cells[1]	Inhibition of target cell lysis[1]
1	B6, B10, C57L	*b b b b b b b b b*	*b*	*a*	*b*	+ +	+ +
	A.BY, BALB.B, C3H.B, AKR.B6	*b b b b b b b b b*				+ +	NT
	D1.LP², 129²	*b b b b b b b b b*				+ +	+ +
2	A, B10.A	*k k k k k d d d d*	*a*	*a*	*a*	−	−
	DBA/2, BALB/c, B10.D2	*d d d d d d d d d*				−	−
	C3H, AKR, B10.BR	*k k k k k k k k k*				−	−
	SJL	*s s s s s s s s s*				−	−
3	I, WB³	*j j j j j j j j j*				+ +	+ +
4	B10.A(4R)	*k k **b b b b b b b***				+ +	+ +
	D2.GD	*d d **b b b b b b b***				+ +	NT
	HTH, B10.A(2R)	*k k k k k d d d **b***				+ +	+ +
	HTG, B10.HTG	*d d d d d d d d **b***				+ +	+ +
	B10.AM	*k k k k k k k k **b***				+ +	NT
5	B10.A(3R)	***b b b b** k d d d d*				−	NT
	B10.(5R)	***b b b** k k d d d d*				−	−
	HTI	***b b b b b b b b** d*				−	NT
6	A.Tlaᵇ	*k k k k k d d d d*	*b*	*a*	*b*	−	−
	B6.Tlaᵃ	*b b b b b b b b b*	*a*	*a*	*a*	+ +	+ +
	B6.K1	*b b b b b b b b b*	*a*	*b*	*b*	+ +	+ +
	B6.K2	*b b b b b b b b b*	*a*	*a*	*b*	+ +	+ +
7	B6D2F$_1$	$K^{b/d}\ D^{b/d}$				−	+
	B6 × C3H, B10 × B10.BR	$K^{b/k}\ D^{b/k}$				−	+
	HTG × B10.D2	$K^{d/d}\ D^{b/d}$				−	+
	B10.A(4R) × B10.A	$K^{k/k}\ D^{b/d}$				−	+
	B10.A(5R) × B10.A	$K^{b/k}\ D^{d/d}$				−	−

[1] + and + + denote reactivity; − denotes absence of reactivity. NT = Not tested.
² $H\text{-}2^{bc}$ variant haplotype instead of $H\text{-}2^b$.
³ $H\text{-}2^{ja}$ variant haplotype instead of $H\text{-}2^j$.

this conclusion was based were not only those of $H\text{-}2D^b$-positive strains (group 4), but also those of $H\text{-}2D^b$-negative $H\text{-}2K^b$-positive mice (group 5). The involvement of genes in the T region was excluded by results obtained with PEC of the four recombinant strains between D and T or intra-T (group 6). Heterozygous F$_1$ hybrid PEC were not significantly lysed even though such cells possess one copy of $H\text{-}2D^b$ and associated D-region genes (group 7 of table I).

The mapping of target determinants to the D region was confirmed by competitive inhibition experiments. Cold PEC of *inbred* mouse strains that were susceptible to direct lysis, including $H\text{-}2^j$-homozygous PEC, were also effective inhibitors of specific lysis and *vice versa* (table I). The ability of $H\text{-}2D^b$-negative PEC to serve as targets or inhibitors in any CML response was verified by control experiments in which appropriate anti-allogeneic CTL replaced anti-parent effectors.

Autoreactivity of F₁ Anti-Parent CTL

PEC syngeneic with B6D2F₁ anti-B6 CTL or, in general, any H-$2D^b$-heterozygous PEC, were not lysed under standard conditions of direct cytotoxic assays (table I, group 7) and even at effector: target cell ratios higher than 40:1. Moreover, F₁ spleen cells did not induce cytotoxicity when used as irradiated stimulators. No evidence for autoreactivity was thus obtained from experiments relying on stimulation or direct lysis. F₁ hybrid PEC were capable, however, of competitively inhibiting specific anti-parental B6 target cell lysis. The inhibition by F₁ PEC was about one half as effective, for given numbers of cells, as that exerted by H-2^b-homozygous PEC (table I; compare groups 1, 4 and 6 with group 7). For inhibition of cytotoxicity to occur, PEC from heterozygotes for recombinant H-2^b haplotypes had to possess one copy of the H-$2D^b$ allele, irrespective of the alleles at other H-2 regions. The critical F₁ hybrids in this group of inhibition tests were (HTG × B10.D2)F₁, whose H-$2D^{b/d}$ cells were inhibitory, and [B10.A(5R) × B10.A]F₁, whose H-$2D^{d/d}$ cells were not inhibitory, although b alleles were present in the genome of these cells at the K, IA, and IB regions.

Two alternative mechanisms, outlined in the scheme of figure 1, were considered to explain the existence of inhibition-positive, lysis-negative F₁ hybrid PEC. Target determinants (controlled by Hh-1 or other H-2D-region gene) would be fully expressed in homozygous parental cells but partially in heterozygous F₁ cells; one could visualize the difference as being quantitative (gene-dose effect on the determinants surface density), qualitative (interallelic interaction modifying parental gene products), or both. Since the determinants on parental and F₁ hybrid cells

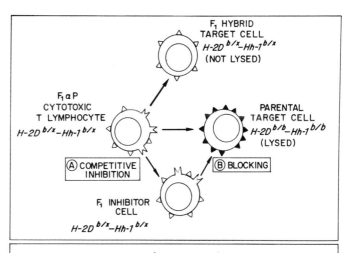

Fig. 1. Two mechanisms explaining the ability of heterozygous F₁ hybrid peritoneal exudate cells to serve as inhibitors but not as targets of F₁ anti-parent cell-mediated lympholysis.

appear to be cross-reactive, one could interpret the results of cold inhibition assays in terms of competition for receptors of F_1 antiparent CTL capable of binding to, and of lysing, parental target cells. Stimulation in culture conferred this competence to responder T lymphocytes. Thus, the differential sensitivity to direct lysis of parental and syngeneic targets would depend on the phenotypic expression of the relevant genes and, as a corollary, F_1 anti-parent CTL would be autoreactive (mechanism A of fig. 1). Consistent with this view is the observation that induction of such F_1 CTL requires parental stimulator T cells endowed with some form of reactivity to alloantigens of responder cells, presumably to provide a back-reaction [7, 8]. This would lead to derepression of autoreactive F_1 cells followed by activation in the presence of 'antigenic' parental cells belonging to T lymphocyte as well as other subpopulations.

Preparations of F_1 hybrid PEC used as inhibitors contained lymphocytes and, thus, an alternative mechanism had to be considered. Nonstimulated F_1 lymphocytes may possess receptors capable of attachment to targets but not of lysis. If so, inhibitory activity of F_1 PEC could have resulted from blocking of interactions between CTL and radiolabeled targets (mechanism B of fig. 1). The blocking mechanism was not consistent with results of additional experiments in which B6 and B6D2F$_1$ embryonic fibroblasts (third serial passage in culture) served as inhibitors of F_1 anti-B6 cytotoxicity. DBA/2 fibroblasts were the noninhibitory control cells. Fibroblasts do not bear surface receptors for recognition and lysis of parental target cells, but they should bear the antigenic products of H-2D-region genes. Thus, the inhibitory activity of fibroblasts favors the competition mechanism; it indicates, moreover, that F_1 anti-parent CML is not likely to be an anti-receptor or anti-idiotype response.

Speculations on the Nature of Target Determinants

F_1 hybrid anti-parent CML *in vitro* was developed under the assumption that its genetic control and effector mechanism were equivalent to those operating *in vivo* for hybrid resistance to parental bone marrow grafts [10]. The mapping of parental determinants to H-2D for both models of F_1 anti-parent cell-mediated reactions [6, 10] lent support to this assumption, and in particular to the view that the relevant gene was *Hh-1* (*hemopoietic-histocompatibility-1*). The gene was so designated because of selective expression in cells of the blood-forming system (including fibroblasts) and the barrier it posed to transplantation; *Hh-1* was distinguished from other *H-2* genes because of noncodominant inheritance. Several distinctive features of the *in vivo* response to *Hh-1* gene products were exhibited also by the *in vitro* induced F_1 anti-parental *H-2^b* CML, notably the late maturation of responsiveness during the fourth week of life, the concomitant induction of specific unresponsiveness, and the critical dependence on macrophage-like cells [10]. However, it soon became apparent that the mediators of hybrid resistance were radioresistant thymus-independent cells, whereas the mediators of anti-parent CML were radiosensitive T lymphocytes [10]. In addition, F_1 anti-parent CML was inducible in strain combinations for which hybrid resistance to parental bone marrow grafts did not materialize [e.g. F_1 anti-parental *H-2^k* CML [4, 9, 12]]. One could explain this type of discrepancy by assuming that the recognitive abilities of T lymphocytes were superior to those of non-T cells. However, two more inconsistencies emerged from this study: (1) The reactivity of B6D2F$_1$ anti-B6 effectors with *H-2^j* targets (table I) would imply that *Hh-1* alleles of the *H-2^b* and *H-2^j* haplotypes are similar or identical, but *H-2$^{b/j}$* hybrids were found to be resistant instead of susceptible to parental grafts [5]. (2) The lack of reactivity of B6D2F$_1$ anti-B6 effectors with *H-2^s* targets (table I) would imply that *Hh-1* alleles of the *H-2^b* and *H-2^s* haplotypes are different, but *H-2$^{b/s}$* hybrids were found to be susceptible instead of resistant to parental grafts [1, 13]. Clearly, the original unitarian hypothesis of control by *Hh-1* of both hybrid resistance and F_1 anti-parent CML needs revision.

The following working hypotheses concerning the nature of parental determinants are presently under investigation:

(1) Determinants are controlled by genes of the *Hh* type clustered as pseudoalleles in the D and K regions of *H-2*. One set of gene products is recognized by non-T cells, and a different set by T lymphocytes, with partial overlap of repertoires. The hypothesis could account

for most of the inconsistencies observed between *in vivo* and *in vitro* F_1 anti-parent reactions. Because of non-codominant inheritance of *Hh* genes, the hypothesis is not predictive of autoreactivity for F_1 anti-parent CTL.

(2) Determinants are controlled by *Hh* genes and recognized as such by non-T cells *in vivo*. For T lymphocytes, *Hh*-gene products are H-2D or H-2K restricted antigens coded for by closely linked polymorphic genes and/or by ubiquitous monomorphic unlinked genes. Recognition of Hh antigens by T cells would only occur in association with H-2D or H-2K antigens, the reason for consistent mapping of target determinants to either the H-2D (table I) or H-2K region [4, 12], regardless of non-H-2-genetic disparities of parental strains. The hypothesis fails to explain competitive inhibition of specific F_1 anti-parental B6 target lysis by *H-2^j* cells, assuming that the *H-2^j* and *H-2^b* haplotypes share serologic specificities but not *Hh* genes. In other systems of dual recognition, inhibition of specific target lysis is only accomplished when inhibitor cells possess both the restricted and the restricting antigens. The hypothesis also fails to predict autoreactivity of F_1 anti-parent CTL, since *Hh*-gene products are lacking from F_1 cells.

(3) Determinants for CML are not controlled by *Hh* but by *H-2* genes coding for private or public specificities. The determinants may represent particular sites of serologically defined H-2 molecules that could become modified *via* gene dose effects or interallelic interactions, independently of the antigenic sites for antibody. Derepression of F_1 T cell clones cross-reactive with the relevant self antigens would be a prerequisite for subsequent differentiation to CTL in the presence of parental antigens. The hypothesis predicts autoreactivity of F_1 anti-parent CTL and accounts for all results obtained so far in competitive inhibition of B6D2F$_1$ anti-B6 CML, including the inhibition by *H-2^j* cells. Were this model applicable to resistance *in vivo* against parental bone marrow and lymphoma cells, one could visualize a role for autoreactivity against *H-2* gene products in the maintenance of homeostasis. Proliferation and differentiation of normal as well as transformed hemopoietic stem cells could be subjected to such regulatory influences.

References

1 Cudkowicz, G.: Discussion; in Cudkowicz, Landy and Shearer Natural resistance systems against foreign cells, tumors, and microbes, pp. 18–19 (Academic Press, New York 1978).
2 Cudkowicz, G. and Bennett, M.: Peculiar immunobiology of bone marrow allografts. I. Graft rejection by irradiated responder mice. J. exp. Med. *134:* 83–101 (1971).
3 Cudkowicz, G. and Bennett, M.: Peculiar immunobiology of bone marrow allografts. II. Rejection of parental grafts by resistant F_1 hybrid mice. J. exp. Med. *134:* 1513–1528 (1971).
4 Ishikawa, H. and Dutton, R. W.: Primary *in vitro* cytotoxic response of F_1 T lymphocytes against parental antigens. J. Immun. *122:* 529–536 (1979).
5 Lotzovà, E. and Cudkowicz, G.: Hybrid resistance to parental WB/Re bone marrow grafts. Association with genetic markers of linkage group IX. Transplantation *13:* 256–264 (1972).
6 Nakano, K.; Nakamura, I., and Cudkowicz, G.: F_1 hybrid anti-parental *H-2^b* cell-mediated lympholysis. I. Target determinants controlled by the H-2D region (submitted for publication).
7 Nakamura, I.: Discussion; in Cudkowicz, Landy, and Shearer Natural resistance systems against foreign cells, tumors and microbes, pp. 121–125 (Academic Press, New York 1978).
8 Nakamura, I.; Nakano, K., and Cudkowicz, G.: F_1 anti-parent cell-mediated lympholysis: autoreactive effectors and requirement of parental T cells for stimulation; in Quastel, Cell biology and immunology of leukocyte function, pp. 669–674 (Academic Press, New York 1979).
9 Schmitt-Verhulst, A. M. and Zatz, M. M.: F_1 resistance to AKR lymphoma cells *in vivo* and *in vitro*. J. Immun. *118:* 330–333 (1977).
10 Shearer, G. M.; Cudkowicz, G.; Schmitt-Verhulst, A. M.; Rehn, T. G.; Waksal, H., and Evans, P. D.: F_1 hybrid antiparental cell-mediated lympholysis: a comparison with bone marrow graft rejection and with cell-mediated lympholysis to alloantigens. Cold Spring Harb. Symp. quant. Biol. *41:* 511–518 (1977).
11 Shearer, G. M.; Garbarino, C. A., and Cudkowicz, G.: *In vitro* induction of F_1 hybrid anti-parent cell-mediated cytotoxicity. J. Immun. *117:* 754–759 (1976).
12 Warner, J. F. and Cudkowicz, G.: F_1 hybrid antiparental *H-2^k* cell-mediated lympholysis. I. Stimulator and target determinants controlled by the H-2K region. J. Immun. *122:* 575–581 (1979).
13 Warner, N. L.: Discussion; in Cudkowicz, Landy and Shearer Natural resistance systems against foreign cells, tumors, and microbes, pp. 12–16 (Academic Press, New York 1978).

Dr. G. Cudkowicz, Department of Pathology, State University of New York at Buffalo, 232 Farber Hall, Buffalo, NY 14214 (USA)

Immunopathology. 6th Int. Convoc. Immunol., Niagara Falls, N.Y., 1978, pp. 36–39 (Karger, Basel 1979)

Selective Action of Cyclosporin A on Lymphoblasts and the Induction of Tolerance to Allografts

A. C. Allison, R. C. Garcia[1], C. Green and P. Leoni[1]

Clinical Research Centre, Harrow

Introduction

For many years, immunologists have attempted to induce tolerance to allografts while leaving intact other immune functions such as resistance to infectious diseases. None of the existing procedures is satisfactory. With the regime of chemotherapy currently in use for renal allograft recipients, the combined use of azathioprine and corticosteroids, patients have to be treated for their life span, and they show increased susceptibility to virus and other infections and to lymphoreticular malignancies. What is needed is a drug that is able to eliminate clones of lymphocytes responding to stimulation by the antigens of the allograft but leaving intact other clones of lymphocytes that can later respond to viral or other antigens. Recent experiments suggest that an antibiotic, Cyclosporin A, is a promising candidate for this role.

Cyclosporin A

Cyclosporin A is a metabolite of the fungi *Cylindrocarpum lucidum* Booth and *Trichoderma polysporum*

[1] Present address: Instituto de Investigaciones Bioquimicas, Obligado 2490, 1428 Buenos Aires, Argentina.

Rifai. It is a cyclic peptide consisting of 11 amino acids, one of which has an unusual structure not previously reported [9]. Cyclosporin A originally attracted interest because of its antifungal activity, but routine screening tests showed it to have antilymphocytic effects, which were further explored. In rodents and guinea pigs, Cyclosporin A inhibits antibody formation, allograft rejection, cell-mediated cytotoxicity, adjuvant arthritis and experimental allergic encephalomyelitis [1, 3, 4, 7]. The *in vitro* response of mouse spleen cells to concanavalin A (Con A) was inhibited by low doses of Cyclosporin A. Cyclosporin A did not inhibit the formation of antibodies to lipopolysaccharide (LPS) in mice, or the *in vitro* responses of spleen cells to LPS [2], from which *Borel and Weisinger* [2] concluded that there is a selective effect on mouse T-lymphocytes, leaving intact the responses of B-lymphocytes to antigens or mitogens.

Since many drugs have immunosuppressive activity, these observations attracted only limited interest. However, studies carried out during the past 2 years have shown a specificity of action of Cyclosporin A which is so far unique and which has important clinical implications. Cyclosporin A in low concentrations acts on human lymphoblasts responding to antigenic or mitogenic stimulation, as well as on leukaemic blasts with T or B cell markers, whereas in the same concentration it has no effect on bone marrow stem cells, leukaemic cells with myeloid markers and a variety of other cell types. Cyclosporin A also has no demonstrable effect on small lymphocytes. These observations suggested that Cyclosporin A might be able *in vivo* to eliminate clones of lymphocytes responding to antigenic stimulation by an allograft. If this were the case, a short course of treatment with Cyclosporin A might be sufficient to induce tolerance to allografts. Our experiments on renal allografts in rabbits show that this aim can be achieved in the majority of recipients.

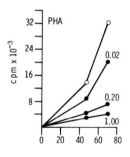 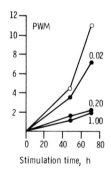 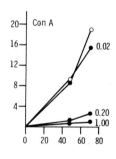

Stimulation time, h

Fig. 1. Effects of different concentrations of Cyclosporin A on responses of human peripheral blood cells to mitogens. [³H]-TdR pulses were given at 47 and 70 h after mitogen addition to the cultures and 5% TCA-insoluble material was determined. Mitogen concentrations were as follows: PHA, 1 μg/ml; Con A, 10 μg/ml; and 1% (v/v) PWM according to the instructions from the manufacturers. The ethanol concentration was 0.2% (v/v) in all cases, which has no effect on lymphocyte growth. Cyclosporin A concentrations (μg/ml) are indicated at the right of the curve.

Effects of Cyclosporin A on Human Peripheral Blood Lymphocytes

The responses of human peripheral blood lymphocyte cultures to phytohaemagglutinin (PHA), Con A and pokeweed mitogen (PWM) were inhibited by Cyclosporin A in a dose-dependent manner (fig. 1) [8]. Inhibition was nearly complete at a concentration of the drug of 1 μg/ml. Similar inhibition was found of mixed lymphocyte reactions (fig. 2).

When Cyclosporin A was added at different times after PHA stimulation, DNA synthesis was inhibited after a short lag period, showing that the drug does not act only on the early events in transformation. Differential counts showed that the number of blasts was selectively reduced. Hence, Cyclosporin A not only inhibits DNA synthesis in blasts, but actually kills these cells.

When human peripheral blood lymphocyte cultures were incubated with Cyclosporin A (1–2 μg/ml), for periods up to 40 h, and removed to medium lacking the drug,

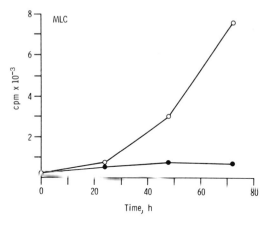

Fig. 2. Effect of Cyclosporin A on mixed lymphocyte reaction. Lymphocytes from pooled buffy coat residues from five donors were cultured and [³H]-TdR incorporation into 5% TCA-insoluble material determined at the times indicated, in the absence (o) or presence (●) of 1 μg of Cyclosporin A/ml.

responses to PHA were nearly normal. This suggests that Cyclosporin A has little effect on small lymphocytes, the inhibition of the response to mitogens being reversible.

Effects of Cyclosporin A on Lymphoblastic Cell Lines, Leukaemic Cells and Other Cell Types

Lymphoblastic cell lines with B or T cell markers and cultured cells from patients with acute lymphoblastic leukaemia were found to be sensitive to Cyclosporin A, marked inhibition being produced by 2 µg/ml (fig. 3). This concentration did not inhibit the proliferation of human leukaemic cells with myeloid markers or human or mouse fibroblastic cell lines. Thus, Cyclosporin A is remarkably specific in its action on lymphoblasts with both T and B cell markers, as opposed to unstimulated lymphocytes and other cell types even when the latter are rapidly proliferating.

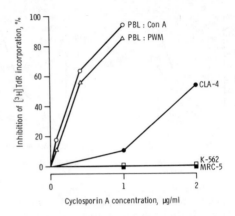

Fig. 3. Inhibition by different concentrations of Cyclosporin A of incorporation of [³H]-TdR in human peripheral blood lymphocytes stimulated with Con A (open circles) or PWM (triangles), a human lymphoblastoid cell line (CLA-4) with B-lymphocyte markers (filled circles), a leukaemic cell line (K-562) with myeloid markers (open squares), and a human fibroblastic cell line (MRC-5, filled squares). Conditions as for figure 1.

Indefinite Rabbit Kidney Allograft Survival after Short-Term Treatment with Cyclosporin A

In experiments already reported [6], rabbits of one outbred strain (Sandy lops) were used as kidney donors and of another outbred strain (New Zealand White) as recipients. The recipients were grafted with a single kidney from the allogeneic donor and the contralateral kidney was removed. Controls and recipients left untreated or given daily doses of olive oil (10 per group) rejected the kidneys usually in 12–16 days after grafting, and in no instance in more than 24 days. In contrast, 8 of our 10 animals receiving Cyclosporin A for 18 or 28 days after grafting (25 mg/kg/day in olive oil by mouth), and thereafter no further treatment, have remained in excellent health with no rejection crises and normal renal function and no infection for the observation period of 10 months. This experiment has been repeated in other groups of rabbits with similar results.

Allogeneic rabbit kidneys are difficult to protect against host responses. Cyclophosphamide, 6-mercaptopurine, azathioprine and antilymphocytic serum in high doses all failed to prevent acute rejection. Only prednisolone acetate at toxic dosage (1.0 mg/kg/day intramuscularly) prolonged graft survival, but the kidneys were always rejected within 12 days of steroid withdrawal, and even if drug administration was continued, renal function fluctuated, many rabbits died with rejected kidneys, often with intercurrent infections or intestinal complications, and all animals lost weight and developed osteoporosis.

The results with Cyclosporin A are clearly superior, with indefinite survival of functioning allografts after a short period of treatment and no side effects, including any demonstrable change in haematological profile.

The blood ureas and creatinines of the animals that have had short-term Cyclosporin A treatment are steadily low whereas those that have received steroids have varied greatly.

The induction of selective tolerance to allografts with Cyclosporin A has been confirmed by suitable experiments. Recipients of renal allografts were treated with Cyclosporin A for 28 days and have had acceptance of their grafts for several months without any treatment. They were then grafted with kidneys or skin from other donors. The second grafts were rejected while the first grafts remained intact and functional.

Calne et al. [5] studied the effects of Cyclosporin A on pigs given orthotopic cardiac allografts from donors mismatched at the major locus. Median survival of 20 control pigs was only 6 days; when 6 animals were given 25 mg/kg/day intramuscularly for 2 days and then orally median survival was greater than 68 days.

Presumably, the long-term survival of functioning allografts after short-term treatment with Cyclosporin A implies that clones of lymphocytes responding to donor antigens have been eliminated or suppressed. If this is so and if the drug behaves similarly in man without serious side effects, Cyclosporin A could be valuable in clinical kidney transplantation. The selective action of Cyclosporin A on lymphoblasts, leaving bone marrow precursors of monocytes, granulocytes, erythrocytes and platelets relatively unscathed, makes it particularly attractive for bone marrow grafting. The effects of the drug on lymphoblasts with both B and T cell markers also raise the possibility that Cyclosporin A, which is structurally unrelated to any known cytotoxic agents, may be useful in the therapy of certain leukaemias of lymphoid origin. Clinical trials are in progress and the results are awaited with interest.

References

1 Borel, J. F.: Comparative study of *in vitro* and *in vivo* drug effects on cell-mediated cytotoxicity. Immunology *31:* 631–641 (1976).

2 Borel, J. F. and Wiesinger, D.: Effect of Cyclosporin A on murine lymphoid cells; in Lucas, Regulatory mechanisms in lymphocyte activation. Proc. 11th Leukocyte Culture Conf., pp. 716–718 (Academic Press, New York 1977).

3 Borel, J. F.; Feurer, C.; Gubler, H. U., and Stahelin, H.: Biological effects of Cyclosporin A: a new anti-lymphocytic agent. Agents Actions *6:* 468–475 (1976).

4 Borel, J. F.; Feurer, C.; Magnée, C., and Stähelin, H.: Effects of the new anti-lymphocytic peptide Cyclosporin A in animals. Immunology *32:* 1017–1025 (1977).

5 Calne, R. Y.; White, D. J. G.; Rolles, K.; Smith, D. P., and Herbertson, B. M.: Prolonged survival of pig orthotopic heart grafts treated with Cyclosporin A. Lancet *i:* 1183–1184 (1978).

6 Green, C. J. and Allison, A. C.: Extensive prolongation of rabbit kidney allograft survival after short-term Cyclosporin-A treatment. Lancet *i:* 1182–1183 (1978).

7 Kostakis, A. J.; White, D. J. G., and Calne, R. Y.: Prolongation of rat heart allograft survival by Cyclosporin A. I.C.R.S. Med. Sci. *5:* 280–282 (1977).

8 Leoni, P.; Garcia, R., and Allison, A. C.: Effects of Cyclosporin A on human lymphocytes in culture. J. clin. Lab. Immunol. *1:* 67–72 (1978).

9 Ruegger, A.; Kuhn, M.; Lichti, H.; Loosli, H. R.; Huguenin, R.; Quiquerez, C., and Wartburg, A. von: Cyclosporin A, a peptide metabolite from *Trichoderma polysporum* Rifai, with remarkable immunosuppressive activity. Helv. chim. Acta *59:* 1075–1086 (1976).

Dr. A. C. Allison, Division of Cell Pathology, Clinical Research Centre, Watford Road, Harrow, Middlesex, HA1 3UJ (England)

Immunopathology. 6th Int. Convoc. Immunol., Niagara Falls, N.Y., 1978, pp. 40–44 (Karger, Basel 1979)

Immunodeficiencies and Autoimmunity

J. C. Allen

State University of New York at Buffalo, School of Medicine, Clinical Center, Buffalo, N.Y.

Recognized interrelationships between immune deficiency states, autoimmune phenomena and malignant disorders form the basis for an ever-expanding body of research on the thesis that their understanding may contribute to mechanistic interpretations of each class of disorder taken alone. It is the purpose of this section to review certain aspects of the associations as observed in man between primary immune deficiency diseases and clinically recognized autoimmunity. Defined deficiencies in human immune systems have by and large been associated with heritable or congenital defects in the T cell, B cell, and complement system and in phagocytic function, with malignant disease, with immunosuppressive (cytotoxic) therapy and with aging. Immune deficiency associated with aging is covered in another section of this volume and pertinent information linking the immunodeficiencies of malignancy and cytotoxic therapy with autoimmunity in man is limited. Our interest, accordingly, will be centered on the first three of these categories.

As will be mentioned subsequently, the classic association of various autoimmune phenomena has been with the hypogammaglobulinemic states, and recent information has significantly increased our understanding of the pathogenesis of these conditions. The classical concept that these disorders represent an absence, or disappearance, of B cells responsible for production of the immunoglobulins has proven to be only relatively true [4, 5]. Thus, subsets of patients may have a normal complement of circulating B cells which are unresponsive to mitogenic stimulation such as by pokeweed mitogen, or which appear normally responsive to mitogen but are unable to release immunoglobulins as a result of that response. Assessment of T cell suppressor populations in these disorders has provided explanations for some of the differences [3, 16, 18, 19]. Thus, among patients with the common variable form of hypogammaglobulinemia, a subset has been defined who have a primary defect in transformation of B cells to antibody-producing plasma cells, and who in addition—and as a defect accentuating their hypogammaglobulinemic disorder—have a population of suppressor T cells which further repress immunoglobulin synthesis. Another subset of this generic group are patients whose primary defect appears to lie in the presence of a suppressor T cell population which depresses immunoglobulin production by B cells. The B cells, however, appear normal when the suppressor cells are removed. This T cell effect is apparently reversed by the use of adrenal cortical steroids *in vivo* or *in vitro*. Similarly, selective IgA deficiency may be associated with a defective transformation of B cells to IgA-producing plasma cells, with apparently normal helper and suppressor T cell populations. A subset of these patients, however, can be shown to have suppressor T cell specifically antagonizing IgA production, either as a primary or secondary abnormality. Thus, the involvement of suppressor cell populations in the pathogenesis of at least some forms of the primary hypogammaglobulinemias now appears well established. This has obvious implications to an understanding of their association with autoimmune disorders in view of data which link abnormal suppressor T cell activity with emergence of systemic lupus erythematosus-like disease in the NZB mouse [10].

What, in fact, is the evidence linking primary immunodeficiency states and autoimmune phenomena in man? Two early reports [6, 8] linked rheumatologic symptomatology to *common variable* and *X-linked hypogammaglobulinemia* in about 36% of the instances. Of those with rheumatic complaints, about three fourths had what was described as 'chronic' or 'classic' rheumatoid arthritis. On the other hand, two more recent papers [11, 12], while reporting a somewhat lower incidence of joint complaints (22%), noted a chronic rheumatologic disease in less than 5% of those afflicted. Though detailed observations are not available, several workers have commented on the amelioration and/or disappearance of rheumatic complaints as a result of γ-globulin treatment, the more intensive use of which in recent times may account for differences in reported frequencies of rheumatologic symptoms. In addition to rheumatic complaints, other manifestations of autoimmunity have been observed in patients with common variable hypogammaglobulinemia [7], including pernicious anemia (19% of those tested) or an abnormal Schilling test (37% of those tested) and keratoconjunctivitis sicca (6% of those tested).

In terms of frequency, the most striking association between autoimmune phenomena and hypogammaglobulinemic disorders has been observed with *selective IgA deficiency*. Our information regarding this association is even more impressive due to the relative frequency of this defect. In one series [1], 23% of the patients with selective IgA deficiency were observed to have autoantibodies of one or more specificities (thyroglobulin, smooth muscle, bile canaliculi, striated muscle, ileal basement membrane). Autoimmune diseases in which selective IgA deficiency has been found include rheumatoid arthritis, thyroiditis, systemic lupus erythematosus, pernicious anemia, vasculitis, dermatomyositis, Sjögren's syndrome and autoimmune hematologic diseases (idiopathic thrombocytopenic purpura, Coombs'-positive hemolytic anemia). Best estimates suggest selective IgA deficiency occurs in 3–12% of such patients, frequencies significantly higher than those with which it occurs in the population at large.

While frequency data are largely unavailable, it seems that in addition to patients with hypogammaglobulinemic disorders, those with primary defects in a variety of other systems classically considered to be important in host defense have an increased frequency of autoimmune phenomena. Patients with *various primary disorders of T cell function* [15] have been shown to have autoantibodies of various specificities (smooth muscle, gastric parietal cells, human thymus) and such autoimmune diseases as Coombs'-positive hemolytic anemia. Patients with various forms of the extensive spectrum of *inherited deficiencies in the complement system* [9] have increased incidence of immune complex glomerulonephritis (deficiencies of C1r, C2, and C̄I inhibitor), dermatomyositis (deficiency of C2), and systemic lupus erythematosus (deficiencies of C1r, C1s, C2, C4, C5 or C̄I inhibitor). Finally, patients with some forms of *defective leukocyte function* [13, 14] have shown either the presence of—or a familial association with—autoimmune disease, such as rheumatoid-like arthritis. The single known common thread tying many of these various deficiency disorders together is increased susceptibility to infection; evidence for their genetic linkage in man is lacking.

Consideration of the clinical picture of those autoimmune diseases associated with the immune deficiencies could expose several facets of importance in understanding this relationship including their identity with 'classical' diseases and relationships between clinical manifestations and the exact immune deficit in the patient involved. Unfortunately, available descriptions often present clinical information incompletely and overemphasize the detailed analyses of the immunologic deficiencies. Furthermore, the presence of frequent intercurrent infections may confuse the clinical picture of autoimmunity. Classic descriptions of rheumatoid complaints associated with the hypogammaglobulinemias reveal in most (but not all) instances some differences from typical rheumatoid arthritis [6, 8]. Thus, involvement of the interphalangeal joints appears to be less frequent, intermittency of symptoms rather than chronicity with progression has (at least in recent times) been the rule [11, 12], and joint effusions without pain and signs of local or systemic inflammation due to the joint involvement appear more common. While classic rheumatoid nodules have been reported, they are the exception rather than the rule. Expected abnormal: ties, such as rheumatoid factor in serum and plasma cell infiltration of the synovium which depend on functions defective in the hypogammaglobulinemic state, are naturally absent. In addition pannus formation, cartilage deterioration and subchondral bony erosions are infrequent or absent. When one considers the possibility that thymus-derived cells may contribute to

the pathogenesis of rheumatoid disease, it is interesting to note that in both classic rheumatoid arthritis and in that associated with the hypogammaglobulinemic disorders, lymphocytic infiltrations of the capsule and periarticular musculature are prominent. Though the average age of onset is lower, pernicious anemia associated with the hypogammaglobulinemic disorders [17] is indistinguishable from the classic disease except for the expected differences (absence of plasma cell infiltration and of autoantibodies against parietal cells and against intrinsic factor), though even these may be present when the anemia is associated with selective IgA deficiency. Though the clinical picture of classic systemic lupus erythematosus is variable, it appears that greater differences may exist when it is associated with immunodeficiency states. Thus, the systemic lupus associated with deficiencies of complement components seems to be associated with an inordinately high frequency of photosensitivity [9], and the autoantibodies associated therewith tend to be of low titer. Lupus seen in mothers whose sons have chronic granulomatous disease is serologically negative and not associated with nephritis [14], but otherwise cannot be distinguished from the classical disease. It is possibly simplistic to ascribe these clinical differences to the underlying immune defects, such as the absence of antibody to promote antigen-antibody complex formation, or complement to promote tissue damage as a result of those complexes (since alternate pathway activation apparently occurs). In any case, cause of clinical differences in the autoimmune diseases associated with immune deficiency disorders is not known.

Finally, it should be mentioned that a recent report describes a child with X-linked hypogammaglobulinemia who died from a chronic, progressive, central nervous system disease diagnosed as encephalitis and who had developed the clinical and histopathologic picture of classical dermatomyositis [2]. Cultures of many tissues at post-mortem examinations revealed the presence of ECHO 24 virus in all of them. While a pathogenetic link between the autoimmune disease and virus infection is appealing, it must be hedged by a report of a similar infection (ECHO 30) in such a child without evidence of dermatomyositis [20], and of dermatomyositis in a child with X-linked hypogammaglobulinemia without clinical evidence of a chronic disseminated viral infection [8].

A number of postulates have been offered to explain the association between immunodeficiency disorders and autoimmune phenomena which may be reasonably collated as follows:

(1) Increased susceptibility to infection predisposes the immunodeficient host to involvement with a microbial pathogen (such as a virus) which is primarily or secondarily responsible for expression of autoimmune phenomena.

(2) There is a quantitative or qualitative alteration in immune complexes in the immunodeficiency diseases which impedes their clearance or enhances their tissue deposition.

(3) Defective host immunity allows absorption from 'external sources' (such as the gut) of antigens which are normally excluded from the body and which may directly or indirectly instigate autoimmunity. This postulate is supported by the observation of a high frequency of anti-milk antibodies in patients with selective IgA deficiency.

(4) There exists an as yet undefined genetic linkage between various limbs of the immune system and factors allowing expression of autoimmunity. Studies to date in man have failed to provide evidence that such a linkage exists, though better evidence exists for the mouse.

(5) There is a delicate balance in the interrelationship between many aspects of host defense, a balance which is key to the suppression of autoimmunity. This is perhaps a less specific way of stating the next postulate.

(6) Associated with the immunodeficiency diseases is a defect in T cell function which is responsible for surveillance against (suppressor)—or an accentuation of T cell function which enhances (helper)—expression of autoimmunity. There is evidence of abnormal suppressor cell activity in some of the hypogammaglobulinemic disorders, but none has been shown for deficiencies in other parts of the immune system with which autoimmune phenomena may be associated.

Obviously, more than one of these mechanisms could be operative in a specific instance, thereby providing a consistent link between autoimmunity and the varied aspects of host immune mechanisms with which it clearly seems entwined.

References

1 Ammann, A. J. and Hong, R.: Selective IgA deficiency: presentation of 30 cases and a review of the literature. Medicine 50: 223–236 (1971).
2 Bardelas, J. A.; Winkelstein, J. A.; Seto, D. S. Y.; Tsai, T., and Rogol, A. D.: Fatal ECHO 24 infection in a patient with hypogammaglobulinemia: relationship to dermatomyositis-like syndrome. J. Pediat. 90: 396–399 (1977).
3 Broom, B. C · DeLaConcha, E. G.; Webster, A. D. B., and Janossy, G. L.: Intracellular immunoglobulin production in vitro by lymphocytes from patients with hypogammaglobulinemia and their effect on normal lymphocytes. Clin. exp. Immunol. 23: 73–77 (1976).
4 Geha, R. S.; Rosen, F. S., and Merler, E.: Identification and characterization of subpopulations of lymphocytes in human peripheral blood after fractionation on discontinuous gradients of albumin. The cellular defect in X-linked agammaglobulinemia. J. clin. Invest. 52: 1726–1734 (1973).
5 Geha, R. S., Schneeberger, E.; Merler, E., and Rosen, F. S.: Heterogeneity of 'acquired' or common variable agammaglobulinemia. New Engl. J. Med. 291: 1–6 (1974).

6 Good, R. A.; Kelly, W. D.; Rotstein, J., and Varco, R. L.: Immunological deficiency diseases. Agammaglobulinemia, hypogammaglobulinemia, Hodgkin's disease and sarcoidosis. Prog. Allergy, vol. 6, pp. 187–319 (Karger, Basel 1962).

7 Hermans, P. E.; Diaz-Buxo, J. A., and Stobo, J. D.: Idiopathic late-onset immunoglobulin deficiency. Clinical observations in 50 patients. Am. J. Med. *61:* 221–237 (1976).

8 Janeway, C. A.; Gitlin, D.; Craig, J. M., and Grice, D. S.: 'Collagen disease' in patients with congenital agammaglobulinemia. Trans. Ass. Am. Physns *69:* 93–97 (1956).

9 Kohler, P. F.: Inherited complement deficiencies and systemic lupus erythematosus: an immunogenetic puzzle. Ann. intern. Med. *82:* 420–421 (1975).

10 Krakauer, R. S.; Waldmann, T. A., and Strober, W.: Loss of suppressor T-cells in adult NZB/NZW mice. J. exp. Med. *144:* 662–673 (1976).

11 Lawrence, J. S.: Hypogammaglobulinemia in the United Kingdom, Medical Research Council Special Report Series 310, pp. 35–44 (HMSO, London 1971).

12 McLaughlin, J. F.; Schaller, J., and Wedgwood, R. J.: Arthritis and immunodeficiency. J. Pediat. *81:* 801–803 (1972).

13 Rodey, G. E.; Park, B. H.; Ford, D. K.; Gray, B. H., and Good, R. A.: Defective bactericidal activity of peripheral blood leukocytes in lipochrome histiocytosis. Am. J. Med. *49:* 322–327 (1970).

14 Schaller, J.: Illness resembling lupus erythematosus in mothers of boys with chronic granulomatous disease. Ann. intern. Med. *76:* 747–750 (1972).

15 Schaller, J. G.: Immunodeficiency and autoimmunity. Birth Defects: Original Article Ser. *11:* 173–184 (1975).

16 Siegal, F. P.; Siegal, M., and Good, R. A.: Suppression of B-cell differentiation by leukocytes from hypogammaglobulinemic patients. J. clin. Invest. *58:* 109–122 (1976).

17 Twomey, J. J.; Jordan, P. H.; Laughter, A. H.; Meuwissen, H. J., and Good, R. A.: The gastric disorder in immunogloublin-deficient patients. Ann. intern. Med. *72:* 499–504 (1970).

18 Waldmann, T. A.; Broder, S.; Blaese, R. M.; Durm, M.; Blackman, M., and Strober, W.: Role of suppressor T-cells in pathogenesis of common variable hypogammaglobulinemia. Lancet *ii:* 609–613 (1974).

19 Waldmann, T. A.; Broder, S.; Krakauer, R.; Durm, M.; Meade, B., and Goldman, C.: Defect in IgA secretion and in IgA specific suppressor cells in patients with selective IgA deficiency. Trans. Ass. Am. Physns *89:* 215–244 (1976).

20 Ziegler, J. B. and Penny, R.: Fatal ECHO-30 virus infection and amyloidosis in X-linked hypogammaglobulinemia. Clin. Immunol. Immunopath. *3:* 347–352 (1975).

J. C. Allen, MD, SUNY Clinical Center, Room 103, 462 Grider St., Buffalo, NY 14215 (USA)

Immunopathology. 6th Int. Convoc. Immunol., Niagara Falls, N.Y., 1978, pp. 45–49 (Karger, Basel 1979)

Induction of Autoimmunity to Inaccessible Tissue Antigens[1]

W. O. Weigle

Department of Immunopathology, Scripps Clinic and Research Foundation, La Jolla, Calif.

Autoimmune phenomena, resulting in disease process, result from an imbalance in the intricate regulatory mechanisms controlling the immune response; this sequence is now a well established fact. Thus, tissue components normally tolerated by an individual's immune system become the targets of attack. Although a number of mechanisms could be responsible for tolerance enjoyed by self antigens, the three most obvious are the dominance of central unresponsiveness, the sequestering of self from the lymphoid tissue and suppressor cells. The interrelationship between the first two possibilities will be the subject of this paper.

Since acquired immunological tolerance to heterologous serum proteins can be induced and maintained in both T and B cells, but need be present only in the T cell for the unresponsive state to exist [3, 19], it is tempting to discuss the nature of unresponsiveness to self antigens in terms of their reactivity at the T and B cell level [17]. Of interest along these lines is that acquired tolerance induced to heterologous serum proteins, when present only at the T cell level (low doses of antigen), can be terminated by bypassing either the

need for or the specificity of helper T cells. The latter requirement can be met by immunizing the tolerant animal (T cell-tolerant but B cell-competent) with cross-reacting antigens. Thus, rabbits tolerant to bovine serum albumin (BSA), immunized with a cross-reacting antigen respond by making antibody reactive with BSA [2].

Thyroiditis, an experimental autoimmune disease that results from immunizing animals with thyroglobulin (Tg) in complete Freund's adjuvant (CFA) [16] is a similar phenomenon in which a tolerated, relatively inaccessible self component becomes antigenic. Tg behaves similarly to a serum protein in that it equilibrates between the intra- and extravascular fluid spaces and persists in the body fluid with a half-life (in rabbits) of 2.5 days [9]. Tg is only partially sequestered and can be detected in the body fluids [7] in concentrations sufficient to maintain tolerance in T cells, but not in B cells [10]. Thus, it is not surprising that injection of an aqueous preparation of heterologous (cross-reacting) Tg into rabbits or mice induces autoantibodies to autologous Tg and, ultimately thyroid lesions [18]. Rabbits were given a series of injections of bovine Tg (cross-reacts 25% with rabbit Tg) and their spleens and thyroid glands were later evaluated by the hemolytic plaque assay for antibody (plaque) forming

[1] This is Publication No. 1542 from the Department of Immunopathology, Scripps Clinic and Research Foundation. This work was supported by United States Public Health Service Grant AI-07007.

cells (PFC) to Tg. The thyroid glands contained PFC to rabbit Tg, the appearance of which preceded by 1 day the appearance of thyroid lesions (fig. 1) [6]. These results strongly suggest that antibodies to autologous Tg are the etiologic agent of disease in this model.

Experimental autoimmune thyroiditis is also readily induced in mice immunized with an aqueous preparation of a mixture of different heterologous Tgs [11]. That these mice are tolerant to autologous Tg at the T cell level but contain competent B cells is supported by the demonstration that their B cells but not T cells bind ^{125}I-labeled syngeneic Tg. Furthermore, B cells incubated with ^{125}I-labeled syngeneic Tg (antigen-induced suicide) and injected into irradiated mice along with normal T cells failed to support the development of thyroiditis or autoantibody. On the other hand, T cells treated in a similar way with radiolabeled Tg and injected along with normal B cells restored, in irradiated mice, the capability of developing thyroiditis and autoantibody (table I) [4]. Further evidence for the B cell nature of this disease is the quality of the histologic lesions in the

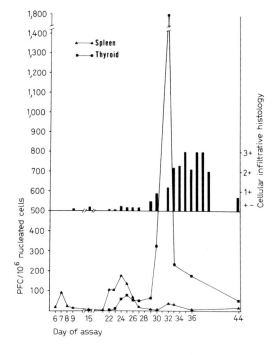

Fig. 1. The plaque-forming cell (PFC) response to rabbit Tg of cells from the spleen (▲) and the thyroid gland (■) of rabbits immunized with aqueous preparations of bovine Tg. The degree of infiltration by mononuclear cells is shown by solid bars.

Table I. Antigen-induced suicide of normal bone marrow cells by ^{125}I-labeled syngeneic Tg in recipients of normal thymus and bone marrow cells

Donor cells		Indirect PFC per spleen to bovine Tg	Incidence of thyroid lesions[a]
T cells	B cells		
100×10^6 normal thymocytes	25×10^6 bone marrow and ^{125}I-mouse Tg	3,385	12/27
100×10^6 normal thymocytes	25×10^6 normal bone marrow	28,037	14/14
100×10^6 thymocytes and ^{125}I-mouse Tg	25×10^6 normal bone marrow	20,693	18/20

[a] Denominator equals total number of animals examined and numerator equals number of animals exhibiting various degrees of inflammation at time of maximal lesions. Reprinted in part from *Clagett and Weigle* [4].

thyroids of these mice [5]. The temporal appearance and quantity of serum autoantibody directly correlates with the formation of complexes between Tg and anti-Tg in the interstitium of the thyroid glands. These complexes were granular to lumpy in appearance and formed at the base of follicular cells in intimate association with the follicular basement membrane. The *in vivo* formation of immune complexes in this model is similar to that in the Arthus reaction. The above data, along with the ability to transfer thyroiditis with serum [1, 12], the evidence for antibody-mediated disease in rabbits immunized with homologous Tg in CFA, and the B cell-associated spontaneous thyroiditis in chickens [20] make a good case for serum antibody in the initiation of thyroiditis.

A similar series of events may be instrumental in the induction of experimental myasthenia gravis. In this model, rats injected with foreign acetylcholine receptor from the electric eel initially produced antibody to eel acetylcholine receptor [8], but responded negatively to the natural rat acetylcholine receptor. Gradually, the responsive rat developed a clone of cells that produced antibody to the rat receptor, causing chronic autoimmune disease. It could be predicted that rat T cells are tolerant to rat acetylcholine receptor, while the B cells are competent.

In contrast to Tg, it appears that basic protein (BP) of myelin is sequestered to such a degree that both the T and B cells are competent (table II). Certainly, both T and B lymphocytes were reactive with ^{125}I-labeled syngeneic BP in the experiments outlined in table II. That cellular immunity is responsible for experimental allergic encephalomyelitis (EAE) has been suggested by numerous workers [15]. T cells were implicated as the effector cells in experiments with irradiated Lewis rats reconstituted with spleen cells from rats immunized 9 days earlier with BP in CFA [13]. Since at this time T cell help was not required for the recipients to form antibody, the treatment of the donor spleen cells with anti-thymocyte serum (ATS) before reconstitution eliminated T cells, but had no effect on the level of serum anti-BP in the recipients. The recipients, however, developed neither the clinical symptoms of paralysis nor the typical lesions in the brain (table III). The role of T and B cells in the induction of EAE in Lewis rats was further defined by

Table II. Antigen-binding cells. Normal T and B cells combining with thyroglobulin (Tg) and basic protein (BP) of myelin

Species	Cell type	Antigen	Antigen-binding cells
Mice	T cell	Tg	—
	B cell	Tg	+
Rat	T cell	BP	+
	B cell	BP	+

Table III. Effect of T cells on induction of experimental allergic encephalomyelitis (EAE) in thymectomized, irradiated rats reconstituted with primed cells[a]

Treatment of transferred cells	EAE		Serum antibody[b]
	clinically	histologically	
None	7/10[c]	10/10	2.3
ATS + C	0/10	0/10	2.3
ATS (abs)[d] + C	5/6	6/6	ND[e]

[a] Lewis rats were thymectomized, irradiated (900 R), and reconstituted with 250×10^6 spleen cells from rats previously sensitized 9 days before with BP-CFA. The transferred cells were either untreated or treated with anti-lymphocyte serum (ATS) + complement (C).
[b] Values represent the μg of BP bound/ml of serum. Mean of animals tested.
[c] Fraction of animals positive.
[d] Absorbed with thymus cells.
[e] ND = Not done.
Reprinted in part from *Ortiz-Ortiz et al.* [13].

antigen-induced suicide experiments, where antigen-binding cells specific for BP, with either T or B cell functions, were specifically eliminated by treatment with BP heavily labeled with [125]I [14]. Thymectomized (Tx) irradiated Lewis rats were readily reconstituted with normal thymus and bone marrow (BM) cells in that such rats subsequently injected with BP-CFA developed typical histological lesions in the brain, clinical symptoms and autoantibody. On the other hand, neither lesions, nor clinical symptoms nor antibody resulted when ^{125}I-BP of high specific activity was incubated with thymus cells subsequently transferred to Tx irradiated rats which were reconstituted with BM and challenged with BP-CFA (table IV). This would indicate that pretreatment with the ^{125}I-BP eliminated specific T cells, and thus abrogated cell-mediated immunity. More precise evidence for cell-mediated immunity in provoking EAE was obtained by preferentially causing suicide of T and B cells. When the BM cells were treated with the heavily ^{125}I-labeled BP and injected into Tx-irradiated recipients along with normal thymus cells, antibody formation to a subsequent challenge with BP-CFA was inhibited. In contrast, both clinical symptoms of

EAE and histological lesions were similar to those observed in rats receiving both normal thymus cells and normal BM cells. These results further indicate that no matter what the enhancing or suppressing effect of antibodies may have after disease is initiated, antibodies are not a requisite for the induction of EAE.

In summary, two experimental autoimmune diseases have been discussed, each differing in the effector mechanism that appears to be dictated by the immune status of the hosts T and B cells. In turn, the immunologic reactivity of T and B cells is determined by the extent to which the antigens in question are sequestered. With thyroiditis, partial sequestering of Tg gives rise to tolerant T cells and competent B cells. The unresponsive state in the T cells can be circumvented by adding cross-reactive Tg resulting in an autoimmune response to Tg that is accompanied by disease. On the other hand, a more effective sequestering of BP of myelin may result in both T and B cells having a certain degree of competency in respect to BP, permitting activation of both cell types. However, in this case, the initiating events are brought about by effector T cells and antibody is not involved.

Table IV. Antigen-induced suicide of rat thymus and bone marrow cells by ^{125}I-syngeneic BP

Bone marrow cells[a]	Thymus cells[b]	EAE		Antibody
		clinically	histologically	
Normal	normal	10/10	10/10	+
Treated with ^{125}I-BP	normal	10/10	10/10	—
Normal	treated with ^{125}I-BP	0/5	0/5	—
Treated with ^{125}I-BP	treated with ^{125}I-BP	0/10	0/10	—

[a] 250×10^6 bone marrow cells.
[b] 200×10^6 thymocytes.
Reprinted in part from *Ortiz-Ortiz and Weigle* [14].

References

1 Anderson, C. L. and Rose, N. R.: Induction of thyroiditis in the rabbit by intravenous injection of papain-treated rabbit thyroglobulin. J. Immun. *107:* 1341–1348 (1971).

2 Benjamin, D. C. and Weigle, W. O.: The termination of immunological unresponsiveness to bovine serum albumin in rabbits. I. Quantitative and qualitative response to cross-reacting albumins. J. exp. Med. *132:* 66–76 (1970).

3 Chiller, J. M.; Habicht, G. S., and Weigle, W. O.: Cellular sites of immunologic unresponsiveness. Proc. natn. Acad. Sci. USA *65:* 551–556 (1970).

4 Clagett, J. A. and Weigle, W. O.: Roles of T and B lymphocytes in the termination of unresponsiveness to autologous thyroglobulin in mice. J. exp. Med. *139:* 643–660 (1974).

5 Clagett, J. A.; Wilson, C. B., and Weigle, W. O.: Interstitial immune complex thyroiditis in mice. The role of autoantibody to thyroglobulin. J. exp. Med. *140:* 1439–1456 (1974).

6 Clinton, B. A. and Weigle, W. O.: Cellular events during the induction of experimental thyroiditis in the rabbit. J. exp. Med. *136:* 1605–1615 (1972).

7 Daniel, P. M.; Pratt, O. E.; Roitt, I. M., and Torrigiani, G.: The release of thyroglobulin from the thyroid gland into thyroid lymphatics; the identification of thyroglobulin in the thyroid lymph and in the blood of monkeys by physical and immunological methods and its estimation by radioimmunoassay. Immunology *12:* 489–504 (1967).

8 Lennon, V. A.; Lindstrom, J. M., and Seybold, M. E.: Experimental autoimmune myasthenia: a model of myasthenia gravis in rats and guinea pigs. J. exp. Med. *141:* 1365–1375 (1975).

9 Nakamura, R. M. and Weigle, W. O.: *In vivo* behavior of homologous and heterologous thyroglobulin and induction of immunologic unresponsiveness to heterologous thyroglobulin. J. Immun. *98:* 653–662 (1967).

10 Nakamura, R. M. and Weigle, W. O.: Induction, maintenance and termination of immunologic unresponsiveness to bovine thyroglobulin in rabbits. J. Immun. *99:* 357–364 (1967).

11 Nakamura, R. M. and Weigle, W. O.: Experimental thyroiditis in complement intact and deficient mice following injections of heterologous thyroglobulins without adjuvant. Proc. Soc. exp. Biol. Med. *129:* 412–416 (1968).

12 Nakamura, R. M. and Weigle, W. O.: Transfer of experimental autoimmune thyroiditis by serum from thyroidectomized donors. J. exp. Med. *130:* 263–283 (1969).

13 Ortiz-Ortiz, L.; Nakamura, R. M., and Weigle, W. O.: T cell requirement for experimental allergic encephalomyelitis induction in the rat. J. Immun. *117:* 576–579 (1976).

14 Ortiz-Ortiz, L. and Weigle, W. O.: Cellular events in the induction of experimental allergic encephaloymelitis in rats. J. exp. Med. *144:* 604–616 (1976).

15 Paterson, P. G.: Autoimmune neurological disease: experimental animal systems and implications for multiple sclerosis; in Autoimmunity, genetic, immunologic, virologic and clinical aspects, pp. 644–691 (Academic Press, New York 1977).

16 Rose, N. and Witebsky, E.: Studies on organ specificity. V. Changes in the thyroid glands of rabbits following active immunization with rabbit thyroid extracts. J. Immun. *76:* 417–427 (1956).

17 Weigle, W. O.: Recent observations and concepts in immunological unresponsiveness and autoimmunity. Clin. exp. Immunol. *9:* 437–447 (1971).

18 Weigle, W. O. and Nakamura, R. M.: The development of autoimmune thyroiditis in rabbits following injection of aqueous preparations of heterologous thyroglobulins. J. Immun. *99:* 223–231 (1967).

19 Weigle, W. O.; Chiller, J. M., and Habicht, G. S.: Effect of immunological unresponsiveness on different cell populations. Transplantn Rev. *8:* 3–25 (1972).

20 Wick, G.; Kite, J. H., jr., and Witebsky, E.: Spontaneous thyroiditis in the Obese Strain of chickens. IV. The effect of thymectomy and thymobursectomy on the development of the disease. J. Immun. *104:* 54–62 (1970).

Dr. W. O. Weigle, Department of Immunopathology, Scripps Clinic and Research Foundation, La Jolla, CA 92037 (USA)

Immunopathology. 6th Int. Convoc. Immunol., Niagara Falls, N.Y., 1978, pp. 50–55 (Karger, Basel 1979)

Immunization against Autologous Immunoglobulins in Allotype-Suppressed Rabbits[1]

S. Dubiski and P. W. Good

Department of Medical Genetics and the Institute of Immunology, University of Toronto, Toronto, Ont.

Introduction

Immunization against autologous immunoglobulins appears to be one of the more important immunological processes in rheumatoid arthritis and perhaps in other related pathological conditions. Sera of rheumatoid arthritis patients contain a wide spectrum of anti-immunoglobulin antibodies including antibodies directed against allotypic specificities of both autologous and isologous origin [5]. The autoimmune character of some of these antibodies has been confirmed by the detection of antigen-antibody complexes in the patients' sera and tissues [10]. The availability of an animal model in which some of the immunological aspects of rheumatoid arthritis could be studied would be of considerable value. Such a model became potentially available when it was learned that antibodies to 'self' allotypic specificities can be raised in rabbits in which phenotypic expression of the corresponding allotype was inhibited as a result of allotype suppression [7].

Allotype suppression is induced by the administration of anti-allotype antibody [2, 3] during a critical period shortly after birth [1]. This treatment has a profound and lasting

effect on immunoglobulin synthesis. Molecules bearing the 'suppressed' specificity are not being synthesized and there is a compensatory increase in the concentration of the 'non-suppressed' immunoglobulin. The duration of suppression depends on the dose of antibodies; it may even last for the entire life of the rabbit. Even if a relatively low dose of antibodies is administered and the suppressed allotype appears in the circulation after a few weeks, its concentration never reaches normal levels.

Lowe et al. [7] injected immunizing material containing the suppressed allotype into suppressed rabbits. The immunized animals made 'autoantibodies' which were indistinguishable in specificity and in potency from alloantibodies raised by conventional methods. A similar observation was later made by *Horng et al.* [6]. These apparent autoantibodies are in fact directed only against antigens which would be autologous had the genetic information for this antigen been phenotypically expressed.

We have induced a true autoimmune process by the immunization of rabbits recovering from allotype suppression. The rabbits were immunized against immunoglobulins which were already present in the circulation at the time the immunizing injections were started. This resulted in the simultaneous

[1] Supported by a grant from the Medical Research Council of Canada.

formation of autoantibodies and of corresponding autoantigen. In the following, we shall describe the specificity of these autoantibodies and their reactions with the autoantigens as well as with normal immunoglobulins carrying the same allotypic marker.

Experimental Design and Results

Heterozygous rabbits whose paternal allotypic specificity was Ab9 were used. The specificities 4, 5, 6 and 9 are all markers of the κ light chain and are controlled by a series of allelic genes at the Ab locus. At birth, the rabbits were injected intraperitoneally with a suppressing dose of anti-Ab9 immune serum. When the rabbits were over 100 days old, we began immunizing them with the Ab9 antigen. The immunizing antigen was prepared by combining antibacterial antibodies of the Ab9 specificity with killed *Proteus vulgaris* organisms [3]. In conventional rabbits, such complexes are a very potent immunogen; strong antibodies to light chain allotypic specificities are produced after 3 weekly injections. In the suppressed rabbits, the outcome of the immunization depended on the extent to which the rabbits had recovered from suppression before the immunization was started

Rabbits still deep in suppression, with no detectable Ab9 immunoglobulin, produced potent anti-Ab9 antibodies which could not be distinguished from antibodies raised in rabbits that lacked the Ab9 gene. On the other hand, rabbits with normal or near-normal levels of Ab9 did not respond to injections with Ab9 immunizing material; we immunized 14 animals which had started their recovery from suppression. Prior to immunization, sera of these rabbits contained low, but measurable concentrations of the 'suppressed' immunoglobulin. Despite the fact that the synthesis of 'self' allotype had already started, all of them eventually produced anti-Ab9 antibody. In general, the higher the concentration of antigen at the beginning of immunization, the slower the rate of subsequent antibody production. After 4 weeks of immunization, most rabbits had antibody titers higher than 1:256 as measured in the hemagglutination reaction, but only a small proportion of them produced antibodies of sufficient concentration to be detectable in the Ouchterlony technique (fig. 1a). The Ab9 antigen present in the sera before the immunization did not necessarily disappear and in some serum samples both antigen and antibody activity could be detected at the same time. This is exemplified in figure 1b where the tested serum reacted

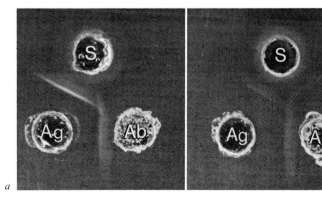

Fig. 1. a Reaction of a serum sample from suppressed-immunized rabbit 1276-4F with normal serum of allotype Ab⁹/Ab⁹. *b* Reactions of a serum sample from suppressed-immunized rabbit 1276-3B with anti-Ab9 antiserum and with Ab⁹/Ab⁹ normal serum. S = Sample (undiluted); Ab = antibody (1:10); Ag = antigen (1:25).

with both Ab9 and anti-Ab9 forming distinct precipitin lines. Similar results were obtained by the hemagglutination assay when the precipitation in gel was insufficiently sensitive.

All these observations indicated strongly that an autoimmune process had been started and was being maintained by the immunization with an autologous antigen. However, the conclusion as to the autoimmune nature of the observed phenomena could only be made if the autoantibodies were shown to react with the autologous antigens. Autologous antigens and antibodies should ideally be isolated from the same serum sample, because showing the reaction between material from the same individual, but obtained at different times, would be open to criticism that the autoantigen was never accessible *in vivo* to the autoantibody. We expected that antigens and antibodies in the same sample might belong to different immunoglobulin classes and attempted to separate them on Sephadex G-200 (table I). Nine serum samples with antibody activity, and 14 samples with both antibody and antigen activity, were chromatographed on Sephadex G-200. Out of 11 samples, in which only antigen was present in both peaks, 4 came from sera which before chromatography contained only antibody. Thus, antibody activity seemed to have disappeared during chromatography. Only partial separation was obtained in 4 samples which contained both antigen and antibody activity before chromatography. Although the first peak contained only antigen, in the second peak again both antigen and antibody activity was present.

In 7 cases, the antigen activity and the antibody activity were recovered in different chromatographic peaks. This made it possible to determine the specificity of the presumed autoantibodies (table II). Five different antibody preparations were tested by the hemagglutination assay before and

Table I. Distribution of Ab9 antigen (Ag) and anti-Ab antibodies (Ab) in protein peaks resolved on Sephadex G-200. The starting material were sera from immunized-suppressed rabbits in which either antibody (9 samples) or antigen and antibody (14 samples) activity was detected

	Peak II		
	Ag	Ab	Ag + Ab
Peak I			
Ag	11	1	4
Ab	6	1	0
Ag + Ab	0	0	0

after neutralization with 8 different antigen preparations. In 2 cases, it was possible to match the antibody preparation with the antigen preparation derived from the same serum sample. Six antigen samples were also autologous, but were prepared from serum samples other than that from which the antibody has been derived. In all cases, autologous antigens neutralized their corresponding antibodies as well as antibodies from other immunized-suppressed rabbits. The activity of antigen preparations was similar to that of normal rabbit sera (in appropriate dilution) and the specificity of all but 1 antibody preparation did not differ from the specificity of conventional anti-Ab9 antibodies. One antibody preparation (rabbit 1141-Z) was neutralized to different degrees by 3 different Ab^9/Ab^9 normal sera. This can possibly be explained by assuming that the specificity spectrum of the antibodies made by this animal was not as wide as that of conventional antibodies.

The autoimmune nature of the observed phenomena made it reasonable to expect the presence of circulating antigen-antibody complexes. To show the presence of these complexes in the sera, we used two approaches. First, we tried to detect IgG in the

Table II. Cross-neutralization of anti-Ab9 antibodies by Ab9 antigens prepared from the sera of immunized-suppressed rabbits by Sephadex G-200 chromatography

	Antigens								
Rabbit	991-3B	991-3E	991-3E	991-3E	1015-4F	1141-Z	1141-Z	1195-B	NRS
Age, days	A 221	A 221	A 221	A 333	A 161	A 151	A 242	A 174	b9/b9
Day[1]	D 24	D 24	D 24	D 136	D 49	D 48	D 139	D 20	
Peak[2]	P II	P I	P II	P II	P II	P II	P II	P II	
Titer[3]	T 64	T 16	T 64	4>T>2	8>T>4	T>256	T>256	4>T>2	
Antibodies									
991-3B A 333 D 136 P II T>256	0[4]	32	0	>256	64	0	0	>128	
991-3E A 333 D 136 P I 32>T>16	0	4>T>2	0	4>T>2	<2	0	0	4>T>2	0
1015-4F A 237 D 125 P II 128>T>64	0	<2	0	0	*0*	0	0	0	0
1141-Z A 151 D 48 P I T 64	0	4>T>2	0	0	0	*0*	*0*	0	0[5] 64>T>32 8>T>4
1195-B A 273 D 119 P II T>256	0	8>T>4	0	128>T>64	0	0	0	*16*	0
Anti-9 T 16	0	0	0	<2	0	0	0	2	*0*

[1] Days after initial immunization.

[2] Sephadex G-200 peak I or II.

[3] Reciprocal of the highest dilution active in hemagglutination or in hemagglutination inhibition test.

[4] The numbers are reciprocals of the hemagglutination titer after neutralization; 0 = no hemagglutinating activity. Numbers in *italics* give results of neutralization with autologous antigen.

[5] The three samples of sera from normal Ab^9/Ab^9 rabbits used gave varying degrees of inhibition with this antiserum.

high molecular weight material excluded on Sephadex G-200; secondly, we used Dr. *Milgrom*'s anti-antibody which has been shown to be specific for antibody bound to antigen [8, 9]. Unfortunately, neither of these two methods gave us unambiguous results. Definitive answers to the question of circulating immune complexes in immunized-suppressed rabbits is therefore not yet available.

Discussion

The foregoing results show clearly that the recognition of self allotypic specificities is determined by the animal's phenotype and not by its genotype. The presence in the circulation of high concentrations of allotypically marked immunoglobulins renders the animal tolerant to this allotype. Absence of a given allotype makes the animal a potential antibody producer irrespective of whether this absence is genetically controlled or whether it is the result of allotype suppression. Animals which had low titers of the suppressed allotype (less than 1% of the normal concentration) could be immunized against this allotype but, as a rule, made less antibody than the rabbits in which this immunoglobulin was absent (i.e. completely suppressed or conventional rabbits). Thus, it seems that low concentrations of the allotype maintain a low level of tolerance, a level which can be overcome by immunization with a potent immunogen. Antibodies produced as a result of such immunization, and detectable either in the whole serum or in serum fractions, do not differ in their specificity from conventional anti-allotype antibodies. Their reactions with the autologous antigen justify their classification as autoantibodies. True autoantibodies should combine with the autoantigen and either be eliminated from the circulation altogether or

circulate as immune complexes. However, we sometimes detected both antigen and antibody activity in the same serum sample, without any fractionation. Most probably, a vast majority of antibody molecules, especially those of high affinity, combine with the autoantigen and disappear from the circulation; the remaining antibody activity can either be attributed to antibodies of very low affinity or to the complexes of such antibodies with the antigen. A low binding constant may cause these complexes to readily dissociate as a result of small changes in molarity, pH, or temperature. Recovery in isolated Sephadex fractions of antigen activity previously undetectable in the starting material may be explained by the dissociation of the antigen-antibody complexes. *In vivo* reactions between antigen and antibody molecules may not only result in the selection of low affinity antibody molecules, but may also lead to changes in specificity. Antibodies produced by the rabbit 1141-Z (table II) seem to differ from conventional antibodies in their reactions with normal Ab9-positive sera. One must mention that the concentration of Ab9 antigen in this particular rabbit was much higher than in any other immunized-suppressed rabbit. The high levels of antigen may have resulted in a more efficient selection of circulating antibody molecules.

Autoimmunization of suppressed rabbits raises the question of whether the autoantibody has any suppressing effect on these animals. Previous reports described immunization of completely suppressed rabbits and stressed the likelihood that such immunization indeed prolongs suppression [1, 6, 7]. A direct proof of such effect would require a very large number of animals. In our experiments, the immunization was started when the suppressed immunoglobulin was already detectable in the circulation. No reversal towards suppression was apparent in any of our rabbits. Even after long periods of immunization, the antigen was detectable in the whole serum or in the Sephadex fractions. It seems, therefore, that in the situation where the synthesis of the antigen precedes the formation of the antibody these two synthetic processes do not interfere with one another.

References

1 Catty, D.; Lowe, J. A., and Gell, P. G. H.: Mechanism of allotype suppression in the rabbit. Transplantn Rev. 27: 157–183 (1975).
2 Dubiski, S.: Synthesis of allotypically defined immunoglobulins in rabbits. Cold Spring Harb. Symp. quant. Biol. 32: 311–316 (1967).
3 Dubiski, S.: Immunochemistry and genetics of a 'new' allotypic specificity A_e14 of rabbit γG immunoglobulins: recombination in somatic cells. J. Immun. 103: 120–128 (1969).
4 Dubiski, S. and Swierczynska, Z.: Allotypic suppression in rabbits. Operational characterization of the target cells. Int. Archs Allergy appl. Immun. 40: 1–18 (1971).
5 Grubb, R.: The genetic markers of human immunoglobulins (Springer, Berlin 1970).
6 Horng, W. J.; Gilman-Sachs, A.; Roux, K. H.; Molinaro, G., and Dray, S.: Auto-antibody to an Ig V_H region allotype: induction of anti-a1 antibody in an a1-suppressed a^1a^2 heterozygous rabbit. J. Immun. 119: 1560–1562 (1977).
7 Lowe, J. A.; Cross, L. M., and Catty, D.: Humoral and cellular aspects of immunoglobulin allotype suppression in the rabbit. III. Production of anti-allotype antibody by suppressed animals. Immunology 28: 469–478 (1975).
8 Milgrom, F.: Rabbit sera with 'anti-antibody'. Vox Sang. 7: 545–558 (1962).
9 Milgrom, F. and Kano, K.: Comparison of various procedures for the detection of antigen-antibody complexes. Int. Archs Allergy appl. Immun. 56: 224–231 (1978).
10 Munthe, E. and Natvig, J. B.: Immunological studies on eluates from rheumatoid inflammatory tissue; in Grubb and Samuelsson Human anti-human gammaglobulins, pp. 101–110 (Pergamon Press, Oxford 1971).

Dr. S. Dubiski, Department of Medical Genetics, University of Toronto, Toronto, Ontario M5S 1A8 (Canada)

Immunopathology. 6th Int. Convoc. Immunol., Niagara Falls, N.Y., 1978, pp. 56–61 (Karger, Basel 1979)

Antibodies to Altered Autologous Antigens[1]

Felix Milgrom

Department of Microbiology, School of Medicine, State University of New York at Buffalo, Buffalo, N.Y.

Introduction

Expression of new antigenic determinants on denatured proteins has attracted the attention of immunologists for many years. *TenBroeck and Wu* [39] and *Rothen and Landsteiner* [37] showed that native oval-bumin and equine serum albumin differ considerably in antigenic structure from their heat-denatured counterparts. Considering that denaturation results in emergence of altered antigenicity, it is not surprising that man and animals form antibodies against altered autologous antigens. Appearance of altered antigens is of great interest and importance in several pathologic states. It is obvious that a short paper cannot give justice to all this extensive field. Therefore, I decided to concentrate my discussion on immune responses to altered immunoglobulins and to heterophile antigens. Admittedly, this decision was prejudiced by my own research interests.

Immunoglobulin G

In our own studies [27], as well as those of other investigators [21a, 41], rabbits injected

[1] Supported by grant IM-24C from the American Cancer Society.

with denatured autologous IgG produced antibodies combining with IgG of foreign species, primarily human IgG, in a variety of serological reactions. The reactions with rabbit IgG were incomparably weaker. Our interpretation of these findings was that denaturation of rabbit IgG exposes hidden configurations or otherwise creates novel antigens. It happens that these novel antigens are not just random structures but they resemble the structure of IgG of other species.

Denaturation of IgG may occur not only under artificial conditions, as in the above described experiments, but also under natural conditions. Over 20 years ago, we [29, 30] postulated that the antibody molecule suffers molecular transformation in the reaction with its corresponding antigen, which results in acquisition of new immunogenic properties. Accordingly, we expected that some human sera would contain 'anti-antibodies' (AA) reacting with antibody molecules denatured in the serological reaction but not with unaltered immunoglobulins. Formation of AA would be stimulated by immune complexes produced *in vivo*, e.g. complexes of microbial antigens and their antibodies. In our original study, we [29] found several AA-containing sera by screening human sera for agglutinins to Rh-positive erythrocytes sensitized by incomplete anti-Rh antibodies. AA became in this way a reagent distinguish-

Table I. Anti-antibody (AA) and rheumatoid factor (RF)

	Ig class	Reactions with			
		IgG fragment	foreign species IgG	allospecific IgG	IgG isolated and aggregated by physical means
RF	mostly IgM	Fc	+	+	+
AA	IgM	F(ab')₂	−	±	−

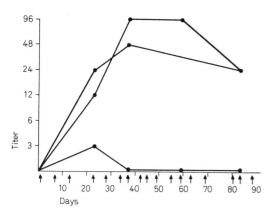

Fig. 1. Antibodies to human IgG in 3 rabbits injected with group A β-hemolytic streptococci. Arrows indicate intravenous injections of a suspension of heat-killed streptococci (bacteria grown for 24 h on one densely inoculated tryptose agar slant were washed off with saline and used for each injection). Antibody titer is expressed as a reciprocal of highest antiserum dilution that produced distinct agglutination of human Rh+ erythrocytes sensitized by incomplete human Rh antibodies.

ing the structural transformation of IgG antibody in serological reaction. Immunochemical studies by *Robert and Grabar* [36] and by *Ishizaka and Campbell* [11] supported the thesis of such a transformation. Furthermore, rabbit sera with AA were also found [22]. With the advent of rheumatoid arthritis serology, it became important to delineate the differences between AA and RF. They are presented in table I. In our recent studies,

AA was successfully employed as a reagent for detection of immune complexes in the circulation and of immune complexes deposited in tissues [15, 23, 26].

We and other investigators have believed that both AA and RF are produced as a result of *in vivo* serological reactions. Therefore, it appeared quite logical that prolonged immunization with any strong antigen will result in the appearance of some anti-γ-globulin factors. Experiments in which rabbits were immunized for 6 months with guinea pig leukocytes supported this contention [25]. This line of investigation was followed by *Eyquem et al.* [8], who observed antibodies to γ-globulins in rabbits injected with streptococci and some anaerobic bacilli. Convincing experiments proving that the reaction of antigen with its corresponding antibody may lead to formation of anti-globulin antibodies resembling rheumatoid factor were performed by *Abruzzo and Christian* [1], who employed coliform organisms for immunization of rabbits.

Our experiments also showed that rabbits injected with streptococci form antibodies to IgG combining primarily with human IgG. These studies were reported at the meeting of the FASEB in 1960 [28]. Figure 1 presents data from some of these old unpublished experiments. In analyzing these results, we were concerned with the speed with which the anti-γ-globulin antibodies were formed by rabbits immunized with streptococci. One hardly could believe that within 3 weeks (or even less), rabbits were able to produce anti-streptococcal antibodies and respond to these antibodies denatured in their *in vivo* reaction with streptococci. A plausible explanation for these findings can be offered now. As shown by *Christensen* and his associates [4–6], as well as by *Schalén et al.* [38], many hemolytic streptococci combine with the Fc piece of IgG of rabbit and human origin. Should such a reaction result in molecular transformation of IgG, then the prompt formation of anti-γ-globulin antibodies becomes understandable. This assumption is at least partially supported by the observations of *Lind* [20] who found that IgG undergoes molecular transformation in its reaction with staphylococcal protein A, which is also caused by binding through the Fc piece.

In finishing this discussion, it might be of interest to mention unpublished experiments performed in collaboration with Drs. *Penner*, *Albini* and *Andres* on dispersion of immune complexes deposited in kidneys of rabbits suffering from chronic serum sickness elicited by injections of BSA. Whereas in acute cases of serum sickness the immune complexes were readily dispersed by BSA, in the chronic cases of several weeks' duration, BSA did not disperse completely the complexes. On the other hand, a mixture of BSA and denatured rabbit IgG readily dispersed such complexes. Apparently, in addition to BSA-anti-BSA complexes, the deposits contained denatured IgG combined with a rheumatoid-like factor.

Cell-Surface Antigens

Formation of heterophile antibodies in the course of infectious mononucleosis has been interpreted [13, 24] as a result of the appearance of a novel antigen due to molec-ular transformation of abnormal cells, possibly those infected by the Epstein-Barr virus (for references, see *Glade* [9]). Direct evidence for the presence of Paul-Bunnell antigen in tissues of patients suffering from infectious mononucleosis has been presented only recently [2]. The formation of heterophile antibodies in infectious mononucleosis and their diagnostic application is discussed in some detail in another presentation of this Convocation [12].

It should be stressed here that Paul-Bunnell antigen appears also in several pathologic conditions other than infectious mononucleosis without any apparent relation to infection by Epstein-Barr virus and without formation of Paul-Bunnell antibodies. Spleen cells from patients with lymphoma and leukemia frequently have Paul-Bunnell antigen, as demonstrated by absorption of Paul-Bunnell antibodies from an IM serum [31, 32], as well as by mixed agglutination reaction [14]. Furthermore, in collaboration with Drs. *Nishimaki* and *Kano*, we showed circulating Paul-Bunnell antigen in sera of some patients suffering from lymphoma, leukemia, and gastrointestinal carcinoma [unpublished observations].

There must be some difference in the presentation of Paul-Bunnell antigen to the immunological apparatus in infectious mononucleosis in which the formation of its corresponding antibodies occurs regularly and in the above-discussed malignant diseases in which this antigen is present in the tissues or even in the circulation without eliciting antibody formation. It seems likely that in infectious mononucleosis, a large amount of Paul-Bunnell antigen is formed and released in immunogenic form in a short period of time. On the other hand, in the above-mentioned malignant conditions, this antigen apparently is formed in relatively small quantities, and it might evoke a low dose tolerance rather than an immune response.

Our recent studies were devoted to another heterophile system, the Hanganutziu-Deicher system. Hanganutziu-Deicher antibodies, originally described under the misnomer 'serum sickness antibodies' [7, 10], had been found in human patients who received injections of foreign species sera such a diphtheria or tetanus antitoxin of horse origin. We [16] found that Hanganutziu-Deicher antibodies may appear in man, under various pathologic conditions, without administration of a foreign serum. Especially interesting appears the formation of Hanganutziu-Deicher antibodies in the course of rheumatoid arthritis, because immune complexes composed of Hanganutziu-Deicher antigen and antibody are quite frequently encountered in sera and synovial fluids of patients suffering from this disease [33, 34].

Interestingly, recent studies have shown that Hanganutziu-Deicher antigen appears in sera and tissues of many patients with malignancies [35]. The significance of this recent observation was not yet explored.

The occurrence of a novel antigen in the course of malignancy is by no means a new discovery; 27 years ago, *Levine* and his associates [17–19] observed an elderly woman belonging to a rare blood group Tj(a−), now called pp, who had a gastric adenocarcinoma apparently containing an 'illegitimate' antigen Tj^a which stimulated, in the patient, formation of antibodies directed to PP_1P^k antigenic complex. In our recent studies, we [21b] observed that antigens acquired by murine tumors appear as normal cell surface structures in mice of other strains.

Comments

The discussed data were used to demonstrate that antigenic alteration of the body's own constituents is a quite frequent event. Antigenic alteration undoubtedly occurs under physiological conditions, but it assumes very significant dimensions under pathologic conditions. Using IgG and heterophile antigens as examples, we demonstrated the important fact that newly derived antigens closely resemble antigenic structures present under physiologic conditions in other individuals of the same species and in members of other species. The appearance of novel antigens may lead to immune response to these antigens. For brevity's sake, we discussed only humoral responses to such antigens. As discussed in other presentations of this Convocation, immune response to altered antigens may play a beneficial role, e.g. by removing aberrant cells [12]; on the other hand, such immune responses may lead to pathologic events [3, 40, 42].

References

1 Abruzzo, J. L. and Christian, C. L.: The induction of a rheumatoid factor-like substance in rabbits. J. exp. Med. *114:* 791–806 (1961).

2 Andres, G. A.; Kano, K.; Elwood, C.; Prezyna, A.; Sepulveda, M., and Milgrom, F.: Immune deposit nephritis in infectious mononucleosis. Int. Archs Allergy appl. Immun. *52:* 136–144 (1976).

3 Beutner, E. H.; Jablonska, S.; Chorzelski, T. P., and Binder, W. L.: A unified concept of autoimmunity and the nature of SCAg conversion phenomenon; in Milgrom and Albini Immunopathology, pp. 142–147 (Karger, Basel 1979).

4 Christensen, P. and Kronvall, G.: Capacity of group A, B, C, D and G streptococci to agglutinate sensitized sheep red cells. Acta path. microbiol. scand. B *82:* 19–24 (1974).

5 Christensen, P. and Oxelius, V.-A.: Quantitation of the uptake of human IgG by some streptococci groups, A, B, C and G. Acta pathol. microbiol. scand. B *82:* 475–483 (1974).

6 Christensen, P.: Agglutinability of some selected streptococci by immune complexes. Acta path. scand. C *83:* 28–34 (1975).

7 Deicher, H.: Über die Erzeugung heterospezifischer Haemagglutinine durch Injektion artfremden Serums. Z. Hyg. Infektkrankh. *106:* 561–579 (1926).

8 Eyquem, A.; Guyot-Jeannin, N. et Podliachouk, L.: Présence dans les immunsérums anti-bactériens de facteurs anti-globuliniques analogues à ceux de la polyarthrite chronique évolutive. Annls Inst. Pasteur, Paris 96: 295–302 (1959).

9 Glade, P. R.: Infectious mononucleosis (Lippincott, Philadelphia 1973).

10 Haganutziu, M.: Hémagglutinines hétérogénétiques après injection de sérum de cheval. C. r. Séanc. Soc. Biol. 91: 1457–1459 (1924).

11 Ishizaka, K. and Campbell, D. H.: Biologic activity of soluble antigen-antibody complexes. V. Change of optical rotation by the formation of skin reactive complexes. J. Immun. 83: 318 (1959).

12 Kano, K.: Infectious mononucleosis: heterophile antibody response; in Milgrom and Albini Immunopathology, pp. 242–246 (Karger, Basel 1979).

13 Kano, K. and Milgrom, F.: Heterophile antigens and antibodies in medicine; in Current topics in microbiology and immunology, pp. 43–69 (Springer, Berlin 1977).

14 Kano, K.; Fjelde, A., and Milgrom, F.: Paul-Bunnell antigen in lymphoma and leukemia spleens. J. Immun. 119: 945–949 (1977).

15 Kano, K.; Nishimaki, T.; Palosuo, T.; Loza, U., and Milgrom, F.: Detection of circulating immune complexes by the inhibition of anti-antibody. Clin. Immunol. Immunopath. 9: 425–435 (1978).

16 Kasukawa, R.; Kano, K.; Bloom, M. L., and Milgrom, F.: Heterophile antibodies in pathologic human sera resembling antibodies stimulated by foreign species sera. Clin. exp. Immunol. 25: 122–132 (1976).

17 Levine, P.; Bobbitt, O. B.; Waller, R., and Kuhmichel, M.: Isoimmunization by a new blood factor in tumor cells. Proc. Soc. exp. Biol. Med. 77: 403–404 (1951).

18 Levine, P.: Illegitimate blood group antigens P_1, A, and MN (T) in malignancy—a possible therapeutic approach with anti-Tj^a, anti-A and anti-T. Ann. N.Y. Acad. Sci. 277: 428–435 (1976).

19 Levine, P.: Comments on hemolytic disease of newborn due to anti-PP_1P^k (anti-Tj^a). Transfusion 17: 573–578 (1977).

20 Lind, I.: The formation of antibodies against hidden determinants of autologous IgG during immunization of rabbits with Staphylococcus aureus. Scand. J. Immunol. 3: 689 (1974).

21a McCluskey, R. T.; Miller, F., and Benacerraf, B.: Sensitization to denatured autologous gamma globulin. J. exp. Med. 115: 253–273 (1962).

21b Merino, F.; Abeyounis, C. J., and Milgrom, F.: Studies on the specificity of cytolytic antibodies to methylcholanthrene-induced sarcomas elicited by immunization of syngeneic mice. Eur. J. Cancer 15: 829–835 (1979).

22 Milgrom, F.: Rabbit sera with 'anti-antibody'. Vox Sang. 7: 545–558 (1962).

23 Milgrom, F.: Immune complex disease; in Int. Symp. on The Nature and Significance of Complement Activation, 1976, pp. 49–56 (Ortho Research Institute of Medical Sciences, Raritan 1977).

24 Milgrom, F.: The unusual serology of syphilis, infectious mononucleosis and rheumatoid arthritis. Transfusion 4: 407–413 (1964).

25 Milgrom, F. and Dubiski, S.: Antigenicity of antibodies of the same species. Nature, Lond. 179: 1351–1352 (1957).

26 Milgrom, F. and Kano, K.: Comparison of various procedures for the detection of antigen-antibody complexes. Int. Archs Allergy appl. Immun. 56: 224–231 (1978).

27 Milgrom, F. and Witebsky, E.: Studies on the rheumatoid and related serum factors. I. Autoimmunization of rabbits with gamma globulin. J. Am. med. Ass. 174: 56–63 (1960).

28 Milgrom, F. and Witebsky, E.: Rabbit antibodies against γ-globulins resembling the rheumatoid factor (abstr.). Fed. Proc. Fed. Am. Socs. exp. Biol. 19: 197 (1960).

29 Milgrom, F.; Dubiski, S., and Wozniczko, G.: Human sera with 'anti-antibody'. Vox Sang. 1: 172–183 (1956).

30 Milgrom, F.; Dubiski, S., and Wozniczko, G.: A simple method of Rh determination. Nature, Lond. 178: 539 (1956).

31 Milgrom, F.; Kano, K., and Fjelde, A.: Studies on heterophile antigen in lymphoma and leukemia spleens by means of absorption of infectious mononucleosis sera. Int. Archs Allergy appl. Immun. 45: 631–637 (1973).

32 Milgrom, F.; Kano, K.; Fjelde, A., and Bloom, M. L.: Heterophile antigens and antibodies in transplantation and tumors. Transplantn. Proc. 7: 201–207 (1975).

33 Nishimaki, T.; Kano, K., and Milgrom, F.: Studies on heterophile antibodies in rheumatoid arthritis. Arthritis Rheum. 21: 634–638 (1978).

34 Nishimaki, T.; Kano, K., and Milgrom, F.: Studies on immune complexes in rheumatoid arthritis. Arthritis Rheum. 21: 639–644 (1978).

35 Nishimaki, T.; Kano, K., and Milgrom, F.: Paul-Bunnell antigen in malignancies and rheumatoid arthritis. Int. Archs Allergy appl. Immun. 60: 115–119 (1979).

36 Robert, B. et Grabar, P.: Dosage des groupements thiol protéiques dans des réactions immunochimiques. Annls Inst. Pasteur, Paris 92: 56 (1957).

37 Rothen, A. and Landsteiner, K.: Serological reactions of protein films and denatured proteins. J. exp. Med. *76:* 437–450 (1942).

38 Schalén, C.; Christensen, P., and Grubb, R.: Lancefield extract of group A streptococci type 15 acts like an anti-human IgG with restricted specificity. Acta path. microbiol. scand. C *86:* 41–43 (1978).

39 TenBroeck, C. and Wu, H.: Chinese J. Physiol. *1:* 277 (1927); quoted by *Rothen and Landsteiner* [37].

40 Vaughan, J. H.; Carson, D. A.; Kaplan, R. A., and Slaughter, L. S.: Anti-IgG in rheumatoid arthritis. Pathogenetic potential and stimulation by Epstein-Barr virus; in Milgrom and Albini Immunopathology, pp. 224–229 (Karger, Basel 1979).

41 Williams, R. C., jr. and Kunkel, H. G.: Antibodies to rabbit γ-globulin after immunizing with various preparations of autologous γ-globulin. Proc. Soc. exp. Biol. Med. *112:* 554–561 (1963).

42 Zvaifler, N. J.: Pathology and pathogenesis of rheumatoid arthritis; in Milgrom and Albini Immunopathology, pp. 217–223 (Karger, Basel 1979).

Dr. F. Milgrom, Department of Microbiology, School of Medicine, State University of New York at Buffalo, Buffalo, NY 14214 (USA)

Ernest Witebsky Memorial Lecture

Immunopathology. 6th Int. Convoc. Immunol., Niagara Falls, N.Y., 1978, pp. 62–69 (Karger, Basel 1979)

Experimental Allergic Encephalomyelitis
New Concepts of Effector Activity and Immunoregulation by Endogenous Neuroantigen with Implications for Multiple Sclerosis

Philip Y. Paterson

Department of Microbiology-Immunology, the Medical and Dental Schools, Northwestern University, Chicago, Ill.

Introduction

The importance of autoantigens and host reactivity as determinants of disease in animals and man has received increasing support during this century [1, 23]. No organ system has figured more prominently than the central nervous system (CNS) in the relentless quest for new insights pertaining to the nature of autoimmune tissue injury and disease [16, 18, 19, 21].

Multiple sclerosis (MS) has remained an enigma ever since its original description more than 100 years ago [11]. Both infectious and immunologic mechanisms have been implicated in this demyelinating disease of world wide importance [2, 11, 16, 18]. At present, accumulated data favor immunologic determinants over other etiologic considerations [16, 18, 19]. Core evidence for immunologic mechanisms in MS are listed in table I.

Organ-specific antigenic constituents in CNS tissue, capable of calling forth host immune responses specifically reactive with brain and spinal cord, have been known for more than 50 years. One of the pioneer investigators in this area was *Witebsky* who this lectureship honors and who might be termed the 'father of studies on autoim-

munity'. Figure 1 is a montage illustrating the first publication in a series of papers by *Witebsky* and his associates concerning brain-specific antigens, published in 1928 [27]. The capacity of mammalian nervous tissue when injected in the form of rabies vaccine to induce disease in man termed acute disseminated encephalomyelitis with histopathologic features bearing a resemblance to MS was known before the present century [19]. Development of experimental allergic encephalomyelitis (EAE) as a reproducible neuro-autoimmunologic disease, produced at will in a variety of species of experimental animals following sensitization to CNS homogenates or defined neuroantigen, i.e. myelin basic protein (MBP), in company with

Table I. Core evidence for immunologic mechanisms in multiple sclerosis (MS)

Nervous tissue is immunogenic and elicits organ-specific immunologic responses
Injection of nervous tissue into man or animals induces disease simulating MS
  (a) Post-rabies vaccine encephalomyelitis
  (b) Experimental allergic encephalomyelitis (EAE)
Common immune responses demonstrable in animals with EAE and patients with MS

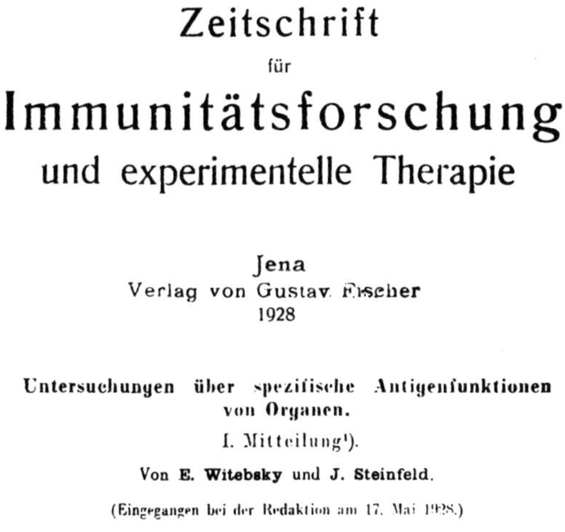

Zeitschrift

für

Immunitätsforschung

und experimentelle Therapie

Jena
Verlag von Gustav Fischer
1928

Untersuchungen über spezifische Antigenfunktionen
von Organen.

I. Mitteilung¹).

Von E. Witebsky und J. Steinfeld.

(Eingegangen bei der Redaktion am 17. Mai 1928.)

Fig. 1. Montage illustrating the first of a series of publications by *Witebsky* dealing with organ-specific antigens published in 1928 [27].

Freund's adjuvant, has been a vital means for probing the MS problem [16, 18, 19]. Probably the most compelling evidence for MS being an immunopathogenetic process, at least in part, has been the finding of common immunologic responses in animals with EAE and patients with MS [15, 16, 18, 19].

As reviewed in detail elsewhere [18, 19], EAE is believed to result from host immune responses, initiated by sensitizing neuroantigen, which cross react with native antigen in the animal's own CNS target tissues. Because the disease can be transferred with sensitized donor lymphoid cells, but has yet to be transferred reproducibly with immune serum, it is generally believed that cell-mediated immune mechanisms engendered by thymus-derived (T) lymphocytes are of paramount importance [10, 12, 13].

My own preoccupation with EAE, which has continued without interruption for more than 25 years, has in the past and even more so now, reflected two deeply rooted convictions. First, EAE is an exceptionally useful

experimental model system for identifying and incisively dissecting the multiplicity of host responses directed against 'self antigens' which cause, prevent or otherwise modulate CNS tissue damage in particular and auto-immune injury in general. Second, while EAE may not be the exact animal counterpart to MS in man, I know of no more meaningful model system for probing this devastating neurologic disease of man. In my opinion, it is time to put to one side discussions as to how well EAE does or does not duplicate the MS process, so as to clear the way for extracting every conceivable clue from the EAE model system that may shed increasing light on central issues concerning the MS problem.

What I wish to summarize briefly here are two recent findings concerning EAE which I believe have pointed meaning for MS: (a) transfer of EAE in Lewis rats with cell-free supernatants derived from sensitized lymphoid cells, and (b) demonstration of an endogenous neuroantigen, indistinguishable from MBP insofar as its capacity to bind reagent MBP antibody is concerned, in the serum and cerebrospinal fluid of normal rats and animals with EAE. This endogenous autoantigen appears to exert an immunoregulatory influence on expression of the disease. In this work, I have been joined by several key associates and collaborators who must share any credit accruing from our research: Dr. *Caroline C. Whitacre*, who has spearheaded the EAE supernatant transfer project, Dr. *Robert S. Fujinami*, my former graduate student whose doctoral research dissertation concerning EAE in suckling Lewis rats led the way for discovering the endogenous neuroantigen and, finally, Drs. *Eugene D. Day* and *Vincent A. Varitek* at Duke University, whose expertise in immunochemistry and radioimmunoassay procedures allowed us to demonstrate and quantitate this circulating neuroantigen.

Transfer of Experimental Allergic Encephalomyelitis with Cell Supernatants

It is of historical interest to mention that the impetus leading to successful transfer of EAE with lymphoid cell supernatants had its roots in work I described at the first of these International Convocations on Immunology, held in 1968 [14]. We reported that when lymph node cells (LNC) from Lewis rats, previously sensitized to spinal cord emulsified in complete Freund's adjuvant (CFA), were incubated with CNS tissue at 37 °C for 1–4 h, they no longer had demonstrable EAE transfer activity. Aliquots of these same LNC suspensions incubated under identical conditions but *without the addition of CNS tissue* were found to have diminished transfer activity. These observations suggested that transfer activity was either destroyed as a result of the incubation procedure or released from the sensitized LNC into the suspending medium.

Using the LNC harvest and incubation procedures described in detail elsewhere [25], we were able to demonstrate that supernatants derived from sensitized LNC of Lewis rats have the capacity to elicit typical lesions of EAE when injected intravenously into normal syngeneic recipients. Clinical neurologic signs were not and still have not been observed in any of our positive supernatant recipients despite some of these animals developing disseminated focal lesions of EAE within their brain and spinal cord. Our overall experience to date with EAE transfer using LNC supernatants is summarized in table II. It is obvious that sensitization of donors via the hindleg footpad, in contrast to injection of the sensitizing neuroantigen over the upper back and anterior neck, is a superior means of securing LNC from which active supernatants can be regularly prepared. Using the footpad route of sensitization, 13 of 14 experiments have proven successful, thereby allowing us to accelerate our efforts to study LNC supernatant activity incisively. Greater reproducibility of EAE transfer with supernatants prepared from lymph nodes draining the lower extremities undoubtedly is due to such tissues having greater EAE effector cell activity vis-à-vis lymph nodes draining the forelegs, upper back and anterior neck of rats [28].

Although several experiments make it abundantly clear that EAE supernatant transfer activity (EAE-STA) cannot be demonstrated in donors sensitized to guinea pig (GP) MBP, recent experience suggests that GPMBP has the capacity to specifically and

Table II. Transfer of EAE in Lewis rats with LNC supernatants

Route of sensitization of LNC donors[1]	EAE in recipients	Successful experiments
Back-neck	45/103	22/38
Hind foot pad	25/42	13/14

[1] Supernatants prepared from LNC collected from donors 9 days after sensitization with GP spinal cord in CFA.

Table III. Specific absorption of EAE-STA by GPMBP

Supernatant[1]	Occurrence of EAE in Lewis recipient rats
Unabsorbed	2/3
Absorbed with	
GPMBP	0/3
Lysozyme	2/3

[1] Supernatant from LNC of donors sensitized to GP spinal cord, with or without addition of either protein 40 μg/ml, held at 6 °C overnight and then injected in volume of 2 ml/recipient.

completely absorb EAE-STA from active preparations derived from donors sensitized to GP spinal cord in CFA. An experiment illustrating this point is shown in table III, using lysozyme as a control as it has a molecular weight and electrostatic charge very similar to that of MBP.

Strenuous efforts are in progress to characterize the properties of the moiety or moieties responsible for EAE-STA. So far, we have found EAE-STA to be stable at 56 °C for at least 1 h and at 4 °C for at least 18 h, to have a molecular weight in excess of 100,000 based on ultrafiltration, and activity remaining in the supernatant after centrifugation at 20,000 g but not at 200,000 g. Experiments designed specifically to determine whether EAE-STA in any way involves immunoglobulin or an immunoglobulin-like moiety have been fraught with frustrating technical problems and have not given definitive results as yet.

The implications of EAE-STA for EAE are obvious, namely an opportunity to isolate and characterize an effector cell product responsible, at least in part, for a disease widely believed to be intimately associated with if not mediated by sensitized T lymphoid cells [10, 12, 13]. The implications of EAE-STA for MS may be equally important. There is no reason to believe that EAE-STA cannot operate across species barriers or that such activity cannot be derived from lymphoid cells of patients with MS. Experiments already are underway in our laboratory to prepare supernatants from incubated peripheral blood leukocytes of MS donors and determine whether they have the capacity to induce EAE or some type of CNS-specific neuropathologic effect in normal Lewis rats. Successful transfer of any neurologic abnormality from MS patients to animals would provide a superb means for directly isolating and defining host factors of etiologic importance in this human disorder.

Endogenous Myelin Basic Protein in Serum and Cerebrospinal Fluid (CSF)

The most important prelude to discovery of endogenous MBP in Lewis rats was our finding that suckling Lewis rats exhibit a striking age-related restriction concerning actively induced EAE as well as the transferred form of the disease [7, 8]. It seemed possible that restricted occurrence of disease in immature animals might be the result of a circulating neuroantigen such as MBP, with the capacity to markedly diminish production of EAE effector cells in numbers required for expression of the disease. It was at this point that Dr. *Eugene Day's* laboratory and my laboratory began to collaborate and focus on this issue.

By converting a standard radioimmunoassay (RIA) utilizing iodinated rat MBP (^{125}I-RMBP) as reagent antigen and rat anti-RMBP antibody as reagent antiserum [4] into a quantitative RIA inhibition, we could look for an inhibitor of MBP binding in sera of both suckling and adult rats [5, 6, 8]. We had no difficulty demonstrating the presence in suckling rat sera of relatively large amounts of a serum factor which additively inhibited binding of ^{125}I-RMBP by reagent antiserum. By four different approaches and methods, it was clear that the serum factor in question was immunochemically indistinguishable from native RMBP with respect to its capacity to bind RMBP reagent antiserum. We therefore designated this serum factor MBP-SF. High MBP-SF levels, of the order of 14–21 ng/ml, were found in a high proportion of suckling Lewis rats. These levels began to decline slowly after weaning and were observed to reach adult levels of ≤ 0.6 ng, the sensitivity limit of the assay, by 8–10 weeks of age [5, 6, 8, 9]. There was a striking inverse correlation between levels of MBP-SF and susceptibility to EAE among rats of widely varying ages

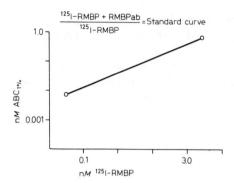

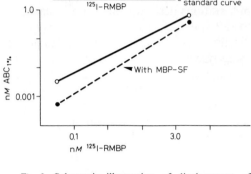

Fig. 2. Schematic illustration of a standard binding curve using dilutions of ^{125}I-RMBP reagent antigen on the abscissa and dilutions of reagent anti-RMBP rabbit antiserum on the ordinate. Capacity of 1 μl of antiserum, of a standard 100 μl volume, to bind nM quantities of ^{125}I-RMBP is expressed in terms of antigen-binding capacity ($ABC_{1\%}$).

Fig. 3. Schematic illustration of displacement of standard binding curve due to serum from a rat with acute EAE which contained MBP factor or inhibitor, designated as MBP-SF, with selective binding for high affinity anti-MBP antibody only.

which were sensitized to RMBP-CFA [8, 9]. We also were able to demonstrate elevated MBP-SF levels in some actively sensitized adult Lewis rats at the time they developed early clinical manifestations of EAE [8].

More recently, *Day et al.* [unpublished data] have developed an inhibition assay that takes into consideration reagent MBP antibody binding affinity as measured at several different concentrations of ^{125}I-RMBP. The assay is based on a quantitative dual dilution technique developed by *Varitek and Day* [24] for measuring MBP-antiMBP systems and reaches a sensitivity approximately 3 orders of magnitude greater than the procedure we employed for the initial phase of our work. A representative standard binding curve, where both antigen and antibody are diluted according to predetermined increments, is illustrated schematically in figure 2. The range of reagent antigen employed was 0.1–3.0 nM ^{125}I-RMBP as shown on the abscissa. The capacity of diluted reagent RMBP antiserum to bind reagent antigen, in terms of 1 μl of a 100-μl volume, is expressed as nM ^{125}I-RMBP antigen binding capacity or $ABC_{1\%}$

on the ordinate. Using this procedure, MBP inhibitor in picomole amounts could be detected and precisely measured in body fluids by means of displacement of the standard curve. Depending on what part of the curve was displaced, we could learn whether we were dealing with endogenous MBP possessing immunodeterminants for either high or/and low affinity reagent antibodies. Presence of endogenous MBP could be recorded as picomoles of inhibitor or/and in terms of standard deviations of displacements of the standard curve at any specific concentration of reagent antigen.

One type of curve displacement we have observed commonly is shown schematically in figure 3. In this instance, the curve is displaced negatively and significantly in the range of 0.1 nM ^{125}I-RMBP, signifying the presence of MBP-SF with determinants for high affinity antibody binding only. No negative displacement of the curve is observed with the largest amount of reagent antigen, i.e. 3.0 nM ^{125}I-RMBP, indicating the absence of any inhibitor binding low affinity RMBP antibody.

Table IV. RMBP inhibitor in CSF and serum of Lewis rats

Status of rats	Fluid assayed[1]	nM RMBP inhibitor detected with reagent ^{125}I-RMBP[2]	
		0.1 nM	3.0 nM
Normal	CSF	− 7(0)	−1,300(−1)
	serum	−17(−1)	− 700(0)
EAE	CSF	−67(−3)	−2,100(−1)
	serum	−52(−3)	−2,900(−2)

[1] Fluid pools from 10 normal rats and 16 paralyzed animals with EAE after sensitization to RMBP or rat cord in CFA.

[2] nM RMBP inhibitor expressed as increments of displacement of ABC 1% binding curve, with SDs in parentheses, using a dual dilution quantitative inhibition assay.

Data pertaining to MBP inhibitors in pooled sera and CSF specimens of normal Lewis rats and animals developing EAE are set out in table IV. Prior to sensitization pooled CSF from normal rats contained significant amounts of MBP binding low affinity antibody. After sensitization and with onset of EAE, pooled CSF now contained a very large amount of MBP binding high affinity antibody. Serum before EAE contained low levels of MBP binding high affinity antibody but considerably more of this type of inhibitor was present after onset of EAE, along with appearance for the first time of MBP binding low affinity antibody. Indirect evidence we have secured so far indicates that the MBP inhibitors in CSF and serum of adult rats exist as fragments of the whole MBP molecule with immunodeterminants for antibody of either high affinity or low affinity but not both. We do not yet have in focus any definitive temporal pattern related to CSF and/or serum MBP inhibitor levels and time- course of EAE. What we have observed to date, however, strongly suggests that we have uncovered an autoneuroantigen of potential importance in terms of regulating host immune responsiveness to MBP.

The implications of this phase of our work as it relates to EAE and MS are as follows. Detection of MBP in CSF of animals with acute episodes of EAE now duplicates what already has been reported in patients suffering acute relapses of MS [3, 26]. In this sense, yet another feature of concordance has been identified for the animal model and its counterpart in human beings. It is unclear whether endogenous MBP fragments in animals with EAE and patients with MS arise within areas of developing injury to myelinated nerve fibers due to the action of proteases released from cells comprising the host inflammatory response or are created as a result of activation of the coagulation, complement or kinin cascades associated with immunologically mediated inflammation. We have detailed evidence elsewhere indicating that activation of the clotting system as reflected by striking perivascular accumulation of fibrin within the CNS of rats developing EAE might be the source of MBP degradation products [17, 20]. Of major importance is learning whether these fragments possess EAE-inducing activity and/or EAE inhibitory activity. Based on studies in experimental animals, it is clear that MBP possesses completely separate immunodeterminants engendering these two opposing types of activity [22]. Conceivably, one gene-specified defect in the MS-susceptible individual might be an inability to degrade MBP properly so as to assure maintenance of critical levels of MBP inhibitory fragments, i.e. neurotolerogens, in host body fluids at all times. The types of investigation and lines of thinking outlined here promise new understanding of EAE as a prototype autoimmune disease of animals and offer new approaches to the enigma of MS.

Summary

Experimental allergic encephalomyelitis (EAE) is a prototypic autoneuroimmunologic model disease with particular promise of identifying immunologic mechanisms operating in multiple sclerosis. Transfer of EAE in rats with cell-free supernatants from sensitized lymphoid cells has been accomplished. Sera of normal Lewis rats contain low and variable levels of a factor which is immunochemically indistinguishable from myelin basic protein in terms of its capacity to bind antibody specific for rat myelin basic protein and has been designated as MBP-SF. High levels of MBP-SF are demonstrable in sera and cerebrospinal fluids of rats developing EAE. Evidence in hand suggests that MBP-SF is an endogenous neuroantigen with regulatory activity concerning susceptibility of rats to EAE and occurrence of clinical remissions of the disease in this host.

Acknowledgements

I wish to express my thanks and debt to Dr. *Lewis Thomas*, who first introduced me to EAE as a model disease for laboratory investigation; to Dr. *Jules Freund*, who never let me stray from my personal quest to transfer the disease; and to Dr. *Ernest Witebsky*, who provided special encouragement when the 'going was rough'. Finally, I express special thanks to Mrs. *Geane Kraus*, my devoted personal secretary of 10 years standing who makes all typescripts expressing my thoughts become a reality.

Supported by United States Public Health Service Grant NS 06262 and Research Grant 147-A-2 from the National Multiple Sclerosis Society. In studies carried out with colleagues, Dr. *Caroline C. Whitacre* was a recipient of a National Multiple Sclerosis Society Postdoctoral Fellowship FG 454-A-1 from 1976–1978; Dr. *Robert S. Fujinami* was supported in his graduate studies through a National Institute General Medical Sciences Training Grant 3T01-GM 00724; and work performed by Drs. *Eugene D. Day* and *Vincent A. Varitek* was supported by United States Public Health Service Grant NS 10237 and Research Grant 833-D-4 from the National Multiple Sclerosis Society.

References

1 Burnet, M.: Autoimmunity and autoimmune disease (Medical and Technical Publishing, Lancaster 1972).

2 Bornstein, M. B.: The immunopathology of demyelinative disorders examined in organotypic cultures of mammalian central nerve tissues. Prog. Neuropath. *II:* 69–90 (1973).

3 Cohen, S. R.; Herndon, R. M., and McKhann, G. M.: Radioimmunoassay of myelin basic protein in spinal fluid. An index of active demyelination. New Engl. J. Med. *295:* 1455–1457 (1976).

4 Day, E. D. and Pitts, O. M.: Radioimmunoassay of myelin basic protein in sodium sulfate. Immunochemistry *11:* 651–659 (1974).

5 Day, E. D.; Varitek, V. A.; Fujinami, R. S., and Paterson, P. Y.: MBP-SF, a prominent serum factor in suckling Lewis rats, that additively inhibits the primary binding of myelin basic protein (MBP) to syngeneic anti-MBP antibodies. Immunochemistry *15:* 1–10 (1978).

6 Day, E. D.; Varitek, V. A., and Paterson, P. Y.: Myelin basic protein serum factor (MBP-SF) in adult Lewis rats: a method for detection and evidence that MBP-SF influences the appearance of antibody to MBP in animals developing experimental allergic encephalomyelitis. Immunochemistry *15:* 437–442 (1978).

7 Fujinami, R. S. and Paterson, P. Y.: Induction of experimental allergic encephalomyelitis in suckling Lewis rats: role of age and type of sensitizing neuroantigen. J. Immun. *119:* 1634–1638 (1977).

8 Fujinami, R. S.; Paterson, P. Y.; Day, E. D., and Harter, D. H.: Circulating myelin basic protein-like antigen in suckling Lewis rat serum (BP-SS): immunodeterminant of age-dependent susceptibility to experimental allergic encephalomyelitis (EAE) (abstr.). Fed. Proc. Fed. Am. Socs exp. Biol. *36:* 1206 (1977).

9 Fujinami, R. S.; Paterson, P. Y.; Day, E. D., and Varitek, V. A.: Myelin basic protein serum factor (MBP-SF): an endogenous neuroantigen influencing development of experimental allergic encephalomyelitis in Lewis rats. J. exp. Med. *148:* 1716–1721 (1978).

10 Gonatas, N. K. and Howard, J. C.: Inhibition of experimental allergic encephalomyelitis in rats severely depleted of T cells. Science *186:* 839–841 (1974).

11 Johnson, R. T.: The possible viral etiology of multiple sclerosis; in Friedlander Adv. Neurol., pp. 1–46 (Raven Press, Hewlett 1975).

12 Ortiz-Ortiz, L. and Weigle, W. O.: Cellular events in the induction of experimental allergic encephalomyelitis in rats. J. exp. Med. *144:* 604–616 (1976).

13 Ortiz-Ortiz, L.; Nakamura, R. M., and Weigle, W. O.: T cell requirement for experimental allergic encephalomyelitis induction in the rat. J. Immun. *117:* 576–579 (1976).

14 Paterson, P. Y.: Sensitized cell-target tissue interactions and autoimmune disease. Approaches using experimental autoimmune encephalomyelitis; in Rose and Milgrom, Int. Convoc. Immunol., pp. 260–264 (Karger, Basel 1969).

15 Paterson, P. Y.: Multiple sclerosis; an immunologic reassessment. J. chron. Dis. 26: 119–126 (1973).

16 Paterson, P. Y.: Experimental autoimmune (allergic) encephalomyelitis: induction, pathogenesis and suppression; in Miescher and Müller-Eberhard Textbook of immunopathology; 2nd ed., pp. 179–213 (Grune & Stratton, New York 1976).

17 Paterson, P. Y.: Experimental allergic encephalomyelitis; role of fibrin deposition in immunopathogenesis of inflammation in rats. Fed. Proc. Fed. Am. Socs exp. Biol. 35: 2428–2434 (1976).

18 Paterson, P. Y.: Autoimmune neurological disease: experimental animal systems and implications for multiple sclerosis; in Talal Autoimmunity, pp. 643–692 (Academic Press, New York 1977).

19 Paterson, P. Y.: Neurological diseases; in Irvine Medical immunology, pp. 361–381 (Teviot Scientific Publications, Edinburgh 1979).

20 Pescovitz, M. D.; Paterson, P. Y.; Kelly, J., and Lorand, L.: Serum degradation of myelin basic protein with loss of encephalitogenic activity: evidence for an enzymatic process. Cell. Immunol. 39: 355–365 (1978).

21 Raine, C.: Experimental allergic encephalomyelitis and related condition; in Zimmerman Prog. in Neuropath., vol. 3, pp. 225–251 (Grune & Stratton, New York 1966).

22 Swanborg, R. H.: Maintenance of immunologic self-tolerance by nonimmunogenic forms of antigen. Clin. exp. Immunol. 26: 597–600 (1976).

23 Talal, N. (ed.): Autoimmunity, genetic, immunologic, virologic and clinical aspects (Academic Press, New York 1977).

24 Varitek, V. A. and Day, E. D.: Relative affinity of antisera for myelin basic protein (MBP) and degree of affinity heterogeneity. Immunochemistry (in press).

25 Whitacre, C. C. and Paterson, P. Y.: Transfer of experimental allergic encephalomyelitis in Lewis rats using supernatants of incubated sensitized lymph node cells. J. exp. Med. 145: 1405–1410 (1977).

26 Whitaker, J. N.: Myelin encephalitogenic protein fragments in cerebrospinal fluid of persons with multiple sclerosis. Neurology, Minneap. 27: 911–920 (1977).

27 Witebsky, E. und Steinfeld, J.: Untersuchungen über spezifische Antigenfunktionen von Organen. Z. ImmunForsch. exp. Ther. 58: 271–296 (1928).

28 Harvey, J. M.; Drobish, D. G., and Paterson, P. Y.: Transfer of experimental allergic encephalomyelitis (EAE) in Lewis rats as a function of peripheral lumphoid tissue effector cell activity (abstr.). Fed. Proc. Fed. Am. Socs exp. Biol. 37: 1473 (1978).

Dr. P. Y. Paterson, Department of Microbiology-Immunology, The Medical and Dental Schools, Northwestern University, Chicago, IL 60611 (USA)

Immunologically Mediated Organ-Restricted Diseases

Immunopathology. 6th Int. Convoc. Immunol., Niagara Falls, N.Y., 1978, pp. 70–73 (Karger, Basel 1979)

The Immunopathology of Multiple Sclerosis[1]

Barry G. W. Arnason

Department of Neurology, University of Chicago and the Pritzker School of Medicine, Chicago, Ill.

The cause of multiple sclerosis (MS) is not known but there is compelling evidence to indicate that immune mechanisms have an important role in the genesis of lesions in this disease. There is general agreement that the pathology of the MS lesion is consistent with either a viral or autoallerigic disorder despite the fact that no known viral or auto-allergic process totally duplicates the pathologic features of MS.

The plaque constitutes the pathologic hallmark of MS. Small plaques are peri-venular in location and larger plaques form by coalescence of smaller ones. Myelin is lost from plaques with relative sparing of axons. Oligodendrocytes disappear from the center of the plaque but can be readily recognized at its margins. In active plaques, ongoing myelin breakdown can be observed at the plaque rim with macrophages constituting the predominant invading cell. Reactive astrocytes are typically seen just beyond the margin of myelin destruction. Perivenular lymphocyte accumulations are characteristic of active plaques—sometimes these accumulations may be located some distance from the regions where myelin is being destroyed.

Plasma cells are frequently present as well, scattered throughout the plaque and sometimes beyond its margins. The active lesion is clearly inflammatory in nature, but the core question remains unanswered. What is the nature of the substance against which the inflammatory response is directed?

The histocompatibility antigens A3, B7, DW2 and DRW2 are overrepresented in MS. The A3–B7 and DW2 antigens are in significant genetic disequilibrium with each other and the putative immune response (Ir) gene associated with susceptibility for MS is most closely tied to the D-locus allele. The A3, B7 and DW2 antigens are particularly prevalent in those North European Caucasian populations in which MS itself is common. These alleles are rare in Negroes and Asiatics in whom MS is rare. American negroes form a special group. DW2 is uncommon in the American negro population as a whole but is found frequently in American negroes with MS [8]. These data go some way towards explaining the varying susceptibilities of different racial groups to MS and the fact that persons of non-susceptible races seldom develop MS even if they live in high risk areas.

While there is reason to believe that an Ir gene is relevant to MS, the search for an antigen has thus far proved fruitless. The

[1] Original investigations reported here were supported by Grant NS 13526 from the National Institute of Health, Bethesda, Maryland and Grant RG 1130-A from the National Multiple Sclerosis Society.

basic protein (BP) of central nervous system myelin has been established as the antigen for experimental allergic encephalomyelitis (EAE) and it was logical to seek evidence for sensitivity to BP in MS patients on the grounds that EAE in animals provided a reasonable experimental model for MS in man. The question of sensitivity to BP in MS patients cannot be considered as resolved but it is, in my opinion, fair to state that consistent sensitivity to BP cannot be demonstrated in MS in the hands of the majority of workers in the field.

There is no agreement as to which white matter structure is first affected in MS. An autoallergic attack directed against some surface component of myelin distinct from basic protein or against a surface structure of the oligodendrocyte could account for the lesions observed. In this regard, *Abramsky et al.* [1] have reported that MS sera do contain anti-oligodendrocyte antibodies but to date rigorous specificity controls for this provocative observation are lacking. Alternatively, a viral infection of oligodendrocytes, perhaps with expression of a virus-coded antigen on the cell surface, could be responsible for MS. All attempts to visualize a virus in MS lesions or to recover virus from MS tissue by fusion or co-cultivation methods have failed to date, but of course viral genome could be incorporated into that of the host in which circumstance it might only be revealed by hybridization techniques.

In mice, the DA strain of polio virus can induce a late onset inflammatory demyelinating disease which shares many morphologic features with MS itself [11, 13]. Polio virus cannot be visualized in the demyelinating lesions and virus can only be recovered with difficulty from them. The mouse polio model for demyelinating disease points up the need for continuing search for an infectious cause for MS.

As is well known, CSF-IgG is increased in MS in the majority of cases, particularly if they are of long standing. Oligoclonal IgG bands are frequently encountered and would seem to indicate ongoing synthesis of antibody directed against a single or at most a few antigens. All attempts to absorb out the oligoclonal bands with viruses, viral antigens or brain components have proven unsuccessful to date. The nature of the antigen which drives oligoclonal responses in MS remains totally unknown. Perhaps the time has come to question whether these immune responses are in fact antigen driven. Clones of B cells passively carried into the CNS during attacks of disease might be freed from normal surveillance mechanisms and capable of expansion even in the absence of antigen drive. If this were the case, oligoclonal bands akin to those found in CSF in MS might be expected to be present in other chronic inflammatory diseases of the CNS, as for example in neurosyphilis, a possibility which, insofar as I am aware, has never been systematically explored.

Any theory of MS must account for the exacerbations and remissions which characterize the disease. Recently, we have studied non-specific T on T suppressor cell (S cell) influence in multiple sclerosis. Con A-pre-activated, mitomycin-blocked lymphocytes are capable of suppressing the response of fresh autologous lymphocytes to Con A. This suppressor T cell response is remarkably deficient during attacks of MS but rises to high normal levels coincident with or just before remission [4, 6]. Between attacks of disease, S cell activity is normal in MS.

Patients beyond the age of 50 seldom have frank flareups of disease. In this age group, the illness is characterized by slow but inexorable progression. Beyond the age of 50, suppressor effect on autologous lymphocytes is increased over that observed in younger adults [3] and MS patients beyond age 50 show normal S cell response for age. Perhaps the 'high-set' of S cell activity in this age group blunts the opportunity for breakdown of suppressor influence. If a loss of suppression, for whatever reason, permits flareups of MS to occur, the high-set of S cell activity in this age group could make sufficient loss of suppressor influence to permit a frank attack of MS difficult to achieve.

S cell activity is believed to be mediated in large part by soluble factors released by the S cells themselves. Supernatants from S cell cultures can block proliferation of target cell lines (e.g. Chang liver cells) and the degree of block can be used as an assay for the quantity of suppressor factor released. Cultured lymphocytes from young MS patients with inactive disease release less soluble suppressor factor than do cultured lymphocytes from young controls; when disease is active, the amount of suppressor factor released rises. No clear correlation exists between the S cell effect on autologous lymphocytes and the S cell supernatant effect on target cells. The data suggest that responder cells of MS patients may vary, at different times, in their susceptibility to suppressive influence. Comparable considerations would seem to apply to the normal population in old age. Soluble suppressor factor release is low in the elderly even though the effect of S cells on autologous lymphocytes is high. We have interpreted the data as seeming to indicate that the elderly are particularly sensitive to suppressive influence whether they have MS or not.

The response of peripheral blood lymphocytes to T cell mitogens is subnormal in MS. The defect is most readily brought out when low doses of Con A are used for stimulation. Response to low dose Con A requires monocyte-T cell cooperation, but when high doses of Con A are employed purified T cells will respond to Con A. Response of purified T cells to high dose Con A is normal in MS [7]. The data would seem to point to a defect in monocytes in MS or more probably to a

defect in a T cell subset which requires monocytes in order to respond to Con A. Interestingly, defective mitogen responsiveness in MS is most readily detected when disease is inactive; during flareups, the response rises to normal control values [4, 7]. Thus, the immune status of MS patients may not be normal even at times when disease seems quiescent. It can be argued, of course, that disease is only seemingly quiescent and there is also some scant evidence to indicate that mitogen responsiveness may be tied to histocompatibility type which, as discussed, is different in the MS population than in the population at large.

Other evidence pointing to T cell subset abnormalities in MS has been brought forward. Avid T cells are decreased in this disease [15, 18] and a subset of T cells capable of binding to B-lymphoblastoid cells (the subset may include suppressor T cells) has been reported as decreased [9]. In contrast, the T_G subset has been reported as increased in MS [16]. Included within the T_G subset are suppressor cells and the effectors of antibody-dependent and spontaneous cytotoxicity.

Levy et al. [12] have reported that lymphocytes from MS patients show an increased binding affinity to measles virus-infected human epithelial cells. The effect may be measles-related or perhaps simply a reflection of the surface properties of lymphocytes, or a lymphocyte subset, in this disease. Since total T cell numbers are normal or only marginally decreased in MS, it is perhaps not totally surprising that if one T cell subset is underrepresented a second should be overrepresented. The relationship of the different T cell subsets just mentioned to each other requires clarification. In addition, study of helper T cell function in MS would be of substantial interest.

T cells increase in CSF during attacks of MS [2]. B cell numbers in CSF and the level of IgG in CSF do not appear to change. While activated T cells are increased during attacks, activated T cells can still be demonstrated in CSF at times when disease appears clinically inactive [14]. It may well be that disease activity smolders subclinically in the vast majority of patients in seeming remission.

Recently, circulating immune complexes have been reported to be present in a substantial proportion of MS patients, albeit in very low titer [10, 17]. In our experience, such complexes are more commonly found when disease is active and suppressor cell activity is low. The significance of this observation is unclear at present.

The evidence presented above points to tantalizing abnormalities in immune regulation in MS. Unfortunately, the basic cause of the disease, despite a substantial amount of new information obtained in recent years, has remained totally elusive.

References

1 Abramsky, O.; Lisak, R.; Silberberg, D. H., and Pleasure, D.: Antibodies to oligodendroglia in multiple sclerosis (abstr.). Annls Neurol. 1: 496 (1977).

2 Allen, J. C.; Sheremata, W.; Cosgrove, J. B. R.; Osterland K., and Shea, M.: Cerebrospinal fluid T and B lymphocyte kinetics related to exacerbations of multiple sclerosis. Neurology, Minneap. 26: 579–583 (1976).

3 Antel, J. P.; Weinrich, M., and Arnason, B. G. W.: Circulating suppressor cell activity in man as a function of age. Clin. Immunol. Immunopath. 9: 134–141 (1978).

4 Antel, J. P.; Weinrich M., and Arnason, B. G. W.: Mitogen responsiveness and suppressor cell function in multiple sclerosis: influence of age and clinical disease activity. Neurology, Minneap. 28: 993–1003 (1978).

5 Antel, J. P. and Arnason, B. G. W.: Correlation of suppressor cell function with disease activity in multiple sclerosis (abstr.). Neurology, Minneap. 28: 394 (1978).

6 Arnason, B. G. W. and Antel, J. P.: Suppressor cell function in multiple sclerosis. Annls Immunol. 129C: 159–170 (1978).

7 Dropcho, E. J.; Richman, D. P.; Antel, J. P., and Arnason, B. G. W.: Mitogenic response of T cells in normals, in multiple sclerosis and myasthenia gravis (abstr.). Fed. Proc. Fed. Am. Socs exp. Biol. 37: 1764 (1978).

8 Dupont, B.; Lisak, R. P.; Jersild C.; Hansen, J. A.; Silberberg, D. H.; Whitsett, C.; Zweiman, B., and Ciongoli, K.: HLA antigens in black american patients with multiple sclerosis. Transplantn Proc. 9: suppl. 11, pp. 181–185 (1977).

9 Goust, J. M.; Carnes, J. E.; Chenais, F.; Haimes, G. G.; Fudenberg, H. H., and Hogan, E. L.: Abnormal T-cell subpopulations and circulating immune complexes in the Guillain-Barré syndrome and multiple sclerosis. Neurology, Minneap. 28: 421–425 (1978).

10 Jacque C.; Davous P., and Baumann, N.: Circulating immune complexes and multiple sclerosis. Lancet ii: 408 (1977).

11 Lehrich, J. R.; Arnason, B. G. W., and Hochberg, F. G.: Demyelinative myelopathy in mice induced by the DA virus. J. neurol. Sci. 29: 149–160 (1976).

12 Levy, N.; Auerbach, P. S., and Hayes, E. C.: A blood test for multiple sclerosis based on the adherence of lymphocytes to measles infected cells. New Engl. J. Med. 294: 1423–1427 (1976).

13 Lipton, H. L.: Theiler's virus infection in mice—an unusual biphasic disease process leading to demyelination. Infec. Immunity 11: 1147–1155 (1975).

14 Noronha, A. B.; Richman, D. P.; Atchley, C. E., and Arnason, B. G. W.: Detection of in vivo stimulated cerebrospinal fluid lymphocytes in multiple sclerosis by flow cytofluorometry. Annls Neurol. (in press).

15 Oger, J. F.; Arnason, B. G. W., and Wray, S. H.: A study of B and T cells in multiple sclerosis. Neurology, Minneap. 25: 444–447 (1975).

16 Santoli, D.; Moretta, L.; Lisak, R.; Gilden, D., and Koprowski, H.: Imbalances in T cell subpopulations in multiple sclerosis patients. J. Immunol. 120: 1369–1371 (1978).

17 Tachovsky, T. G.; Lisak, R. P.; Koprowski, H.; Theofilopoulos, A. N., and Dixon, F. J.: Circulating immune complexes in multiple sclerosis and other neurological diseases. Lancet ii: 997–999 (1976).

18 Utermohlen, V.; Farmer, J.; Kornbluth, J., and Kornstein, M.: The relationship between direct migration inhibition with measles antigen and E-rosettes in normals and patients with multiple sclerosis. Clin. Immunol. Immunopath. 9: 63–66 (1978).

Dr. B. G. W. Arnason, Department of Neurology, University of Chicago, Chicago, IL 60637 (USA)

Immunopathology. 6th Int. Convoc. Immunol., Niagara Falls, N.Y., 1978, pp. 74–77 (Karger, Basel 1979)

Immunological Disorders of the Eye

A. H. S. Rahi

Department of Pathology, Institute of Ophthalmology, London

The ocular tissues behave as an immunological microcosm which can initiate and sustain allergic insult, not only by participating in systemic hypersensitivity reactions but also in mounting immune responses to antigens peculiar to the eye. There are a number of unique anatomical, physiological and biochemical features of the eye which impart to it a distinctive character which tends to modify and modulate the ocular immune responses [5]. It is important, therefore, to consider these factors before attempting to understand the nature of the immunological disorders of the eye.

Factors Modifying Ocular Immune Reactions

The lens and the cornea are devoid of any blood vessels. There is no lymphatic drainage to the intraocular structures and the eye like the brain has evolved to develop a strong blood-tissue barrier for high molecular weight proteins, which is exerted by the tight junction at the level of the retinal capillaries, the pigment epithelium of the retina, and the ciliary epithelium. These anatomico-physiological characteristics lead to a state of immunological isolation which at times the eye enjoys but on occasions seems to suffer from,

depending upon whether or not the products of the immune responses are harmful or beneficial to the ocular structures.

Furthermore, any antigen released into the eye locally, in the absence of a lymphatic drainage, may gain access to the systemic circulation and lead to a generalized immune response. Alternatively, there may develop a state of immunological tolerance. It is of interest that the spleen plays a vital role in both these effects, since it can provide not only B lymphocytes with plasma cell potential, but also suppressor T cells which are known to inhibit immunological responses and are believed to be involved in the development of immune tolerance.

The ocular tissues, especially the vitreous and the cornea, are rich in polyanions, which along with an active blood-ocular barrier can impart an immunoadsorbent property to the eye. The antigens thus retained may be slowly released to produce an enhanced and prolonged immune reaction leading to a chronic eye disease. Furthermore, the uveal vessels, either by chance or by design, may trap circulating antigen-antibody aggregates and thus may act as a repository for immune complexes of endogenous or exogenous origin.

There is evidence that several ocular tissues, especially the lens, the retina and the cornea, contain organ-specific antigens which may participate in eye diseases initiated by some physical, chemical or microbial insult. Autoimmunity in this situation may maintain if not initiate an intraocular inflammation.

Since there are no regional lymph nodes which drain intraocular structures, the antigen-sensitive cells may migrate into the eye to produce antibody locally and thus in this way the uvea may act as an accessory lymph node. Lymphocytic infiltration of the uvea may therefore signify a physiological rather than a pathological response. It should be realized, however, that the ocular structures are richly innervated by autonomic nerves and therefore show an abnormal vasomotor sensitivity. It is not surprising, therefore, that mild immunological adventures which may be ignored in other parts of the body are given cognizance in the eye.

Allergic Diseases of the Eye

The immunological disorders of the eye can be divided into six distinct categories, each consisting of a group of diseases having similar pathogenetic mechanisms (table I).

The space allotted to me does not permit description of every condition listed in table I and therefore I will briefly describe one disease from each category; it is hoped that this will not only stimulate further reading but also create interest for further research in this relatively underinvestigated field of ocular immunology.

IgE-Mediated Disease. The conjunctiva like the skin is richly supplied with mast cells. It is not surprising therefore that a large group of conjunctival diseases are manifestations of IgE-mediated allergy to a variety of airborne exogenous allergens. Vernal catarrh is of wide geographical distribution. Typically, the conjunctiva lining the upper lid becomes hyperaemic and hyperplastic and forms a mosaic of flat papillae. The stroma is infiltrated by eosinophils, lymphocytes and plasma cells; sometimes, basophils and mast cells are also prominent. A significant proportion of patients with this condition show high levels of IgE in the blood and also in the tears [unpublished personal observations] which may also contain increased amounts of IgG, IgM and IgA [2]. Although the majority of the patients respond to local treatment with disodium cromoglycate, a pro-

Table I. Some examples of possible immune disorders of the eye

1. *IgE-mediated reactions*	4. *Cell-mediated hypersensitivity*
Hay fever conjunctivitis	Herpetic keratitis
Atopic conjunctivitis	Sympathetic ophthalmitis
Vernal catarrh	Optic neuritis
Drug allergy	Corneal graft rejection
2. *Ig and complement-dependent cytotoxicity*	Certain microbial infections of the eye
Mooren's ulcer	Drug allergy
Ocular pemphigus and pemphigoid	5. *Stimulatory hypersensitivity*
Experimental immune retinitis	Endocrine exophthalmos
Corneal graft rejection	6. *Neutralization or inactivation reaction*
3. *Toxic immune-complex reactions*	Myasthenia gravis
Corneal immune rings	
Erythema multiforme	
Endogenous uveitis	
Phaco-allergic endophthalmitis	
Scleritis and episcleritis	

portion remain unresponsive and it is possible that in these patients the pathogenetic mechanism is either an immune complex-mediated reaction or a delayed tissue allergy. It is of interest that eosinophils are also prominent in the retest reaction, and basophils are the main constituent of cutaneous basophil hypersensitivity (CBH), both of which are variants of type IV allergy.

Antibody and Complement-Mediated Disease. As with the other organs of the body, it is often difficult to assign a particular eye disease as being specifically due to type II allergy, because in tissue destruction more than one immune mechanism plays a conjoint phlogistic role.

The degeneration of the pigment epithelium of the retina and the photoreceptors is the hallmark of retinitis pigmentosa. The aetiology of this disease is obscure and for want of a better explanation an autoimmune hypothesis has been proposed. Although it seems unlikely that autoimmunity is the cause of retinitis pigmentosa, it is of interest that animals immunized experimentally with retinal extracts show impaired activity of the retina both *in vivo* and *in vitro*. Histological examination of the eyes from immunized animals shows evidence of lymphocytic infiltration of the choroid and degeneration of the photoreceptors [7, 11]. Apart from antibody response there is also evidence of a T cell response to immunization with photoreceptor cells [3, 9]. In a recent immunofluorescent study, it was possible to show the presence of antiphotoreceptor cell antibodies in the blood from patients with retinitis pigmentosa [10]; it was, however, difficult to exclude the possibility of a heterophile antibody reactive against some antigen in the visual cells which are also found in a variety of tissues in several species.

Immune Complex Disease. The number of occasions when a specific aetiology of endogenous uveitis can be demonstrated or reasonably assumed is rarely more than 50%. Intravenous injection of large doses of horse serum in rabbits leads to the formation of circulating antigen-antibody aggregates which may be deposited in susceptible vascular beds to produce immune complex uveitis in conjunction with lesions in the renal glomeruli. It is therefore generally believed that uveitis in man is also an immune complex disease. In a recent study, it was possible to demonstrate, by ^{125}IC1q binding assay, the presence of immune complexes in the blood of about 11% of patients with uveitis [6]. The failure to demonstrate immune complexes in the remainder does not exclude this aetiology since these aggregates may be formed intermittently in very small amounts and sometimes even locally thus producing uveitis without ever reaching the circulation.

Cell-Mediated Allergy. A large number of eye diseases are believed to develop following a delayed hypersensitivity reaction to a variety of exogenous and endogenous antigens. Sympathetic ophthalmitis is often considered as the prototype. It is a rare bilateral granulomatous uveitis which follows perforation of the globe. It is believed that the uveal inflammation is initiated by an occult virus infection and perpetuated by an autoimmune reaction involving antigens native to the uvea and the retina [8].

It is of interest that photoreceptors which contain strong soluble antigens [4] have now been shown to induce granulomatous uveitis in rabbits which simulates very closely the histological appearance of sympathetic ophthalmitis in man [12].

Stimulatory Hypersensitivity. About 50% of thyrotoxic individuals at some stage of the disease develop signs of ocular involvement in the form of exophthalmos which is usually progressive and bilateral. The anatomical basis for this is principally an increase in orbital fat and mucopolysaccharides, and lymphocytic infiltration and oedema of the orbital muscles and of the surrounding tissues.

Blood from these patients is often found to contain two types of non-complement fixing antibody which exert a stimulatory effect on the thyroid. Long-acting thyroid stimulator (LATS) belongs to the IgG class of immunoglobulin and is present in the serum of up to 40% of patients with thyrotoxicosis and is believed to have a stimulatory effect on orbital fat. Human-specific thyroid stimulator (HTS) known in the past as LATS protector is the second antibody and seems to correlate more closely with the hyperthyroid state and exophthalmos than does LATS. The exophthalmos-producing substance (EPS) is a fragment of thyroid-stimulating hormone which appears to bind to orbital tissues through an IgG autoantibody possibly identical to HTS, and to stimulate the orbital contents which become oedematous and accumulate fat and mucopolysaccharides.

Neutralization and Inactivation Reactions. Myasthenia gravis is a form of immunological disorder in which the characteristic feature is weakness and readily provoked fatigue of voluntary muscles which is believed to be produced at least in part by the blocking of the acetylcholine receptors on the motor endplate by an autoantibody which is demonstrable by ^{125}I-α-bungarotoxin binding assay in about 90% of the patients [1]. Ocular symptoms are almost invariable in this disease and may take the form of external ophthalmoplegia, paresis of accommodation, inadequate convergence and diplopia. Occasionally, the disturbance may be limited to a degree of ptosis.

References

1 Lindstrom, J.: An assay for antibodies to human acetylcholine receptors in serum from patients with myasthenia gravis. Clin. Immunol. Immunopath. 7: 36–43 (1977).

2 McClellan, B. H.; Whitney, C. R.; Newman, L. P., and Allansmith, M. R.: Immunoglobulins in tears. Am. J. Ophthal. 76: 89–101 (1973).

3 Meyers, R. L.: Experimental allergic uveitis. Mod. Probl. Ophthal., vol. 16, pp. 12–20 (Karger, Basel 1976).

4 Rahi, A. H. S.: Autoimmunity and the retina. Br. J. Ophthal. 54: 441–444 (1970).

5 Rahi, A. H. S. and Garner, A.: Immunopathology of the eye (Blackwell, London 1976).

6 Rahi, A. H. S.; Holborow, E. J.; Perkins, E. S., and Dinning, W. J.: What is endogenous uveitis? in Silverstein and O'Connor, Proc. 2nd Int. Symp. Immunopath. Eye, San Francisco (Masson, New York 1979).

7 Rahi, A. H. S.; Lucas, D. R., and Waghe, M.: Experimental immune retinitis. Mod. Probl. Ophthal., vol. 16, pp. 41–50 (Karger, Basel 1976).

8 Rahi, A. H. S.; Morgan, G.; Levy, I., and Dinning, W. J.: Immunological investigations in post traumatic granulomatous and non-granulomatous uveitis. Br. J. Ophthal. 62: 722–731 (1978).

9 Rahi, A. H. S.; Otiko, G., and Winder, A. F.: Evaluation of macrophage electrophoretic mobility test as an indicator of cellular immunity in ocular tumours. Br. J. Ophthal. 60: 589–593 (1976).

10 Spalton, D. J.; Rahi, A. H. S., and Bird, A. C.: Immunological studies in retinitis pigmentosa associated with retinal vascular leakage. Br. J. Ophthal. 62: 183–187 (1978).

11 Wacker, W. B. and Kalsow, C. M.: The role of uveal and retinal antigens in experimental autoimmune ocular pathology. Mod. Probl. Ophthal., vol. 16, pp. 12–20 (Karger, Basel 1976).

12 Wacker, W. B.; Rao, N. A., and Marak, G. E.: Experimental sympathetic ophthalmia; in Silverstein and O'Connor, Proc. 2nd Int. Symp. Immunopath. Eye, San Francisco (Masson, New York 1979).

Dr. A. H. S. Rahi, Department of Pathology, Institute of Ophthalmology, Judd Street, London WC1 H9QS (England)

Immunopathology. 6th Int. Convoc. Immunol., Niagara Falls, N.Y., 1978, pp. 78–84 (Karger, Basel 1979)

Immune Response to Spermatozoa

J. A. Andrada, E. Comini and O. Vilar

Instituto de Investigaciones Médicas, University of Buenos Aires, Buenos Aires

Definitive demonstration of antigenic properties of spermatozoa or of whole semen in heterologous sensitization was first presented by *Metchnikoff* [17] in 1900. In an attempt to establish methods of contraception, efforts were made to produce damage to the seminiferous epithelium in the male or to inhibit fertility in the female by eliciting formation of sperm antibodies. In the last 20 years, it was shown that testis, sperm, seminal plasma and the accessory glands possess antigenic capacity to induce formation of antibodies which can render the male organism temporarily or permanently sterile.

Experimental Allergic Orchitis

A selective destruction of germinal epithelium was obtained in guinea pigs by autologous or homologous sensitization with one injection of homogenate prepared from testis, semen, or spermatozoa emulsified in complete Freund's adjuvant (CFA) [26]. The appearance of specific humoral and cellular immunity accompanied the histologic lesions in the testis. A similar immune response to antigens of the testis, but of lower incidence and magnitude could be elicited by repeated injections of testis homogenate without adjuvant for several months [9]. Although testicular tissue cross-reacts with brain tissue, the allergic orchitis has a high degree of organ and species specificity. It was suggested that prepuberal testis does not contain the antigen responsible for aspermatogenesis [10].

Guinea pigs are apparently the most susceptible laboratory animal for induction of allergic orchitis. Other species such as mice, rats and monkeys show similar responses. Six of 8 rhesus monkeys sensitized with testicular homogenates emulsified in CFA developed, after 6–8 weeks, patchy lesions in the testes characterized by congestion, edema and mild mononuclear infiltration of the intertubular spaces [2]. Changes in the germinal epithelium were pronounced; some tubules were atrophic and exhibited sloughing of the germinal cells and vacuolization of the cytoplasm of the Sertoli cells. These alterations were most pronounced between 10 and 13 weeks after the sensitizing injection. Four monkeys developed oligo- or azoospermia. Specific circulating antibodies were detected in two animals at very low titers; following castration, however, titers increased. Tissue specificity was detected by IF. Cross-reaction between interstitial cells of the testis and ovary on the one hand and zona fasciculata and reticularis of the adrenal gland on the other was also shown by IF. No cell-mediated immunity could be detected.

The production and pathway of steroid hormones were studied in these monkeys by *in vitro* incubation of the damaged tissue with labeled steroid precursors. The output of testosterone by the testicular tissue of the sensitized animals was somewhat decreased as compared with non-sensitized animals. The difference was not statistically significant and the result reflected the lack of damage of the Leydig cells. Partial recovery of spermatogenesis, after the last immunization, occurred in these animals in period ranging from 360 to 400 days [5].

In most experiments, adjuvant is needed in addition to sperm or testicular antigens to induce allergic orchitis. An experimental model that did not use adjuvants was reported, however, in guinea pigs [19] and monkeys [3]. Severe thermal damage to the testis may be followed by lesions similar to those obtained in allergic orchitis, in the contralateral gland. An immunological response of the delayed type, as shown by skin tests, has been obtained [11].

Histopathology. Slight vascular changes and mononuclear cell infiltration appear around the second week and may precede the germinal cell lesion. The cellular basis of the tubular lesion has been investigated. Sertoli cells cytoplasm shows numerous vacuoles giving the impression that many of them belong to germinal cells (spermatocytes, spermatids) liberated into the tubular lumen. Cellular debris or dead cells are phagocytized by Sertoli cells. This coincides with the appearance of abundant bodies showing acid phosphatase-positive reaction (lysosomes). When spermatogenesis develops during puberty, permeability barriers appear between the blood and the seminiferous epithelium. Not only capillary endothelium and basal membrane, lymphatic drainage, connective tissue and tubular wall, but also the occluding junction between adjacent Sertoli cells can act as a diffusion barrier for antibodies. Under ordinary circumstances, existing antibodies should not traverse this barrier. Therefore, response to sperm antibodies rarely occurs. Autoallergic orchitis is, consequently, the result of the failure of the blood-testis barrier either in the seminiferous tubules or in other parts of the germinal tract. This produces some leakage of immunoglobulins into the tubules. Sertoli cells may or may not be altered, but

they can act as a transporting 'bridge' between the intertubular spaces and the most advanced types of germinal cells.

Antigens. The site of localization of testicular antigens was assessed by immunohistochemical methods. Specific antitestis antibodies react with the acrosomes of spermatozoa and spermatids [14, 24], as seen in figure 1. The antigenic complexity of semen emphasized the importance of considering sperm and seminal plasma antigens separately. By using seminal or epididymal sperm for immunization, an allergic orchitis was obtained in various laboratory animals. Cross reactivity was observed between testis and epididymal or testicular spermatozoa. Spermatozoal antigens, like testicular antigens, have a polysaccharide or a glycoprotein structure and, when injected along with CFA, are capable of producing humoral and cellular immune response, along with testicular damage.

Antibodies and Cellular Immunity. Humoral and cell-mediated immune responses have been described in laboratory animals sensitized with testicular material and CFA. Humoral antibodies are of low titers and can be detected by most of the serological techniques as well as systemic and local anaphylaxoid procedures. Besides, the immune serum shows *in vitro* cytotoxic activity [25], immobilization [27] of spermatozoa and a lytic effect on the acrosome of the spermatid and the spermatozoa (fig. 2) [16, 24]. The titers are low and there is no strict correlation between them and the degree of histological damage. Cell-mediated immunity, which appears around the 6th day after immunization, may be revealed by the presence of a typical granuloma after intradermal injection of antigen alone (skin test). Cell-mediated immunity has been demonstrated by several *in vitro* and *in vivo* test. Circulating antibodies can be detected 3 days later but are not constantly present.

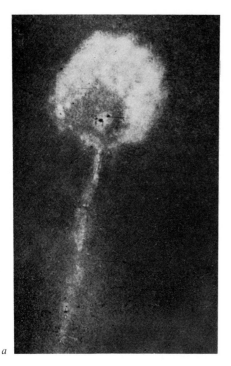

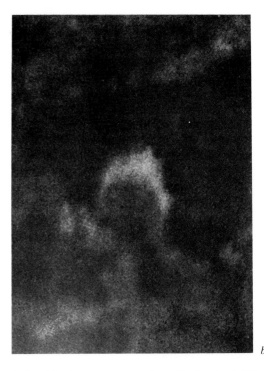

a

b

Fig. 1. Smears of a cell suspension of germinal cells from guinea pig showing immunofluoescent reaction of the acrosome of a spermatozoon (a) and a spermatid (b) induced by immune serum of sensitized animal. HE. × 1,000.

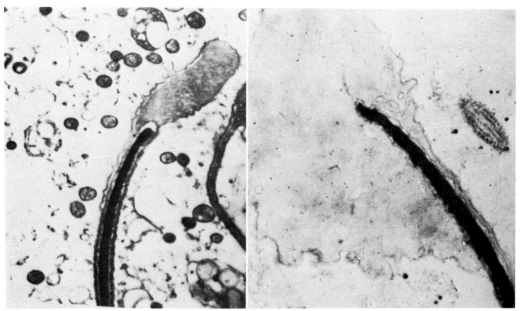

2a

Experimental Studies in Man

Testis. In an attempt to induce allergic orchitis in man, the antigenicity of human testis was studied during auto- and allo-sensitization. 29 volunteers with prostate carcinoma were selected according to age, previous treatment and findings in the testicular biopsies. The first group of patients was autosensitized or allosensitized with testicular homogenate in CFA. Other groups were sensitized with testicular homogenate with incomplete Freund's adjuvant or with CFA without testicular homogenate and served as controls. Humoral and cell-mediated immune responses were assayed, and testicular biopsies were performed during and at the end of the experiment, which was followed by therapeutic castration. Four patients of the experimental group exhibited low titer circulating antibodies and positive skin tests. Biopsies of the testis showed patchy lesions, with numerous foci of tubular damage with sloughing of germinal cells (fig. 3). Immunofluorescence, with each patient's own serum showed staining of the head of spermatozoa and perinuclear area of spermatids [15].

Semen and Adnexal Glands. Human spermatozoa obtained from a spermatocele lacked the antigens which characterize the seminal spermatozoa [29]. Experimental evidence indicated that, as in animals, a substantial part of the antigenic material is taken up during 'transit'. Histoimmunochemical studies demonstrated several antigens in the heads, the necks and the tails of human seminal spermatozoa, whereas only one antigen was demonstrable in testicular sperm cells. Antibodies against prostate and seminal plasma may be responsible for agglutination of seminal spermatozoa, and produce higher hemagglutination titers than antibodies against testis, epididymis, seminal vesicles or spermatozoa [7]. Therefore, we can assume that the testis contributes few sperm-specific antigens, as they are present in washed epididymal ans seminal spermatozoa, but not in seminal plasma, whereas the prostate and seminal vesicles supply the major part of secondary sperm antigens.

Clinical Findings. The existence of spermagglutinins in the serum or the sperm of patients with infertility of unknown etiology suggested an immunopathogenesis for this condition [22]. Spermagglutination techniques using the patients' own spermatozoa (or those from normal donors) were performed in various studies. The sera of approximately 3% of 2,015 infertile males gave positive agglutination tests, while all serum samples from 416 fertile subjects were negative [23]. From various studies in the literature, one [12] demonstrated that 7% of man in infertile matings had significant titers of spermagglutinins. The titers correlated with reduced cervical mucous-penetrating ability of the sperm. There is evidence that azoospermia is not due to the action of spermagglutinins since *per se* these antibodies are not capable of producing any damage in spermatogenesis. On the other hand, in our recent, as yet unpublished studies, there was a correlation between the presence of autoantibodies and obstruction of vasa deferentia.

Appearance of antibodies in patients who have undergone vasectomy for fertility control has received, in the last years, increasing attention. Sperm antibodies appear within 2 weeks of vasectomy in man [6] and rhesus

Fig. 2. a Guinea pig testis incubated with homologous normal serum and complement. No gross modifications are observable in the acrosome and nucleus. Fragments of Sertoli cell cytoplasm are seen. × 8,000 before reduction. *b* Guinea pig testis incubated with homologous antisperm serum and complement. Hypertrophy of the acrosome, numerous infoldings of the acrosomal membrane, and areas of low electron density adjacent to the inner acrosomal membrane. × 8,000 before reduction.

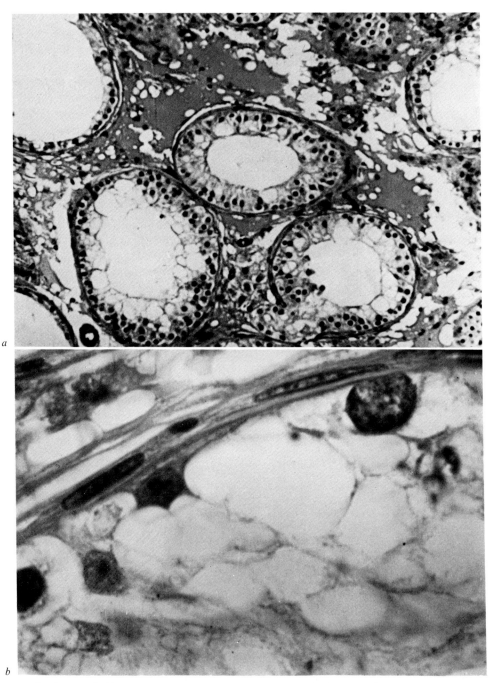

Fig. 3. a Testis biopsy of a patient 40 days after sensitization. Seminiferous tubules show variable degrees of sloughing of germinal cells. HE. × 130. *b* Same specimen at higher magnification (× 1,000). The cytoplasm of Sertoli cells is extremely vacuolated. Few spermatogonia are seen.

monkeys [1]. A more detailed experimental study showed that 6 months after vasectomy, half of the treated rabbits exhibited antisperm antibodies. Few of them, however, developed orchitis associated with deposits of sperm antigens, IgG and C3 in the basement membrane of seminiferous tubules, presumably in form of antigen-antibody complexes [8].

The antibodies in vasectomized patients produce agglutination and immobilization of human spermatozoa and give positive passive hemagglutination tests. Cell-mediated immunity to sperm, however, did not develop in man and guinea pigs even 1 year after vasectomy [18]. Scattered reports [20, 21] suggested a correlation between vasectomy and long-term systemic diseases as a result of cross-reactivity of testicular with non-genital antigens. Nevertheless, no clinical evidence of major disturbances or the appearance of any autoimmune disorders have been reported [13].

The testicular lesions of lepromatous leprosy may have an immunological basis, since there is evidence in this condition of production of antibodies and sensitized T lymphocytes leading to testicular damage. In leprosy, antibodies against germinal cells were found in 70% of patients [28]. Leprous orchitis may be a model for an organ-specific autoimmune disease in which an infection induces the autoimmune disorder. Another inflammatory condition of the testis appears in young males during mumps infection. Using four serological techniques and skin tests [4], we found that the histological damage of the tubules was more closely correlated with cellular medlated immunity than with circulating antibodies to spermatozoa.

Conclusions

From the experimental background and the clinical investigations, we can postulate that immunological factors may affect human fertility. Oligo- or azoospermia might reflect the immunological destruction of germinal cells or the halting of spermatogenesis, whereas immobilization and agglutination of seminal sperm probably predominantly depend on allergic reactions to antigens of the adnexal glands of the male tract.

References

1 Alexander, N. J.; Wilson, B. J., and Patterson, G. D.: Vasectomy: immunologic effects in rhesus monkeys and man. Fertil. Steril. 25: 149–156 (1974).
2 Andrada, J. A.; Andrada, E. C., and Witebsky, E.: Experimental allergic orchitis in rhesus monkeys. Proc. Soc. exp. Biol. Med. 130: 1106–1113 (1969).
3 Andrada, J. A.; Comini, E., and Hoschoian, J. C.: Effect of thermal injury on monkey testis. Endocrine and immune response. Medicina, Buenos Aires 37: 133–138 (1977).
4 Andrada, J. A.; Walde, F. van der; Hoschoian, J. C.; Comini, E., and Mancini, R. E.: Immunological studies in patients with mumps orchitis. Andrologia 9: 207–215 (1977).
5 Andrada, J. A.; Comini, E.; Hoschoian, J. C., and Walde, F. van der: Experimental autoimmune orchitis. Recovery of spermatogenesis. 4th Int. Symp. on Immunology of Reproduction, Varna 1978.
6 Ansbacher, R.: Vasectomy: sperm antibodies. Fertil. Steril. 24: 788–792 (1973).
7 Barnes, G. W.; Soanes, W. A.; Mamrod, L.; Gonder, M. J., and Shulman, S.: Immunologic properties of human prostatic fluid. J. Lab. clin. Med. 61: 578–591 (1963).
8 Bigazzi, P. E.; Kosuda, L. L.; Hsu, K. C., and Andres, G. A.: Immune complex orchitis in vasectomized rabbits. J. exp. Med. 143: 382–404 (1976).
9 Bishop, D. W.: Aspermatogenesis induced by testicular antigen uncombined with adjuvants. Proc. Soc. exp. Biol. Med. 107: 116–120 (1961).
10 Bishop, D. W.; Narbaitz, R., and Lessof, M.: Induced aspermatogenesis in adult guinea-pigs injected with testicular antigen and adjuvant in neonatal stages. Devl. Biol. 3: 444–485 (1961).
11 Fernandez Collazo, E.; Thierer, E., and Mancini, R. E.: Immunological and testicular response in guinea-pig after unilateral thermal orchitis. J. Allergy clin. Immunol. 49: 167–173 (1972).
12 Fjalbrandt, B.: Sperm antibodies and sterility in men. Acta obstet. gynec. scand. 47: suppl. 4, pp. 1–37 (1968).
13 Houk, J. L.; Herman, J. H.; Smiddy, B. A.; Troiano, P., and Hess, E. V.: Immunological consequences of human vasectomy. Workshop on Immunology in Human Reproduction. Newcastle 1977.
14 Mancini, R. E.; Davidson, O. W.; Vilar, O.; Nemirovsky, M., and Bueno, M. P.: Acrosomal antigenicity in rat testis. Fertil. Steril. 15: 695–700 (1964).
15 Mancini, R. E.; Andrada, J. A.; Saraceni, A.; Bachmann, A. E.; Lavieri, J. C., and Nemirovsky, M.: Immunological and testicular response in man

sensitized with human testicular homogenate. J. clin. Endocr. Metab. *25:* 859–875 (1965).

16 Mancini, R. E.; Monastirsky, R.; Fernandez Collazo, E.; Seiguer, A. C., and Alonso, A.: Cytotoxic effect of antispermatic antibodies on guinea-pig germinal cells *in vitro*. Fertil. Steril. *20:* 779–798 (1969).

17 Metchnikoff, E.: Sur la spermatotoxine et l'antispermatotoxine. Annls Inst. Pasteur, Paris *14:* 1–5 (1900).

18 Muir, V. Y.; Turk, J. L., and Hanley, H. G.: Comparison of allergic aspermatogenesis with that induced by vasectomy. Clin. exp. Immunol. *28:* 461–466 (1977).

19 Rapaport, F. T.; Sampath, A.; Kano, K.; McCluskey, R. T., and Milgrom, F.: Immunological effects of thermal injury. I. Inhibition of spermatogenesis in guinea-pigs. J. exp. Med. *130:* 1411–1425 (1969).

20 Roberts, H. J.: Delayed thrombophlebitis and systemic complications after vasectomy: possible role of diabetogenic hyperinsulinism. J. Am. Geriat. Soc. *16:* 267–272 (1968).

21 Roberts, H. J.: Letters to the editor. Perspect. Biol. Med. *14:* 176–178 (1970).

22 Rümke, P.: The presence of sperm antibodies in the serum of two patients with oligospermia. Vox Sang. *4:* 135–140 (1954).

23 Rümke, P. and Hellinga, G.: Autoantibodies against spermatozoa in sterile men. Am. J. clin. Path. *32:* 357–361 (1969).

24 Spooner, R. L.: Cytolytic activity of the serum of normal male guinea pigs against their own testicular cells. Nature, Lond. *202:* 915–919 (1964).

25 Toulett, F. and Voisin, G. A.: Spermatotoxic, spermagglutinating and cytotoxic activities of guinea pig autoantibodies to sperm auto-antigen. J. Reprod. Fert. *37:* 299–313 (1974).

26 Voisin, G. A.; Delaunay, A. et Barber, M.: Sur les lesions testiculaires provoquées chez les cobayes par iso et autosensibilisation. Annls Inst. Pasteur, Paris *81:* 48–63 (1961).

27 Voisin, G. A.; Toulett, F., and Maurer, P.: The nature of tissular antigens with particular reference to autosensitization and transplantation immunity. Ann. N.Y. Acad. Sci. *73:* 726–744 (1958).

28 Wall, J. R. and Wright, D. J. M.: Antibodies against testicular germinal cells in lepromatous leprosy. J. clin. Immunol. *17:* 51–59 (1974).

29 Weil, A. J. and Rodenburg, J. M.: Immunological differentiation of human testicular (spermatocele) and seminal spermatozoa. Proc. Soc. exp. Biol. Med. *105:* 43–45 (1960).

Dr. J. A. Andrada, Instituto de Investigaciones Médicas, University of Buenos Aires, Donato Alvarez 3000, Buenos Aires (Argentina)

Immunopathology. 6th Int. Convoc. Immunol., Niagara Falls, N.Y., 1978, pp. 85–90 (Karger, Basel 1979)

Immunological Aspects of Diabetes mellitus[1]

W. James Irvine

Endocrine Unit/Immunology Laboratories and University Department of Medicine, Royal Infirmary, Edinburgh

Clinical observation established that ketosis-prone, insulin-dependent diabetes, but not diabetes that can be controlled by diet or oral hypoglycaemic agents, is associated with the organ-specific group of autoimmune disorders [11]. There is a markedly increased prevalence of thyroid cytoplasmic and of gastric parietal cell cytoplasmic antibodies especially in young female diabetics compared to age- and sex-matched controls, even when all patients are excluded who had any clinical features or past history of thyroid disease, atrophic gastritis or anaemia. When insulin-dependent diabetics were compared with those who were non-insulin-dependent, it was found that the increased prevalence of these cytoplasmic antibodies (which was highly significant statistically) was solely confined to the insulin-dependent group [20].

Cell-Mediated Immunity to Islet Cell Antigens

Evidence for cell-mediated immunity to porcine, bovine [32] and to human [30] pancreatic antigen was obtained by the migration inhibition test using leucocytes from the peripheral blood of diabetics, although there is some uncertainty as to how specific this test is for type IV immune reactions [14].

Statistically significant positive findings were again confined to insulin-dependent diabetics. That the pancreatic antigen in question was in the islets was shown by using an antigen of very high islet-cell content derived from calf pancreas in which atrophy of the exocrine tissue had been induced by surgical ligation of the pancreatic duct 8 weeks before the organ was removed [32], and by using appropriate fresh human insulinoma tissue [17].

The findings reported with insulinoma cells that had been in culture for many years [10] and which were probably no longer secreting insulin must be viewed with circumspection.

Islet Cell Antibodies (ICAb) in Diabetics

It was in the sera of patients with insulin-dependent diabetes plus autoimmune polyendocrine disease that ICAb was first independently described in late 1974 by the Middlesex [4] and Edinburgh [29] groups, using the indirect immunofluorescence technique and unfixed cryostat sections of fresh group 0 human pancreas. The antibody or antibodies react with the cytoplasm of all the cells of the pancreatic islets. Rarely, a serum may only react with A cells or D cells, but this does not seem to be characteristic of diabetes in any of its forms [3, 12].

[1] This work is supported by grants from the British Diabetic Association, the British Medical Research Council, and the American Juvenile Diabetes Federation.

ICAb occurs in about 60–70% of newly diagnosed Caucasian insulin-dependent (ketosis prone) diabetics [25, 28], irrespective of age [25]. Some diabetics only have ICAb detectable in the serum for a few weeks or less (ICAb transients) while others retain ICAb in the serum for many years (ICAb persisters) [25]. The short duration of ICAb in most insulin-dependent diabetics is in contrast to the long duration of other organ-specific antibodies such as gastric parietal cell, thyroid and adrenocortical antibodies that characterise pernicious anaemia, primary atrophic hypothyroidism and idiopathic (autoimmune) Addison's disease, respectively [15].

In contrast to insulin-dependent (ketosis prone) diabetes, the prevalence of ICAb in what used to be referred to as 'maturity onset' diabetics (who are insulin-independent and can be controlled by diet or by oral hypoglycaemic agents) is very much less. In those controlled by diet alone, the prevalence is very similar to that in a control Caucasian population at about 0.5%. However, a significant minority of diabetics controlled on OHA have ICAb in the serum [25]. Such patients have a very high tendency towards becoming insulin-dependent in subsequent years, indicating that they are at an earlier stage of the same disease process that culminates in insulin-dependent ketosis prone (type I) diabetes [18].

ICAb as a Marker for Potential Diabetes. Some 6% of patients with organ-specific, autoimmune disease, some 3% of first degree relatives (without clinical diabetes) of ICAb-positive diabetics and 0.5% of the normal Caucasian population have ICAb in the serum [25]. A substantial number of these subjects go on to develop diabetes, sometimes acutely as ketosis-prone, insulin-dependent diabetes but sometimes only reaching this stage by going more slowly through milder stages of what would appear to be the same disease process that culminates in insulin-dependent diabetes [16]. These findings therefore point to the value of ICAb as a marker for type I diabetes, especially in its less severe forms, and suggest that not all diabetics controlled by diet or oral hypoglycaemic agents have the 'maturity onset' type of the disease (type II). At the present time, ICAb is the only *in vitro* marker for potential type I diabetes.

Other Autoantibodies

Antibodies in the sera of type I diabetics reactive with the cell surface of rat islet cells in culture have been described using the indirect immunofluorescence technique [27].

It is not yet clear whether these antibodies are the same as ICAb. Their lower prevalence in type I diabetes compared to ICAb could be due to the relatively poor antigenicity of rat compared to human islet cells. Autoantibodies to insulin receptors have been described in the rare clinical situation of insulin resistance associated with acanthosis nigricans, but they are not characteristic of the common type I or type II diabetes [8].

Classification of Diabetes

It would now appear to be established that the syndrome referred to as primary diabetes consists of two principal and distinct diseases which may be referred to as type I and type II [13]. In addition, there is a multiplicity of rare disease processes that also may produce primary diabetes [35]. The separation of primary diabetes into two main distinct types is also supported by the HLA studies described below.

Type I diabetes is characterised by the state of insulin dependency. Although this condition most commonly develops in young people, it is by no means confined to them, so that the term 'juvenile-onset' diabetes is no longer appropriate. Likewise, type II diabetes, while occurring predominantly in older persons, is not confined to them. As mentioned above, it is important to realise that a significant minority of diabetics controlled by diet or especially by oral hypoglycaemic agents belong not to type II but to type I, and that such patients are indicated by the presence of ICAb in the serum. Therefore, patients on oral hypoglycaemic agents should only be called type II diabetics if their serum is negative for ICAb at the time of diagnosis. Type II diabetics may be obese or non-obese, and may be treated by their physicians with insulin without them being insulin-dependent. They are not prone to ketosis.

Genetics of Diabetes

The use of the age at onset of diabetes as a basis for classifying primary diabetes into two main types ('juvenile onset' and 'maturity onset') lead to much confusion in the analysis of its familial and therefore of its genetic aspects [36]. However, when the criterion of insulin dependency compared to non-insulin dependency was used and the age at onset of diabetes ignored in relation to classification, results were obtained that strongly suggest that the two main types of primary diabetes as so defined breed true [22].

HLA. The three series of HLA alleles which appear to be in linkage disequilibrium with three immune response (Ir) genes and which are associated with type I diabetes in Caucasians are shown in figure 1. It is probable that the Ir genes are located near to the D locus or to the DR locus [31]. The series A1, B8, DW3 and DRW3 and the series A2, CW3, B15, DW4 and DRW4 have a positive and additive risk factor for type I diabetes, while the series A3, B7, DW2 and DRW2 has a protective effect associated with a resistance to type I diabetes [6, 34]. Type II diabetes is not associated with any known HLA type.

The series which includes B8 is associated with persistence of ICAb and with the occurrence of other clinical autoimmune disorders (fig. 2). In turn, the persistence of ICAb (even in the absence of other clinical immunological disorders) is associated with an increased prevalence of thyroid and of gastric autoantibodies (fig. 3), indicating that persistence of ICAb is associated with an increased diathesis towards organ-specific autoimmunity in general [24].

The series which includes B15 is associated with an

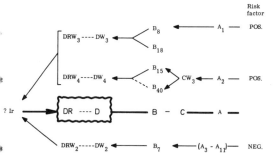

Fig. 1. The three series of HLA antigens, each probably in linkage disequilibrium with an immune response (Ir) gene associated with type I diabetes; two with a positive and one with a negative risk factor. From *Irvine* [14], by kind permission of the editor of Medical Immunology (Teviot Scientific Publications).

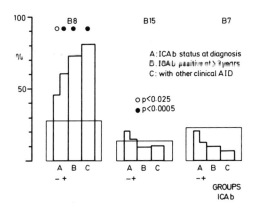

Fig. 2. The positive association of the autoimmune aspects of type I diabetes with HLA-B8 and the lack of it with B15 and with B7. From *Irvine et al.* [24], by kind permission of the editor of J. Clin. Lab. Immunol.

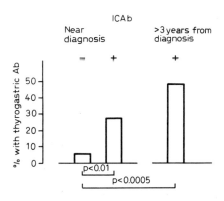

Fig. 3. The increased prevalence of thyroid and of gastric antibodies in type I diabetics with persistence of ICAb. From *Irvine et al.* [24], by kind permission of the editor of J. Clin. Lab. Immunol.

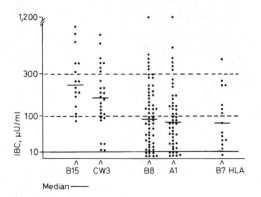

Fig. 4. The association of higher titres of insulin antibodies with HLA-B15 and CW3 than with HLA-B8 or B7 in insulin-treated diabetics. From *Irvine et al.* [19], by kind permission of the editor of J. Clin. Lab. Immunol.

increased titre of antibodies to coxsackie B viruses [7] and to heterologous conventional insulin given as regular therapy (fig. 4) [2, 19]. Allergic reactions (type I and type III) to conventional therapeutic insulin have been reported to be associated with B7 [1].

Immune Complexes

The occurrence of immune complexes in the serum, detected by Clq-SP at diagnosis, shows a significant correlation with the occurrence of ICAb [21]. This suggests that some, if not most, of these complexes consist of islet cell antigen and antibody to it, in the antibody excess. This could be important in the pathogenesis of type I diabetes through the immune mechanism of antibody-dependent cell-mediated cytotoxicity (ADCC). In preliminary studies, there was no significant correlation with viral antibody titres, including those to the coxsackie B group.

When type I diabetics have been treated with conventional heterologous insulin for some months, they generally form antibodies to insulin [33]. Immune complexes have been shown to be present in patients who have been

treated with insulin for many years and some of these complexes may be insulin-anti-insulin. However, type II diabetics who have been treated for a comparably long time with oral hypoglycaemic agents may also have evidence of immune complexes in the serum [23]. It is possible that impaired clearing mechanisms which would normally remove such complexes may be responsible for their presence [26]. In this way, immune complexes may aggravate the development of vascular complications [23].

The Possible Role of Autoimmunity in the Pathogenesis of Type I Diabetes

ICAb is unlikely on its own to be a main pathogenic agent [9]. Experiments whereby glucose intolerance was induced in nu/nu mice by the transfer of washed leucocytes from the peripheral blood of insulin-dependent diabetics are suggestive that immunological mechanisms that are cell-dependent may be important [5]. Exactly what immune mechanisms may be operative will have to await improved islet cell culture techniques so that such mechanisms can be analysed more precisely *in vitro*.

In type I diabetes autoimmunity may uncommonly be the only pathogenic mechanism (type Ia), in which case the patient is likely to have polyendocrine autoimmune disease. In other cases (type Ic), other genetically determined factors, such as susceptibility to viral infection of the islets, may be the main factor without there being any significant autoimmune reaction to the islet cells. However, it is tempting to speculate that more commonly (type Ib) there is both a greater susceptibility to a pancreatotropic viral infection and to islet cell autoimmunity which augment the damage done by the virus [13]. This would fit the observations described above that there are two HLA-related positive risk factors for type I diabetes that are additive in their effects and that only one of these is associated with autoimmunity. It would also fit with the transient nature of islet cell antibodies in the majority of type I diabetics. It is to be stressed, however, that type Ia, b and c are stages in the continuing spectrum of interaction between autoimmunity and some other agent such as viral infection.

References

1 Bertrams, J. and Gruneklee, D.: Association between HLA-B7 and allergic reactions to insulin in insulin-dependent diabetes mellitus. Tissue Antigens 10: 273–277 (1977).

2 Bertrams, J.; Jansen, F. K.; Gruneklee, D.; Reis, H. E.; Drost, H.; Beyer, J.; Gries, F. A., and Kuwert, E.: HLA antigens and immunoresponsiveness to insulin in insulin-dependent diabetes mellitus. Tissue Antigens 8: 13–19 (1976).

3 Bottazzo, G. F. and Lendrum, R.: Separate auto-antibodies to human pancreatic glucagon and somatostatin cells. Lancet ii: 873–876 (1976).

4 Bottazzo, G. F.; Florin-Christensen, A., and Doniach, D.: Islet cell antibodies in diabetes mellitus with autoimmune polyendocrine deficiencies. Lancet ii: 1279–1283 (1974).

5 Buschard, K.; Madsbad, S., and Rygaard, J.: Passive transfer of diabetes mellitus from men to mouse. Lancet i: 908–910 (1978).

6 Cudworth, A. G. and Woodrow, J. C.: Genetic susceptibility in diabetes mellitus: analysis of the HLA association. Br. med. J. ii: 846–848 (1976).

7 Cudworth, A. G.; Gamble, D. R.; White, G. B.; Lendrum, R.; Woodrow, J. C., and Bloom, A.: Etiology of diabetes. A prospective study. Lancet i: 385–388 (1977).

8 Flier, J. J.; Kahn, C. R.; Roth, J., and Bar, R. S.: Antibodies that impair insulin receptor binding in an unusual diabetic syndrome with severe insulin resistance. Science 190. 63–65 (1975)

9 Gamlen, T. R.; Aynsley-Green A.; Irvine, W. J., and McCallum, C. J.: Immunological studies in the neonate of a mother with Addison's disease and diabetes mellitus. Clin, exp. Immunol. 28: 192–195 (1977).

10 Huang, S-W. and MacLaren, N. K.: Insulin-dependent diabetes: a disease of autoaggression. Science 192: 64–66 (1976).

11 Irvine, W. J.: Autoimmunity in endocrine disease. Proc. R. Soc. Med. 67: 548–555 (1974).

12 Irvine, W. J.: Organ-specific autoimmunity in diabetes mellitus and correlation with other endocrine disorders. Proc. 9th Congr. Int. Diabetic Federation, Delhi 1976, pp. 260–272 (Elsevier, Amsterdam 1977).

13 Irvine, W. J.: Classification of idiopathic diabetes. Lancet i: 638–642 (1977).

14 Irvine, W. J.: Basic immunology; in Irvine Medical immunology, chap. 1 (Teviot Scientific Publications, Edinburgh 1979).

15 Irvine, W. J.: Endocrine disorders; in Irvine Medical immunology, chap. 6 (Teviot Scientific Publications, Edinburgh 1979).

16 Irvine, W. J.; Gray, R. S., and McCallum, C. J.: Pancreatic islet cell antibody as a marker for asymptomatic and latent diabetes and prediabetes. Lancet ii: 1097–1102 (1976).

17 Irvine, W. J.; MacCuish, A. C.; Campbell, C. J., and Duncan, L. J. P.: Organ-specific cell-mediated autoimmunity in diabetes mellitus. Acta endocr., Copenh. suppl. 205, pp. 65–67 (1976).

18 Irvine, W. J.; McCallum, C. J.; Gray, R. S., and Duncan, L. J. P.: Clinical and pathogenic significance of pancreatic islet cell antibodies in diabetics treated with oral hypoglycaemic agents. Lancet i: 1025–1027 (1977).

19 Irvine, W. J.; Mario, U. Di; Gray, R. S., and Morris, P. J.: Insulin antibodies in relation to islet cell antibodies and HLA antigens in type I diabetes. J. clin. Lab. Immunol. 1: 111–114 (1978).

20 Irvine, W. J.; Clarke, B. F.; Scarth, L.; Cullen, D. R., and Duncan, L. J. P.: Thyroid and gastric autoimmunity in patients with diabetes mellitus. Lancet ii: 163–168 (1970).

21 Irvine, W. J.; Di Mario, U.; Guy, K.; Gray, R. S., and Duncan, L. J. P.: Immune complexes in newly diagnosed insulin-dependent (Type I) diabetics. J. clin. Lab. Immunol. 1: 183–186 (1978).

22 Irvine, W. J.; Toft, A. D.; Holton, D. E.; Prescott, R. J.; Clarke, B. F., and Duncan, L. J. P.: Familial studies of type I and type II idiopathic diabetes mellitus. Lancet ii: 325–328 (1977).

23 Irvine, W. J.; Di Mario, U.; Guy, K.; Iavisoli, M.; Pozilli, P.; Lumbroso, B., and Andreani, D.: Immune complexes and diabetic microangiopathy. J. clin. Lab. Immunol. 1: 187–191 (1978).

24 Irvine, W. J.; Di Mario, U.; Gray, R. S.; Feek, C M.; Ting, A.; Morris, P. J., and Duncan, L. J. P.: Autoimmunity and HLA antigens in type I diabetes. J. clin. Lab. Immunol. 1: 107–110 (1978).

25 Irvine, W. J.; McCallum, C. J.; Gray, R. S.; Campbell, C. J.; Duncan, L. J. P.; Farquhar, J.; Vaughan, H., and Morris, P. J.: Pancreatic islet cell antibodies in diabetes mellitus correlated with the duration and type of diabetes, coexistent autoimmune disease and HLA type. Diabetes 26: 138–147 (1977).

26 Lambert, P. H.; Dixon, F. J.; Zubler, R. H.; Agnello, V.; Cambiaso, C.; Casali, P.; Clarke, J.; Cowdery, J. S.; McDuffie, F. C.; Hay, F. C.; MacLennan, I. C. M.; Masson, P.; Müller-Eberhard, H. J.; Penttinen, K.; Smith, M.; Tappeiner, G.; Theofilo-

poulos, A. N., and Verroust, P.: A WHO collaborative study for the evaluation of 18 methods for detecting immune complexes in serum. J. clin. Lab. Immunol. *1:* 1–15 (1978).

27 Lernmark, A.: Islet cell surface antibodies in diabetes; in Irvine, Int. Symp. Immunology of Diabetes mellitus (Teviot Scientific Publications, Edinburgh 1979).

28 Lendrum, R.; Walker, G.; Cudworth, A. G.; Theophanides, C.; Pyke, D. A.; Bloom, A., and Gamble, D. R.: Islet cell antibodies in diabetes mellitus. Lancet *ii:* 1273–1276 (1976).

29 MacCuish, A. C.; Barnes, E. W.; Irvine, W. J., and Duncan, L. J. P.: Antibodies to pancreatic islet cells in insulin-dependent diabetics with coexistent autoimmune disease. Lancet *ii:* 1529–1531 (1974).

30 MacCuish, A. C.; Jordan, J.; Campbell, C. J.; Duncan, L. J. P., and Irvine, W. J.: Cell-mediated immunity to human pancreas in diabetes mellitus. Diabetes *23:* 693–697 (1974).

31 Morris, P. J.: HLA and disease; in Irvine, Medical immunology, chap. 3 (Teviot Scientific Publications, Edinburgh 1979).

32 Nerup, J.; Andersen, O. O.; Bendixen, G.; Egeberg, J.; Gunnarsson, R.; Kromann, G., and Poulsen, J. E.: Cell-mediated immunity in diabetes mellitus. Proc. R. Soc. Med. *67:* 506–513 (1974).

33 Ortved Andersen, O.: Insulin antibody formation, I. The influence of age, sex, infections, insulin dosage and regulation of diabetes. Acta endocr., Copenh. *71:* 126–140 (1972).

34 Platz, P.; Jakobsen, B.; Dickmeiss, E.; Ryder, L. P.; Thomson, M., and Svejgaard, A.: Ia and HLA-D typing of patients with multiple sclerosis (MS) and insulin dependent diabetes (IDD) (abstr.). Tissue Antigens *10:* 192 (1977).

35 Rimoin, D. L. and Schmike, R. N.: Genetic disorders of the endocrine glands (Mosby, St. Louis 1971).

36 Smith, C.; Falconer, D. S., and Duncan, L. J. P.: A statistical and genetical study of diabetes. II. Heritability and liability. Ann. hum. Genet. *35:* 281–299 (1972).

Dr. W. J. Irvine, Endocrine Unit, Immunology Laboratories and University Department of Medicine, Royal Infirmary, Edinburgh (Scotland)

Immunopathology. 6th Int. Convoc. Immunol., Niagara Falls, N.Y., 1978, pp. 91–95 (Karger, Basel 1979)

Genetic Regulation of Autoimmune Thyroiditis in the Mouse[1]

N. R. Rose, Y. M. Kong, P. S. Esquivel, M. Elrehewy, A. A. Giraldo and C. S. David

Department of Immunology and Microbiology, Wayne State University School of Medicine, Detroit, Mich., and Department of Immunology, Mayo Clinic Medical School, Rochester, Minn.

A recent upsurge of interest in a genetic predisposition toward autoimmune disease arose from two sorts of clincal observations. First is the aggregation of several autoimmune disorders in the same family [5]. It may be seen as several cases of autoimmune thyroid disease, such as Graves' thyrotoxicosis or Hashimoto's thyroiditis, or overlaps between autoimmune diseases of different organs, such as pernicious anemia, thyroid disease, and Addison's disease of the adrenal. Epidemiological investigations have shown a statistical association of various forms of human autoimmune disease with genetic markers, such as particular HLA alleles [9]. A prominent association within Caucasian populations is found between HLA-B8 and Graves' and Addison's diseases, myasthenia gravis, and juvenile diabetes mellitus. It is interesting that in other populations where the distribution of HLA alleles differs, the association with autoimmunity is also different. For example, in Japan, HLA-B8 is relatively uncommon and Graves' disease is more commonly linked to HLA-Bw35 [4].

Experimental autoimmune thyroiditis in the mouse provides a valuable avenue for exploring the genetic

control of autoimmune disease. Studies initiated on this topic many years ago in Buffalo with Drs. *Frank Twarog, Adrian Vladutiu,* and *Vesna Tomazić* have been pursued more recently at Wayne State University.

As an initial step in an investigation on genetic control of the autoimmune response, many different inbred strains of mice were tested for their response to a standard injection of mouse thyroid antigen given with complete Freund's adjuvant (CFA). In most experiments, mouse thyroid extract or purified mouse thyroglobulin (MTg) was used. Sometimes, thyroglobulin was prepared from a given inbred strain. Individual strains of inbred mice were then tested for responsiveness in terms of production of autoantibodies to thyroglobulin and development of typical inflammatory lesions in the thyroid.

Mouse strains vary greatly in response, some producing high titers of antibody and severe thyroiditis, others developing lower antibody titers and very mild disease. It was found that the relative responsiveness of mice to MTg was related to their H-2 type [8]. For example, all nine inbred strains of mice having the H-2^k haplotype were good responders with high titers of antibody and severe disease. It should be emphasized that the only point in common among these nine strains was their H-2 type. They differed in virtually all other genetic characteristics. Similarly, three strains sharing the H-2^s haplotype and three strains with H-2^q were good responders, despite many other different genetic traits. On the other hand, the six strains of mice that bore the H-2^b haplotype were all poor responders. Their antibody titers were relatively low and their thyroids only mildly inflamed after immunization by the standard method. Similarly, three strains of the H-2^d haplotype were poor responders. A few inbred strains of mice seemed to be intermediate. For example, H-2^a mice had moderate titers of antibody and mild thyroid lesions. We will discuss these intermediate responders later.

[1] This work was supported by PHS Research Grants AMAI-20023 and CA-18900 from the National Institutes of Health.

These results strongly suggested that a major genetic element controlling the immune response of mice to MTg is closely linked to or part of the *H-2* histocompatibility complex. Further evidence solidifying this genetic association was obtained from two sorts of experiments [10]. In the first, SJL (*H-2^s*) mice were crossed with BALB/c (*H-2^d*) poor responders; the F$_1$ hybrids responded to immunization with MTg just as well as their good responder SJL parents. Similarly, RF (*H-2^k*) mice were crossed with BALB/c (*H-2^d*) animals; the F$_1$ hybrids resulting from this cross responded as well as their RF progenitors. The results indicate that an important gene controlling susceptibility of mice to thyroiditis is a Mendelian dominant. These F$_1$ hybrid animals were then backcrossed with the poor responder parental line and the F$_2$ offspring classified for *H-2* type. All mice carrying the *H-2^k* allele were good responders, in contrast to those that were *H-2^d*, which were poor responders. Within the limited group of F$_2$ offspring examined, no instances of separation between *H-2* type and susceptibility to thyroiditis were encountered.

The second experimental approach consisted of employing congenic mice that were genetically identical except for their *H-2* regions [8]. For example, C3H.SW/J mice are *H-2^b*, but in every other respect identical to the congenic C3H/HeJ (*H-2^k*) line. These C3H.SW/J mice proved to be poor responders following immunization with MTg, giving responses comparable to other *H-2^b* mice. Similarly, A.SW/J mice, bearing the *H-2^s* haplotype, are significantly better responders than the congenic A/WySn parental line which, like all *H-2^a* strains, is an intermediate responder. Together with the backcross experiment described above, the investigations with paired congenic mice support the view that response to MTg is controlled to a great extent by one or more genes within the *H-2* complex.

In nearly all crosses tested, F$_1$ hybrid mice obtained by mating good responder with poor responder strains were good responders, statistically identical to the good responder progenitor. However, an exception was seen in a cross between two related strains of mice derived at the Rockefeller University and bred for resistance or susceptibility to bacterial and viral infection. A cross between BSVS and BRVR mice gave rise to F$_1$ hybrids that were intermediate in response between the two parental lines [6]. This result emphasizes that additional genes, perhaps even located outside of the *H-2* complex, may influence the response of mice to MTg.

In addition to mice with defined *H-2* haplotypes, geneticists can supply us with animal strains in which recombination has occurred within the *H-2* complex. Such intra-*H-2* recombinants have been tested for responsiveness to MTg [7]. In general, mice bearing good responder (*k*) alleles at the *K* end or *I-A* subregion produce high titers of antibody and significant lesions following immunization with MTg. In contrast, animals with *H-2^b* or *H-2^d* alleles in these regions are poor responders. This result suggests that a major degree of genetic responsiveness is controlled by one or more genes located at *K* or *I-A*. Because most well-defined immune response (*Ir*) genes are located in the *I-A* subregion, it is logical to suggest that there is an *Ir* gene controlling responsiveness of mice to antigenic determinants of MTg located in the *I-A* subregion. This gene has tentatively been designated *Ir-Tg* [1b].

It was pointed out above that, although most mouse strains with good responder *k* alleles at *K* or *I-A* produce high titers of antibody similar to those found in usual *H-2^k* strains, the degree of thyroiditis may be only moderate. A similar observation was described with *H-2^a* mice, which represent a recombination of *H-2^k* and *H-2^d* [8]. This observation suggests that there may be additional controls to the right of the *I-A* subregion that modify the immune response of mice to MTg, particularly as far as the development of pathologic changes in the thyroid is concerned.

In the experiments described above, CFA was always injected with MTg. It seemed possible, therefore, that genetic regulation might depend upon the adjuvant used rather than upon antigenic determinants of thyroglobulin itself. Therefore, immunization was undertaken using two additional adjuvants whose mode of action is quite different from that of CFA—bacterial lipopolysaccharide (LPS) [3] and synthetic polynucleotides, polyadenylic-polyuridylic acid (poly A:U) [2]. In most of these experiments, congenic pairs differing only in the *H-2* region were compared [1a, 1b]. B10.BR mice are

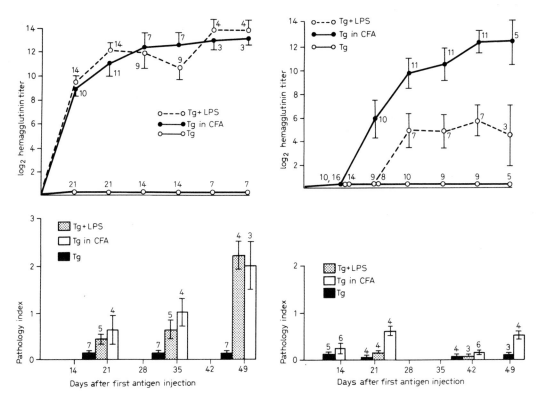

Fig. 1. Effect of LPS on the antibody responses to MTg and thyroid pathology in good responder (B10.BR) mice. LPS was given in a dose of 20 μg i.v. at 3 h after 250 μg of MTg i.v. on days 0 and 7. Control groups received MTg alone or MTg incorporated in CFA. The data are represented as the mean of the indicated number of animals ± SE. Reprinted from *Esquivel et al.* [1b] with the kind permission of the publisher.

Fig. 2. Effect of LPS on the antibody response to MTg and thyroid pathology in poor responder (B10.D2) mice. See legend of figure 1 for immunization protocol. Reprinted from *Esquivel et al.* [1b] with the kind permission of the publisher.

H-2^k and proved to be good responders to MTg, whereas B10.D2 mice, being H-2^d, were poor responders. As seen in figure 1, when B10.BR mice were injected intravenously on two occasions 1 week apart with a saline solution of MTg, no response was observed. Injection with CFA evoked high titers of antibody by day 14 which continued to rise through day 49. These animals showed severe thyroiditis when they

were killed on the 49th day. An intravenous injection of MTg followed by an injection of LPS also resulted in production of high antibody titers and severe thyroiditis characterized by the infiltration with mononuclear cells. When LPS and CFA were compared as adjuvants in low responder B10.D2 (H-2^d) mice, the induction period was lengthened (fig. 2). In mice given CFA, antibody levels approached those found in good res-

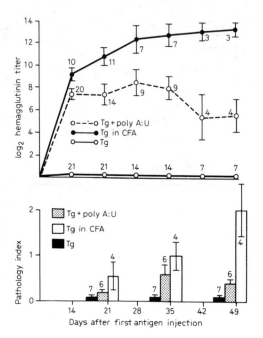

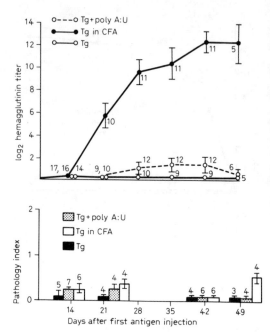

Fig. 3. Effect of poly A:U on the antibody response to MTg and thyroid pathology in good responder (B10.BR) mice. Poly A:U was given in a dose of 300 μg i.v. at 3 h after 250 μg of MTg on days 0 and 7. Control group received MTg alone or MTg emulsified in CFA. The data are presented as the mean of the indicated number of animals ± SE. Reprinted from *Esquivel et al.* [1a] with the kind permission of the publisher.

Fig. 4. Effect of poly A:U on the antibody response to MTg and thyroid pathology in poor responder (B10.D2) mice. See figure 3 legend for experimental procedure. Reprinted from *Esquivel et al.* [1a] with the kind permission of the publisher.

ponder B10.BR mice and mild thyroiditis was observed in some of the animals. In contrast, relatively low levels of antibody were detected in mice given LPS adjuvant and thyroid infiltration was not evident.

Poly A:U as an adjuvant was also compared in the same strains of congenic mice. Antibodies and transient cellular infiltration were observed only in good responder B10.BR mice (fig. 3). No significant levels of antibody and infiltration were present in poor responder B10.D2 animals (fig. 4).

The above studies led us to conclude that

both LPS and poly A:U are effective adjuvants in mice when given with MTg. Furthermore, the genetic control of the immune response to MTg as seen with the CFA regimen is mirrored in immunization using LPS and poly A:U as adjuvants. It is of considerable interest that LPS induces antibody production in both good and poor responder strains, but lesions are found only in the good responder mice. LPS and CFA are the only adjuvants known to induce an immunologic response associated with production of lesions of thyroiditis in mice. It should further be noted that poly A:U acts as adjuvant only in good responder strains of mice, and gives rise neither to significant antibody levels nor to lesions in the poor responder strain.

Further studies on the fine structure of genetic control were performed in intra-*H-2* recombinant strains, using both LPS and poly A:U adjuvants. As was the case when CFA was used, strains with good responder alleles at the *K* or *I-A* subregion were good responders using LPS and poly A:U adjuvants. Animals with poor responder (*d*) alleles at the *K* or *I-A* subregion produced very low titers or no antibody and no lesions. These experiments show that the differentiation between good and poor responders is much the same as when CFA was employed, and the differences are even more clear-cut with LPS or poly A:U adjuvants.

Additional experiments were carried out to assign the cellular basis of good and poor response to thyroglobulin [1b, 10]. For this purpose, 'B' mice were prepared by thymectomy plus lethal irradiation, followed by reconstitution with bone marrow cells treated by anti-Thy-1 serum plus complement. Sometimes thymus cells were also given. The bone marrow or thymus cells were taken from good or poor responder donors. It was found first that irradiated, reconstituted recipients not given thymus cells at all failed to respond to immunization with MTg in CFA, regardless of the source of their marrow cells. If thymus cells were taken from poor responder parents, the reconstituted chimeras also failed to respond or responded with only low titers of antibody and very mild lesions of thyroiditis. On the other hand, chimeras reconstituted with thymic cells taken from good responder progenitors were good responders regardless of whether their marrow cells came from good or poor responder donors. These experiments demonstrate that the genetic basis of good or poor response to thyroglobulin in mice is the thymus-derived (T) lymphocyte.

References

1a Esquivel, P.S.; Kong, Y. M., and Rose, N. R.: Evidence for thyroglobulin-reactive T cells in good responder mice. Cell Immunol. *34:* 14–19 (1978).

1b Esquivel, P. S.; Rose, N. R., and Kong Y. M.: Induction of autoimmunity in good and poor responder mice with mouse thyroglobulin and lipopolysaccharide. J. exp. Med. *145:* 1250–1263 (1977).

2 Johnson, A. G.: The adjuvant action of synthetic polynucleotides on the immune response; in Cohen, Immune RNA, pp. 17–35 (CRC Press, West Palm Beach 1976).

3 Johnson, A. G.; Gaines, S., and Landy, M.: Studies on the O antigen of *Salmonella typhosa*. V. Enhancement of antibody response to protein antigens by the purified lipopolysaccharide. J. exp. Med. *103:* 225–246 (1956).

4 Nakao, Y.; Kishihana, M.; Baba, Y.; Kuma, K.; Fukunishi, T., and Imura, H.: HLA antigens in Japanese patients with autoimmune thyroid diseases. Archs intern. Med. *138:* 567–570 (1978).

5 Roitt, I. M. and Doniach, D.: A reassessment of studies on the aggregation of thyroid autoimmunity in families of thyroiditis patients. Clin. exp. Immun. *2:* 727–736 (1967).

6 Rose, N. R.; Vladutiu, A. O.; David, C. S., and Shreffler, D. C.: Autoimmune murine thyroiditis. V. Genetic influence on the disease in BSVS and BRVR mice. Clin. exp. Immunol. *15:* 281–287 (1973).

7 Tomazić, V.; Rose, N. R., and Shreffler, D. C.: Autoimmune murine thyroiditis. IV. Localization of genetic control of the immune response. J. Immunol. *112:* 965–969 (1974).

8 Vladutiu, A. O. and Rose, N. R.: Autoimmune murine thyroiditis. Relationship to histocompatibility (H-2) type. Science *174:* 1137–1139 (1971).

9 Vladutiu, A. O. and Rose, N. R.: HL-A antigen: association with disease. Immunogenetics *1:* 305–328 (1974).

10 Vladutiu, A. O. and Rose, N. R.: Cellular basis of the genetic control of immune responsiveness to murine thyroglobulin in mice. Cell. Immunol. *17:* 106–113 (1975).

Dr. N. R. Rose, Department of Immunology and Microbiology, Wayne State University School of Medicine, 540 E. Canfield Avenue, Detroit, MI 48201 (USA)

Immunopathology. 6th Int. Convoc. Immunol., Niagrara Falls, N.Y., 1978, pp. 96–100 (Karger, Basel 1979)

The Immune Response of Obese Strain Chickens[1]

J. H. Kite, jr., J. Tyler and J. Pascale

Departments of Microbiology and Pathology, School of Medicine, State University of New York at Buffalo, Buffalo, N.Y.

The Obese strain of White Leghorn chickens is an excellent animal model for studies on the development of spontaneous autoimmune thyroiditis. The disease develops shortly after hatching and leads to a severe destruction of the thyroid gland with a concomitant decrease in circulating thyroxine. Because of the reduction in thyroid hormones, phenotypic signs develop that are easily recognizable and include reduction in size of the skeletal structure, changes in the appearance of the feathers, a smaller comb and wattle, increased subcutaneous fat and poor laying ability. Selection for these phenotypic signs and development of a strain was made by Dr. *R. K. Cole* [3, 10]. We gave the term 'Obese strain' to these chickens as a simplified term for the hypothyroid condition [6, 14], although the name reflects only one phenotypic characteristic.

A few of the principal findings which we and others have demonstrated in Obese strain (OS) chickens are presented in table I. In our first paper on the immunological aspects of this disease, appearing in 1968 [4], the autoimmune nature of the disease was established for the first time by the demonstration of autoantibodies to thyroglobulin,

recognition of pathological changes in the thyroid gland similar to Hashimoto's disease of humans, and the finding that bursectomy can prevent the development of the disease. Shortly thereafter, we demonstrated that autoantibodies could be produced to several nonthyroid tissue antigens, in particular liver and kidney, and rarely to pancreas and lung tissue extracts [5b]. Although we recognize this disease as an organ-specific autoimmune disease, it is interesting that autoantibodies are formed to other tissue antigens but without producing pathology.

Table I. Principal characteristics of OS chickens

Spontaneous autoimmune thyroiditis—presence of autoantibodies to thyroglobulin; mononuclear cell infiltration and thyroid cell destruction [4]

B cell-mediated disease—bursectomy prevents thyroiditis [4]

Autoantibodies produced to non-thyroid tissue antigens [5b]

Thymectomy increases severity of thyroiditis [12]

Thyroiditis under genetic control—correlation of genotype at B locus (major histocompatibility complex) with severity of thyroiditis [1, 2, 8]

Endocrine abnormalities—decrease of T_3, T_4, and free T_4 hormones in serum; increase in uptake of iodine [9, 13]

Early morphological changes in thyroid membranes [11]

Increase with age of thyroglobulin-binding lymphoid cells in spleen and thymus [7]

[1] Supported by USPHS NIH Grant CA-02357 and 5-SO7-RR7066, BRSG from State University of New York at Buffalo.

Thymectomy of OS chickens leads to an increased severity of thyroiditis, apparently reflecting a loss of suppressor cells [12]. The expression of thyroiditis is determined genetically since correlations can be made between genotype and severity of thyroiditis [1, 2, 8]. Endocrine abnormalities have been noted [9, 13] as well as morphological changes in thyroid membranes by electron microscopy [11]. As the disease progresses, there is an increase of thyroglobulin-binding lymphoid cells in the spleen and thymus [7].

In this report, studies will be presented which sought to determine if the autoimmune disease could be due partially to a generalized hyperactive immune response to autologous, and consequently heterologous, antigens through some fault in the regulatory mechanism. Three approaches were employed to examine antibody responses to sheep red blood cells (SRBC), the immune response to tumor growth, and finally the proliferative responses of lymphocytes to T-cell mitogens.

Figure 1 depicts the peak titers of hemagglutinating antibody detected in groups of OS and the parent C-strain chicks injected

with different doses of SRBC at 4 and 11 days of age. C-strain chicks exhibit a typical dose response profile, but OS chicks are uniformly responsive over the dose range of 10^8 to 2×10^9 SRBC. Thus, at moderate doses OS chicks exhibit enhanced antibody responses. Since comparable titers of antibody can be produced by C-strain chicks at the high dose, the results suggest that OS chicks are overreactive to antigen or that, in some way, antibody responses are abnormally regulated in OS chicks. If the injection series was delayed until 4 weeks of age, enhanced responses were no longer observed in OS chickens. These findings suggest that enhanced antibody responses are a transient phenomenon restricted to young OS chicks. Antibody responses to SRBC were also compared with two unrelated strains of normal White Leghorn chickens (NWL). When chicks were immunized at 4 and 11 days with 10^8 SRBC, OS chicks exhibited enhanced responses as compared to KSU-C and line G chicks, as well as C-strain chicks. Thus, enhanced antibody responses appear to be a unique characteristic of OS chickens.

Since autoimmune thyroiditis occurs early in the life of OS chicks, the question may be raised as to whether enhanced antibody responses are simply a reflection of the increased cellular activity due to the autoimmune disease. To examine this question, OS chickens were thyroidectomized on the day of hatching, so as to prevent the development of autoimmune disease. Thyroidectomy does not impair the ability of OS chicks to mount enhanced antibody responses to SRBC. Only thyroidectomized chicks which were shown to be athyroid and free of autoantibodies to thyroglobulin were included in these results. Thus, enhanced antibody responses appear to be a primary trait of young OS chicks.

A second approach used to study the immune response of OS chickens was their

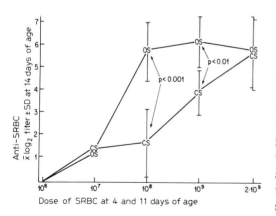

Fig. 1. Peak titers of hemagglutinating antibody in groups of chicks injected with different doses of SRBC at 4 and 11 days of age.

reaction to the development of a tumor. When Rous sarcoma virus (RSV) was injected 5 days after hatching, no significant reduction in tumor growth occurred in OS or C-strain or in normal strains of chickens (table II). However, when RSV was injected at 2.5 or 6 weeks following hatching, then there was considerably less growth of tumors. In additional experiments, thyroidectomy did not prevent the enhanced immune response.

Since the magnitude of antibody responses to the T-dependent antigen, SRBC, appeared to be abnormally regulated in OS chicks, examination was made for T-cell reactivity. For this purpose, experiments compared *in vitro* proliferative responses of OS and normal strain lymphocytes to T-cell mitogens, phytohemaglutinin (PHA) and concanavalin A (Con A). Proliferation of lymphocytes was determined by ^{3}H-thymidine uptake. Figure 2 depicts the proliferative response to PHA of peripheral blood lymphocytes (PBL) from OS, C-strain and random-bred NWL during the first 5 weeks after hatching. For control purposes, proliferation is expressed as a percent of the response of adult C-strain PBL. PBL from OS chicks are significantly more responsive than normal controls. The increase in proliferative response with age probably reflects T-cell maturation. Therefore, enhanced OS responses may be indicative of precocious T-cell maturation. Similar findings were made when Con A was employed, and when lymphocytes from the thymus were stimulated with PHA or Con A. Enhanced responses to mitogens were independent of autoimmune disease, since lymphocytes from neonatally thyroidectomized chicks showed no impairment of hyperactivity. Thus, enhanced mitogen-induced proliferation appears to be a primary characteristic of OS T-cells. Antibody responses to the T-independent antigen, lipopolysaccharide of *Escherichia coli*, were not significantly elevated in

Table II. Growth in chickens of tumors induced by RSV: variation in time of RSV injection

Chicken strain	Time of RSV[1] injection after hatching		
	5 days	2.5 weeks	6 weeks
OS	10.3[2]	2.1	1.5
C strain	15.2	48.0	19.4
Line G	25.3	41.8	20.1

[1] RSV, lot No. 1, 10^{-3} dilution.
[2] Size of tumor produced in wing web, measured in ml, 3 weeks after RSV injection. This figure is the mean value from 5 chickens.
From [5a].

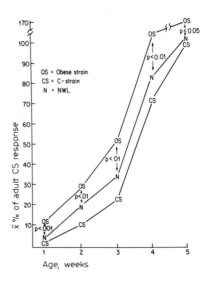

Fig. 2. Proliferative response of PBL to PHA.

OS chicks, suggesting that OS B-cells are not intrinsically hyperactive to antigen.

One approach to evaluate the qualitative properties of OS and C-strain lymphocytes was to analyze the effect of co-culturing lymphocytes from the two strains in the presence of mitogen. The OS and C-strain chicks

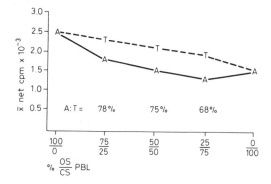

Fig. 3. Inhibition of proliferative responses of OS lymphocytes to PHA by CS lymphocytes.

Table III. Inhibition of proliferative responses of OS lymphocytes to PHA by CS lymphocytes: age dependence

Age, weeks	Source of PBL [1]	$\bar{x}$ net CPM $\pm$ SD		A : T [2]
		actual	theoretical	
2	OS	1,305 ± 220		
	CS	450 ± 46		
	OS + CS	454 ± 64	879 ± 133	0.52
3	OS	2,362 ± 158		
	CS	1,035 ± 105		
	OS + CS	883 ± 109	1,698 ± 122	0.52
5	OS	7,740 ± 713		
	CS	4,680 ± 473		
	OS + CS	6,413 ± 493	6,210 ± 593	1.03

[1] PBL were cultured alone or together (1:1) at 10^6 cells/ 0.2 ml culture with 2.5 μl/ml PHA. The same 3 chicks of each strain were used at each age.
[2] A : T = Actual response/theoretical response.

share the same B^1B^1 genotype at the major histocompatibility locus and their lymphocytes exhibit very little, if any, mixed lymphocyte reactivity. If the enhanced OS response is entirely due to quantitative differences in the number of mitogen responsive T-cells, then the proliferative response of co-cultures should be predictable based on the respective qualitative response of lymphocytes from the two strains.

Figure 3 depicts the PHA-induced proliferative response at 2 weeks of age, of OS and C-strain lymphocytes cultured alone, or co-cultured in varying proportions. The actual response (A) of co-cultured lymphocytes is considerably less than theoretically predicted (T). The ratio of the actual to theoretical response (A:T) is inversely proportional to the degree of apparent inhibition. Inhibition increases with higher proportions of C-strain PBL in the co-cultures. Since CS PBL are less responsive than OS PBL, one might speculate that CS PBL are endowed with greater suppressor activity than OS PBL. We have determined that inhibition in OS-CS co-cultures requires the presence of CS T-cells. Thus, enhanced OS responses may be due to a deficiency of suppressor T-cells. Inhibition of OS lymphocyte responses to PHA could also be accomplished by the addition of cell-free supernatant fluids from PHA-activated CS lymphocytes. Thus, inhibition appears to be mediated by soluble factors.

When co-culture responses are examined at different ages, an interesting finding is observed (table III). At 2 or 3 weeks of age, co-culture responses to PHA are markedly inhibited, as evidenced by low A:T ratios However, by 5 weeks of age, co-cultivation no longer results in inhibition. The actual and theoretical responses are essentially equivalent. Of importance is the fact that OS chicks still exhibit an enhanced response at this age. Additional experiments not reported here also support the hypothesis that in addition to decreased suppressor activity, there is a concomitant increase in stimulatory activity.

In hypothesizing a mechanism for autoimmune thyroiditis in OS chickens, evidence indicates a primary defect in the immune system. One may speculate that possible alterations in the membranes of thymus or bursa cells could change viral receptors, permitting infection leading to an autoimmune response; on the other hand, an immunological reaction of one subpopulation of lymphocytes against another could lead to destruction of suppressor lymphocytes or stimulation of helper cells. Our data support the view for both reduction in suppressor cells and an increase in helper cell activity. Such occurrences would lead to an enhanced immune reactivity that may predispose the birds to autoimmune disease. In addition to this postulated defect in the immune system, it would appear that another defect must occur in the thyroid gland, perhaps associated with the recognition of thyroglobulin, in order to enable an autoimmune disease of the thyroid to develop. A reason for this hypothesis comes from a failure to produce thyroiditis in CS (B^1B^1) birds with spleen cells transferred from OS (B^1B^1) chickens. The mechanism finally proposed for the autoimmune response to thyroid antigens should also account for the production of autoantibodies to non-thyroid tissue antigens. Thus, it would appear that a combination of several genetic defects is necessary for the final expression of autoimmune disease in OS chickens.

References

1 Bacon, L. D.; Kite, J. H., and Rose, N. R.: Immunogenetic detection of B-locus genotypes in chickens with autoimmune thyroiditis. Transplantation *16:* 591–598 (1973).
2 Bacon, L. D.; Kite, J. H., and Rose, N. R.: Relation between the major histocompatibility (B) locus and autoimmune thyroiditis in obese chickens. Science *186:* 274–275 (1974).
3 Cole, R. K.: Hereditary hypothyroidism in the domestic fowl. Genetics, N.Y. *53:* 1021–1033 (1966).
4 Cole, R. K.; Kite, J. H., and Witebsky, E.: Hereditary autoimmune thyroiditis in the fowl. Science *160:* 1357–1358 (1968).

5a Kite, J. H.: Genetic control of thyroiditis; in Friedmann et al., Infection, immunity and genetics, pp. 157–176 (University Park Press, Baltimore 1978).
5b Kite, J. H.: Unpublished findings.
6 Kite, J. H.; Wick, G.; Twarog, B., and Witebsky, E.: Spontaneous thyroiditis in the obese strain of chickens. II. Investigations on the development of the disease. J. Immun. *103:* 1331–1341 (1969).
7 Richter, E.; Wick, G., and Schauenstein, K.: The nature of active and passive thyroglobulin binding lymphoid cells in Obese strain (OS) chickens. Eur. J. Immunol. *5:* 554–559 (1975).
8 Rose, N. R.; Bacon, L. D., and Sundick, R. S.: Genetic determinants of thyroiditis in the OS chicken. Transplantn Rev. *31:* 264–284 (1976).
9 Sundick, R. S. and Wick, G.: Increased ^{131}I uptake by the thyroid glands of Obese strain (OS) chickens derived from non-protamone-supplemented hens. Clin. exp. Immunol. *18:* 127–139 (1974).
10 Tienhoven, A. van and Cole, R. K.: Endocrine disturbances in obese chickens. Anat. Rec. *142:* 111–118 (1962).
11 Wick, G. and Graf, J.: Electron microscopic studies in chickens of the Obese strain with spontaneous hereditary autoimmune thyroiditis. Lab. Invest. *27:* 400–411 (1972).
12 Wick, G.; Kite, J. H., and Witebsky, E.: Spontaneous thyroiditis in the obese strain of chickens. IV. The effect of thymectomy and thymo-bursectomy on the development of the disease. J. Immun. *104:* 54–62 (1970).
13 Witebsky, E.: The clinical pathology of autoimmunization. Am. J. clin. Path. *49:* 301–311 (1968).
14 Witebsky, E.; Kite, J. H.; Wick, G., and Cole, R. K.: Spontaneous thyroiditis in the obese strain of chickens. I. Demonstration of circulating autoantibodies. J. Immun. *103:* 708–715 (1969).

Dr. J. H. Kite, jr., Department of Microbiology, School of Medicine, State University of New York at Buffalo, Buffalo, NY 14214 (USA)

Immunopathology. 6th Int. Convoc. Immunol., Niagara Falls, N.Y., 1978, pp. 101–106 (Karger, Basel 1979)

The Nature of Effector Cells in Experimental and Spontaneous Autoimmune Thyroiditis[1]

G. Wick, R. Kofler, R. Gundolf, P. U. Müller and R. Boyd

Institute for General and Experimental Pathology, University of Innsbruck, Medical School, Innsbruck

The exact effector and regulatory mechanisms operative in autoimmune diseases are still far from being elucidated. The understanding of these mechanisms would be both of theoretical interest and practical importance. Thus, a more refined diagnosis of autoimmune disease in man based on the effector mechanism involved would facilitate a more selective immunosuppressive therapy. For a long time, experimentally induced autoimmune diseases have been the only animal models used to investigate this problem [29]. Most of this work was perhaps done on experimental autoimmune thyroiditis (EAT) [22]. However, it becomes increasingly apparent that the effector mechanisms thought to be active in EAT may be different from those in human Hashimoto thyroiditis. In contrast, it seems that the spontaneous hereditary autoimmune thyroiditis (SAT) which arises in chickens of the Obese strain (OS) corresponds more closely to the human situation [8, 33]. In this paper only short allusion will be made to EAT, as the general topic of experimentally induced autoimmune diseases will be covered by several other authors during this Convocation. The major part of the following discussion will be devoted to the OS. Figure 1 summarizes some of the conceivable effector mechanisms in EAT and SAT.

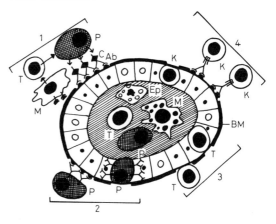

Fig. 1. Schematic representation of some possible pathogenetic immunologic effector mechanisms in autoimmune thyroiditis. Modified from *Allison* [5]. Mechanism 1: Cytotoxic antibody needs T cell help for its formation and complement for induction of damage. Mechanism 2: Periopolesis by plasma cells. These cells produce antibody (with T cell help?) and act like K cells. Mechanism 3: Direct cytotoxicity by sensitized T cells. Mechanism 4: Antibody-dependent cellular cytotoxicity (ADCC). K cells either attached to thyroid autoantibodies *in situ* or sensitized by immune complexes in antibody excess in circulation. Penetration of antibodies or effector cells through basement membrane and periopolesis entail damage of epithelial cells. All types of cells may be found in lumen of destroyed follicles. P = Plasma cell; T = T cell; M = macrophage; Ep = thyroid epithelial cell; Ab = autoantibody to thyroglobin or other thyroid antigen; C = complement; BM = basement membrane.

[1] This work was supported by a grant from the Austrian Research Council (Project No. 3120).

Experimentally Induced Autoimmune Thyroiditis

Experimentally induced autoimmune diseases have long been considered to be mediated by T-cells (mechanism 3 in fig. 1). Thus, delayed type skin reactions to thyroglobulin (Tg) can consistently be evoked in guinea pigs with EAT and precede the onset of disease [11]. This observation could, however, not be confirmed in rabbits [28]. In rodents successful transfer of EAT has first been possible with lymph node cells, but not with serum [10]. Furthermore, EAT cannot be produced in neonatally thymectomized chickens [14] or rats [4], nor in nude mice [9, 32]. However, more recent data clearly speak for the assumption that EAT is a result of a termination of the normal T cell unresponsiveness to Tg in the presence of autoreactive B cells. Bypassing of specific T cells can be achieved by the injection of altered (arsanil-sulfanil) autologous Tg [27] or complexed homologous Tg [12]. Via the bypass of specific T cells, the T cells so activated may provide the second signal to Tg-reactive B cells for further differentiation into effector cells. Reconstitution of thymectomized, lethally irradiated mice with syngeneic bone marrow cells alone before immunization with heterologous Tg does not lead to the development of EAT or Tg-autoantibodies, but thymus plus bone marrow reconstitution restores responsiveness [5]. In addition, antigenic suicide experiments with heavily labelled autologous ^{125}I-Tg lead to a prevention of EAT and Tg-autoantibody production in mice, if bone marrow cells are so treated, but not if thymus cells are incubated [13].

After many unsuccessful attempts in the past, *Nakamura and Weigle* [17] and *Vladutiu and Rose* [25] were able to achieve transfer of EAT with serum in rabbits and mice, respectively.

The light and electron microscopical analysis of thyroid glands from animals with EAT reveals Ig-deposits along the follicular basement membrane. In mice, these deposits consist of IgG and Tg and contain complement [4] (mechanism 1 in fig. 1). In contrast to SAT in OS chickens and to Hashimoto thyroiditis (discussed below), periopolesis of plasma cells cannot be observed in EAT, while small lymphoid cells are constantly found to disrupt the follicular epithelial lining. The T or B cell nature of these latter cells has not yet been elucidated. An additional difference to the human situation is the absence of germinal centers and of autoantibodies to microsomal thyroid antigens in EAT. Nevertheless, Tg-producing cells can be demonstrated in cell suspensions of infiltrated thyroid glands of rabbits with EAT using Tg-coated sheep red blood cells in a plaque assay [7]. The peak number of Tg plaque-forming cells (PFC) precedes the maximal degree of thyroid infiltration. However, in spite of the evidence for an important role of humoral Tg-autoantibody in EAT, it has been shown that animals depleted of C3 or C5 are perfectly able to develop the disease [2]. Recent studies rather imply the importance of antibody-dependent cellular cytotoxicity (ADCC) as a possible, or even the most probable, effector mechanism in EAT (mechanism 4 in fig. 1) [2, 7]. These data will have to be supplemented by more detailed studies on the role of direct cytotoxicity in order to elucidate the possible proportional contribution of T cells as effectors for thyroid damage in EAT.

In conclusion, it seems that K cell activity of the ADCC type may be the major effector mechanism in EAT, and T cell help is needed for the production of Tg-autoantibodies. If, and to what extent, direct cytotoxicity represents an alternative or additional effector mechanism (mechanism 3 in fig. 1) still remains to be clarified.

Spontaneous Autoimmune Thyroiditis

In contrast to EAT, SAT in OS chickens resembles human Hashimoto's disease very closely in its histopathological and serological characteristics [33]. The fact that this disease arises in an avian species provides unique possibilities for the investigation of the role of B and T cells in its development, and for manipulation of the embryos. The availability of OS lines homozygous at the B-locus will also enable cell transfer experiments to test different hypotheses concerning the effector mechanisms involved in SAT. Current experiments implicate the B cell nature of the effector cells.

Evidence for B-Cell Nature of Effector Cells
Morphological Evidence. Histologically, plasma cells are the main elements within the massive cellular thyroid infiltrate, and the high number of germinal centers is a characteristic feature. Plasma cells are among the first lymphoid cells to be found in the early stage of thyroid infiltration at about 1 week of age. They not only abut the follicular basement membrane, but can also be found between epithelial cells (periopolesis), thus disrupting the continuous lining. In immunofluorescence and electron microscopical preparations these plasma cells are surrounded by Ig and electron-dense deposits, respectively. Besides plasma cells, smaller lymphoid cells can also be found both in the interstitium and penetrating between epithelial cells. The B or T cell nature of these latter cells, however, has not yet been determined.

Serological Evidence. Tg-autoantibodies can be demonstrated in the sera of most OS birds and their occurrence and titers, especially of precipitating antibodies, show a good correlation with the severity of disease. *In situ* production of Tg-autoantibodies by the above-mentioned plasma cells and germinal centers has also been demonstrated.

Detailed studies on the occurrence of autoantibodies to additional thyroid antigens have so far provided no evidence for antibodies to the second colloid antigen, CA2. Recently, however, antibodies to microsomal thyroid antigens were detected by *Khoury and Bottazzo* [personal commun.] in some OS sera.

Tg-autoantibody has been found to be vertically transmitted from the mother hen via the egg yolk into the newly hatched OS chicken and granular Ig deposits can also be identified along the follicular basement membrane of OS embryos or chicks. Severe degenerative changes can already be observed in the untreated thyroid glands of newly hatched OS birds.

Bursectomy-Thymectomy. In contrast to the findings in EAT, the incidence and severity of SAT is significantly reduced, or even completely abolished, in neonatally or —even more so—*in ovo* bursectomized OS chickens [34]. Neonatal thymectomy, however, leads to more severe disease [31]. Similar observations have been made in rats which develop SAT after neonatal thymectomy [18].

From these data, it was concluded that B cells play a major role in the development of SAT and that the underlying immunologic defect in this strain may rest in the suppressor T cell population.

Analysis of Antigen-Binding Cells. OS chickens have an increased number of B cells identified by specific turkey anti-chicken B cell sera (ABS) in their peripheral blood, spleen and thymus as compared to sex- and age-matched normal controls [1]. Subsequent experiments were aimed at the demonstration of Tg-binding cells (Tg-BC) in the peripheral blood and spleen of OS chickens. In a chronological study using a rosette assay with Tg-coated chicken red blood cells, Tg-BC could be demonstrated with a peak preceding the maximum degree of SAT and the highest titers of Tg-autoantibodies [20]. Inhibition assays with ABS and anti-T cell sera (ATS) showed that the total number of Tg-BC consists of two populations, active (B) and passive (T) Tg-BC. Active Tg-BC possess Tg receptors of IgM nature synthesized by themselves, passive Tg-BC are T cells which acquire Tg-receptors—again IgM—via Fc receptors from the serum [19]. A similar approach in humans has shown that Tg-BC also occur in the peripheral blood of Hashimoto patients and that their identification may be a better diagnostic parameter than conventional thyroid serology [21].

From these results, it was assumed that the occurrence of Tg-BC is a prerequisite for the subsequent development of SAT and that they may be precursors of effector cells. For functional studies of Tg-BC, methods for their enrichment were devised which allow the harvest of larger numbers of cells for *in vitro* analysis and *in vivo* transfer studies which are currently under way.

Previous immunofluorescence studies on the possible sites of Tg-autoantibody synthesis have shown the *in situ* production in the thyroid glands themselves, but were not successful in the central and peripheral lymphoid organs [15, 23]. In view of the fact that circulating Tg-autoantibodies can also be found in OS chickens with minor thyroid disease, these data are being reinvestigated using a PFC assay.

*Different Pathogenic Effector Mechanisms
Underlying Experimental Allergic Encephalomyelitis
and SAT*

To investigate the possibility of different effector mechanisms underlying an experimentally induced autoimmune disease and SAT, the following experiments were performed: experimental allergic encephalomyelitis (EAE), known to be T-dependent in chickens, was induced in 6- to 11-week-old OS chickens which had been bursectomized *in ovo*, thymectomized at hatching, or left unoperated. Thus, both types of diseases could be studied in the *same* animal and it was shown that EAE and SAT developed independently from each other in untreated OS birds. Bursectomy and thymectomy had the same effect on SAT as in chickens not simultaneously afflicted with EAE. In contrast to EAE in normal White Leghorn chickens we found, however, that while thymectomy entailed a strong reduction of the susceptibility of OS chickens for EAE, bursectomy also had a, albeit less pronounced, suppressive effect. It seems therefore that EAE may be mediated both by T and B cells in the OS [4].

K-Cell Activity

To analyze further the nature of the effector cells, an *in vitro* ^{51}Cr-release assay was established, utilizing Tg-coated chicken erythrocytes and, for ADCC, anti-Tg-containing serum from OS chickens. Although the results are still preliminary, 3 main points are emerging. First, ADCC activity of peripheral blood leukocytes appears lower in younger (5-week) than older (28-week) birds. It is interesting to speculate that this early depressed level may reflect a preoccupation of such cells in the thyroid gland (thus accounting for the previously noted maximal influx of mononuclear cells into the thyroid at this age). Secondly, significant direct cellular cytotoxicity to Tg-coated cells occurs only in OS chickens, compared to normals as expected; again, this appears generally higher in the older birds. Thirdly, there does not appear to be any correlation between these forms of cytotoxicity and serum antibody levels.

Suppressor Cell Defect

It has been hypothesized that neonatal thymectomy preferentially depletes chickens of suppressor cells while enough helper cells, if necessary for the development of SAT, may already have reached the periphery before the operation. In this respect, it may also be of interest that sublethal whole body X-irradiation (without surgical manipulation) results in more severe disease [33] and that T suppressor cells are known to be more sensitive to irradiation as compared to the helper cells [2]. This concept is further supported by the fact that thymectomy also leads to the occurrence of autoantibodies to non-

thyroid antigens, such as liver, kidney and erythrocyte nuclear antigens [33]. Recent studies have also revealed circulating autoantibodies to stomach parietal cells in OS sera [*Khoury et al.*, personal commun.]. The fact that autoimmune disease only involves the thyroid gland may be due to a primary thyroid abnormality manifested already before the first sign of lymphoid infiltration, i.e. in the embryo and newly hatched OS chicks. Thus, while older OS chickens show the typical symptoms of hypothyroidism, the thyroid glands of OS embryos or newly hatched chicks incorporate significantly more ^{131}I than those of normal White Leghorn controls [24].

Immunogenetic Aspects

Bacon et al. [3] first studied a possible correlation between the development of SAT and the occurrence of Tg-autoantibodies and the MHC-type of OS chickens. Such a correlation had been described by *Vladutiu and Rose* [26] for EAT in mice. In the studies of *Bacon et al.* the presence of the *B1* allele was found to be correlated with high responsiveness in respect to both SAT and Tg-autoantibody production, while *B4* was associated with low responsiveness. *B1B4* heterozygotes appeared as intermediate responders [29]. In our own OS colony, *B1B1* chickens *and B4B4* birds display severe mean degrees of SAT and high Tg-autoantibody titers, while a line developed in our laboratory with the genotype *B3B3* appears to be low responding [30]. However, this correlation was not absolute as there were always several *B1B4* birds with mild SAT and low Tg-autoantibody titers and also some *B3B3* chickens with severe disease. The hypothesis summarized in table I was put forward to accommodate the divergent results obtained with different colonies of OS chickens so far. According to this concept, the development of SAT is dependent on the action of genes at (at least) three loci. Ir-1 genes associated with the *B* locus code for high (*B1, B4*) or low

Table I. Schematic outline of possible genetic basis for the development of SAT in OS chickens

Respon-siveness		
High	Ir-1^a	B1
High	Ir-1^b	B4	I (B-locus)
Low	Ir-1^c	B3
High	Ir-2^a	nB (non-B)	II (non B-locus)
	Thyroid abnormality		III (thyroid locus)

(*B3*) responsiveness, respectively. Ir-2, localized at a non-*B* locus, are also responsible for high responsiveness; this may, e.g. be operative via a decreased number and (or) function of T suppressor cells. Finally, the development of SAT is dependent on a primary thyroid defect genetically determined by a separate locus. This latter assumption could also explain the hitherto unsuccessful attempts to transfer SAT from OS to normal white Leghorn chickens by sera or cells. Thus, *B1B1* chickens which possess Ir-1[a], Ir-2[a] and the gene(s) at the third locus should develop severe SAT, while *B1B1* birds lacking Ir-2[a] will rank as low responders.

Summary of Possible Effector Mechanisms in OS Chickens. Tg-autoantibodies of the IgG class are vertically transferred into the OS chicken embryo. They bind to the primarily altered thyroid gland and lead to damage by complement-mediated cytotoxicity (mechanism 1 in fig. 1). Tg leaking from damaged follicles binds (directly or via macrophage) to Tg-BC and triggers their differentiation into plasma cells. Free Tg or Tg/anti-Tg complexes may be bound by reticular cells thereby trapping Tg-BC (B-cells) evoking further differentiation and proliferation within germinal centers. Tg-autoantibody production may need T cell help as in the mouse. The Tg-autoantibodies produced are both of the IgG and IgM class. Destruction of target cells occurs either by the antibody-producing cells themselves acting as effector cells without the need of Fc receptors (because they are associated with the target cells by their own antibody; chicken plasma cells showing membrane-associated Ig in contrast to the situation in mammals: mechanism 2 in fig. 1) or by Fc receptor-positive K cells (mechanism 4 in fig. 1). These K cells may have receptors for either IgG or IgM [16]. Direct, antibody-independent T cell cytotoxicity may also be operative, but seems to play a minor role (mechanism 3 in fig. 1). Immune responses of B cells and the quantitative or qualitative lack of T suppressor cells in the OS is coded for by genes associated both with the *B* and a non-*B* locus.

References

1 Albini, B. and Wick, G.: Proportional increase of bursa-derived cells in chickens of the Obese strain. Nature, Lond. *249:* 653–654 (1974).

2 Allison, A. C.: Autoimmune diseases: concepts of pathogenesis and control; in Talal Autoimmunity. Genetic, immunologic, virologic and clinical aspects, pp. 91–139 (Academic Press, New York 1977).

3 Bacon, L. D.; Kite, J. H., jr., and Rose, N. R.: Immunogenetic detection of B-locus genotypes in chickens with autoimmune thyroiditis. Transplantation *16:* 591–598 (1973).

4 Busci, R. A. and Strausser, H. R.: The effect of neonatal thymectomy in the induction of experimental autoimmune thyroiditis in the rat. Experientia *28:* 194–195 (1972).

5 Clagett, J. A. and Weigle, W. O.: Roles of T and B lymphocytes in the termination of unresponsiveness to autologous thyroglobulin in mice. J. exp. Med. *135:* 643–660 (1974).

6 Clagett, J. A.; Wilson, C. B., and Weigle, W. O.: Interstitial immune complex thyroiditis in mice. J. exp. Med. *140:* 1439–1456 (1974).

7 Clinton, B. A. and Weigle, W. O.: Cellular events during the induction of experimental thyroiditis in the rabbit. J. exp. Med. *136:* 1605–1615 (1972).

8 Cole, R. K.; Kite, J. H., jr., and Witebsky, E.: Hereditary autoimmune thyroiditis in the fowl. Science *160:* 1357–1358 (1968).

9 Esquivel, P. S.; Rose, N. R., and Kong, Y.-C. M.: Induction of autoimmunity in good and poor responder mice with mouse thyroglobulin and lipopolysaccharide. J. exp. Med. *145:* 1250–1263 (1977).

10 Felix-Davies, D. and Waksman, B. H.: Passive transfer of experimental immune thyroiditis in the guinea pig. Arthritis Rheum. *4:* 416–417 (1961).

11 Flax, M. M.; Janković, B. D., and Sell, S.: Experimental allergic thyroiditis in the guinea pig. I. Relationship of delayed hypersensitivity and circulating antibodies to the development of thyroiditis. Lab. Invest. *12:* 119–129 (1963).

12 Habicht, G. S.; Chiller, J. M., and Weigle, W. O.: in Sterzl and Řiha Developmental aspects of antibody formation and structure, p. 893 (Academic Press, New York 1970).

13 Humphrey, J. H. and Keller, H. U.: in Šterzl and Řiha Developmental aspects of antibody formation and structure, p. 485 (Academic Press, New York 1970).

14 Janković, B. D.; Išvaneski, M.; Popesković, L., and Mitrović, K.: Experimental allergic thyroiditis (and parathyroiditis) in neonatally thymectomized and

bursectomized chickens. Participation of the thymus in the development of disease. Int. Archs. Allergy appl. Immun. *26:* 18–33 (1965).

15 Kofler, R. and Wick, G.: Immunofluorescent localization of thyroglobulin autoantibody producing cells in various organs of Obese strain (OS) chickens. Z. Immun Forsch. Immunobiol. *154:* 88–93 (1978).

16 Lamon, E. W.; Shaw, M. W.; Goddson, S.; Lidin, B.; Walia, A. S., and Fuson, E. W.: Antibody-dependent cell-mediated cytotoxicity in the Moloney sarcoma virus system: differential activity of IgG and IgM with different subpopulations of lymphocytes. J. exp. Med. *145:* 302–313 (1977).

17 Nakamura, R. M. and Weigle, W. O.: Passive transfer of experimental autoimmune thyroiditis from donor rabbits injected with soluble thyroglobulin without adjuvant. Int. Archs. Allergy appl. Immun. *32:* 506–520 (1967).

18 Penhale, W. J.; Farmer, A.; McKenna, R. P., and Irvine, W. J.: Spontaneous thyroiditis in thymectomized and irradiated Wistar rats. Clin. exp. Immunol. *15:* 225–236 (1973).

19 Richter, E. and Wick, G.: The nature of active and passive thyroglobulin binding lymphoid cells in Obese strain (OS) chickens. Eur. J. Immunol. *5:* 554–559 (1971).

20 Richter E. and Wick G.: Thyroglobulin binding lymphoid cells in Obese strain (OS) chickens. J. Immun. *114:* 757–761 (1975).

21 Richter, E.; Wick, G.; Zambells, N.; Ludwig, H., and Schernthaner, G.: Demonstration and characterization of thyroglobulin binding peripheral blood cells in Hashimoto patients by fluoroimmunocytoadherence (FICA). Clin. Immunol. Immunopath. *11:* 178–189 (1978).

22 Rose, N. R. and Witebsky, E.: Changes in the thyroid glands of rabbits following active immunization with rabbit thyroid extracts. J. Immun. *76:* 417–427 (1956).

23 Schauenstein, K. and Wick, G.: Local production of immunoglobulin in the thyroid gland of Obese strain (OS) chickens. Clin. exp. Immunol. *17:* 637–646 (1974).

24 Sundick, R. S. and Wick, G.: Increased ^{131}I uptake by the thyroid glands of Obese strain (OS) chickens derived from non-Protamone-supplemented hens. Clin. exp. Immunol. *18:* 127–139 (1974).

25 Vladutiu, A. O. and Rose, N. R.: Transfer of experimental autoimmune thyroiditis of the mouse by serum. J. Immun. *106:* 1139–1142 (1971).

26 Vladutiu, A. and Rose, N. R.: Autoimmune murine thyroiditis: relation to histocompatibility (H-2) type. Science *174:* 1137–1139 (1971).

27 Weigle, W. O.: The production of thyroiditis and antibody following injection of unaltered thyroglobulin without adjuvant into rabbits previously stimulated with altered thyroglobulin. J. exp. Med. *122:* 1049–1062 (1965).

28 Weigle, W. O. and Romball, C. G.: Humoral and cell-mediated immunity in experimental progressive thyroiditis in rabbits. Clin. exp. Immunol. *21:* 351–361 (1975).

29 Wick, G.: Experimental animal models in autoimmune endocrine disease. Clin. Endocr. Metab. *4:* 241–266 (1975).

30 Wick, G.: Gundolf, R., and Hala, K.: Major histocompatibility (B) antigens and spontaneous autoimmune thyroiditis in OS chickens. Folia. biol., Praha *23:* 408–411 (1977).

31 Wick, G.; Kite, J. H., jr., and Witebsky, E.: Spontaneous thyroiditis in the Obese strain of chickens. IV. The effect of thymectomy and thymo-bursectomy on the development of the disease. J. Immun. *104:* 54–62 (1970).

32 Wick, G.; Schwarz, S., and Müller, P.-U.: No development of experimental autoimmune thyroiditis in nude mice. Z. Immun Forsch. Immunobiol. *154:* 162–168 (1978).

33 Wick, G.; Sundick, R. S., and Albini, B.: Review. The Obese strain (OS) of chickens. An animal model with spontaneous autoimmune thyroiditis. Clin. Immunol. Immunopath. *3:* 272–300 (1974).

34 Wick, G.; Kite, J. H., jr.; Cole, R. K., and Witebsky, E.: Spontaneous thyroiditis in the Obese strain of chickens. III. The effect of bursectomy on the development of the disease. J. Immun. *104:* 45–54 (1970).

Dr. G. Wick, Institute for General and Experimental Pathology, University of Innsbruck Medical School, Fritz-Pregel-Strasse 3, A-6020 Innsbruck (Austria)

Immunopathology. 6th Int. Convoc. Immunol., Niagara Falls, N.Y., 1978, pp. 107–111 (Karger, Basel 1979)

Human Autoimmune Thyroid Disease

I. M. Roitt, D. Doniach and G. F. Bottazzo

Department of Immunology, Middlesex Hospital Medical School, London

It is now many years since the first reports of thyroid autoimmunity in human disease [18] and experimental animal models [19] were published.

Human thyroid disorders which are considered to have an autoimmune pathogenesis, include the goitrous and atrophic forms of thyroiditis (Hashimoto's disease and primary myxoedema respectively) and thyrotoxicosis. These diseases are closely related and may occur together in families, in pairs of identical twins and even within a given individual as evidenced by progression from Hashimoto goitre to thyroid atrophy and the frequent finding of thyroiditis in the glands of patients with Graves' disease. Several comprehensive reviews on the subject have been published (3, 7–9) and the reader is referred to these for more detailed discussion.

Thyroid Autoantigens and Their Antibodies

The antigen systems which have been recognised are listed in table I, and of these, thyroglobulin and the TSH-receptor are the only ones whose functional significance has been identified.

In the clinical immunology laboratory, antibodies to thyroglobulin and the microsomal antigen are routinely detected by the agglutination of antigen-coated erythro-cytes rather than by immunofluorescence. The haemagglutination test is altogether simpler and has been greatly improved by the introduction of turkey red cells which are stable and, because of their size, settle quickly; a further advantage is the relatively low incidence of heteroagglutinins in the general population. For diagnostic purposes it is important to include the test for microsomal antibodies since up to 30% of thyroiditis patients give positive reactions only with this antigen and fail to react with thyroglobulin (fig. 1). Antibodies to the 'second colloid' antigen do not appear to be of major significance.

There is considerable interest in the complexity of interactions with cell surface antigens. The involvement of the TSH receptor will be discussed later but, in addition, there are one or more antigens present on the surface of the thyroid cell in sufficient density to be detectable by immunofluorescent staining [11] and to make the cell susceptible to complement-dependent lysis by sera from thyroiditis patients. A correlation between the titres of cytolytic and cytoplasmic microsomal antibodies originally suggested that common antigenic specificities might be implicated [12], but this is clearly not so, since cytotoxic

Table I. Thyroid autoantigens and the most useful tests currently employed for detection of their autoantibodies

Antigen	Autoantibody test
Thyroglobulin	passive haemagglutination
Microsomal	passive haemagglutination
Cell surface	immunofluorescence on viable cells
Second colloid	immunofluorescence on fixed thyroid section
TSH receptor	radioligand binding/ adenyl cyclase stimn.

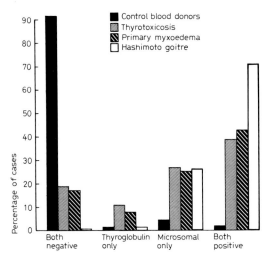

Fig. 1. Haemagglutination tests for thyroglobulin and microsomal antibodies in thyroid autoimmune disease and normal controls.

antibodies can be absorbed with a plasma membrane fraction without affecting the reaction with cytoplasmic antigens [23]. The introduction of techniques such as the separation of membrane proteins in undenatured form by isoelectric focusing in non-ionic detergents, which gives multiple bands with thyroid preparations [4], should permit more effective dissection of the antigen systems concerned in these surface reactions.

Thyrotoxicosis

The breakthrough in our understanding of the pathogenesis of Graves' disease came with the finding that injection of serum from the patients into animals led to stimulation of thyroid activity [1]. The term 'long-acting thyroid stimulator' (LATS) was introduced to describe the relatively prolonged course of this stimulation if compared to that evoked by TSH. Subsequent studies, showing that activity was confined to the IgG fraction, retained in the $F(ab')_2$ fragment and specifically absorbed by thyroid, established LATS as a thyroid autoantibody. The sim-

plest hypothesis that LATS was directly responsible for the characteristic thyroid metabolism in Graves' disease was unacceptable to many on the grounds that a significant proportion of the patients' sera were LATS-negative despite strenuous efforts to boost activity by concentrating the IgG fraction. Nearly all thyrotoxic patients have, however, IgG antibodies which block the ability of human thyroid membranes to absorb LATS activity [2]. It would, therefore, appear that antibodies to human thyroid are the rule with many, but not all, giving the cross-reaction with animal thyroids which is expressed as LATS activity.

There is considerable evidence to support the view that these antibodies stimulate the human gland: *in vitro* they stimulate colloid droplet formation and adenyl cyclase activity while *in vivo* they cause a discharge of radioiodinated material from the thyroid upon injection into euthyroid volunteers and are responsible, through the transplacental passage of IgG, for the transient symptoms of neonatal thyrotoxicosis (cf. review by *Doniach and Marshall* [7]). This stimulation of the thyroid is closely associated with the ability of the serum IgG to displace radiolabeled TSH from its receptor in the plasma membrane and it seems likely that these anti-receptor antibodies mimic the action of TSH much in the way that anti-Ig can behave like antigen in causing B-lymphocyte proliferation, and some antibodies to insulin receptors can simulate the action of the hormone itself. Furthermore, cross-reaction of the human thyroid-stimulating antibodies with receptors in other tissues might account for some of the extrathyroidal symptoms which are associated with thyrotoxicosis. However, not all the antibodies are stimulatory and indeed there is evidence that occasional sera contain immunoglobulins which inhibit the augmentation of adenyl cyclase activity induced by TSH or by other autoantibodies, a situation more reminiscent of the blocking action of the anti-receptor antibodies in myasthenia gravis and rare cases of insulin-resistant diabetes.

Yet other biological effects may be induced by antibodies directed to particular components on the cell surface. *Doniach and Marshall* [7] have postulated a growth-promoting effect of some antibodies, which is independent of functional stimulation, to account for the difference between goitrous and atrophic forms of thyroiditis, and the existence of a new variant of euthyroid Graves' disease. Preliminary evidence for effects on thyroid cells, which are distinct from those induced by TSH, has been obtained by *Philip Penfold* in our laboratory who has shown that injection into mice of IgG from the sera of thyrotoxic patients induces not only the colloid droplet formation seen after TSH, but also a dramatic dilatation of the cisternae of the rough endoplasmic reticulum.

Pathogenesis of Autoimmune Thyroiditis

It is curious that despite the multiplicity of potentially destructive immunological mechanisms which have been recognised, we are still uncertain about the precise pathogenetic events leading to loss of acinar thyroid cells in Hashimoto's disease and primary myxoedema. Probably combinations of different mechanisms will be found to operate and the variety of histological forms of thyroiditis will be seen to reflect different combinations. The complement-dependent cytotoxic antibodies offer the most direct route to tissue damage but their failure to cause discernible change on placental transfer to the fetus, or to affect explants, or collagenase-derived cell cultures suggests that cooperating factors are required. These might take the form of effectors of antibody-dependent cell-mediated cytotoxicity (ADCC) but our efforts to damage isolated thyroid cells by this mechanism *in vitro* have not been conspicuously successful and it is conceivable that the acinar basement membrane might prevent access of ADCC effectors to their target *in vivo*. Thyroid cells do become susceptible to cytotoxic antibodies after treatment with trypsin and this raises the possibility that proteolytic enzymes generated *in vivo* could provide the cooperating factor which permits complement-mediated cell killing to occur. Different immunological processes could trigger the release of such enzymes from tissue macrophages. For example, thyroglobulin is known to be released from thyroid acini under normal circumstances [6] and appropriately sensitized cytotoxic T cells

could disrupt macrophages bearing this protein on their surface. Immune aggregates, which have been demonstrated on the acinar basement membranes, could also induce lysosomal enzyme release from macrophages by reaction with the Fc receptors. It is perhaps worth noting that damage to the basement membrane in these circumstances is not a precondition for IgG cytotoxic antibodies to reach the surface of the acinar cells since we know that thyroid-stimulating antibodies are effective in normal animals, but it might facilitate access by ADCC effectors or plasma cells which are often seen in close proximity to thyroid cells to which they may bind through specific surface Ig receptors and produce cytopathic effects.

The composition of the basement membrane deposits of immunoglobulin and complement, which are most conspicuous in selected areas of glands removed for thyrotoxicosis [22], has still not been fully established. We have failed to detect thyroglobulin or microsomal antigen in these deposits using direct conjugates of the human autoantibodies; one should not exclude the possibility that, though present initially, thyroid antigens may be broken down more readily than the Ig or complement components of a complex and therefore be more difficult to demonstrate, or even that the complexes consist essentially of idiotype-anti-idiotype antibodies.

Genetic Influences

Thyroid antibodies are present in nearly half the sibs of patients with Hashimoto's disease or thyrotoxicosis [13]. The association with gastric autoimmunity in such families strongly indicates a genetic predisposition to the development of organ-specific autoimmune phenomena [16] and it is likely that this trait is linked to the 'HLA-B8-DW3 (DRw3) axis'.

A clear association between HLA-B8 and thyrotoxicosis has been established, but no such relationship was found in Hashimoto's disease although thyroiditis presenting with other autoimmune endocrine disorders does show an increased tendency to HLA-B8 [5]. It will be of particular interest to know the incidence of DRw3 in Hashimoto patients since the HLA-D locus may well provide the dominant factor which makes an individual susceptible to the development of organ-specific autoimmunity, just as the DRw4 type (rather than HLA-A, B or C locus specificities) greatly increases the risk of developing rheumatoid arthritis [21].

Autoimmune diseases are almost certainly under multifactorial control (see review by *Rose et al.* [20]) and in organ-specific autoimmune diseases there appears to be a factor which influences the selection of the target organ. Thus, although thyroid and gastric autoimmunity are frequently associated, the first-degree relatives of Hashimoto probands show more thyroid autoimmunity, whereas the converse is true in the families of patients with pernicious anaemia where gastric autoantibodies predominate. Typing for Gm allotypes would also be of interest in connection with possible linkage to different Ig variable gene repertoires.

Factors controlled by the sex-chromosomes are also implicated in the susceptibility to develop thyroid autoimmunity as evidenced by the high female to male sex ratio and the raised incidence of thyroid antibodies in patients with X-chromosome abnormalities [10]. Whether it is the sex hormone pattern or some other factor regulated by these chromosomes which exerts the critical influence on the immune system is unknown.

Conclusions

There are many exciting pathways to follow in the study of human autoimmune thyroid disease. The range of specificities covered by antibodies to cell surface components remains to be analysed, especially in relation to function. The production of EB virus stabilized clones of cells producing individual antibodies would help in this respect and would also provide reagents for the radioassay of these antibodies in patients' sera which could be of practical benefit particularly in Graves' disease.

HLA markers may help to delineate defined clinical subgroups within the thyroiditis spectrum and to segregate pathogenetically different forms of severe endocrine exophthalmos. Within families, prospective studies could be carried out to follow the evolution of the disease in terms of the onset of antibodies to surface as compared with the other thyroid antigens and to look for a possible segregation of HLA-type and some basic thyroid abnormality in different family members.

The 'state of the art' with respect to the study of regulation of lymphocyte self-reactivity has not yet advanced to a stage at which significant application to autoimmune thyroiditis patients can be made. It will be intriguing to see whether the production of prostaglandins by lymphocytes grown in contact with thyroid monolayers [14] represents a product of suppressor T-lymphocytes acting to inhibit potentially autoreactive T-helper cells.

The development of methods by which antibody responses in mice can be inhibited by antigens on thymus-independent carriers or by anti-idiotype sera has raised expectations that patients may be manipulated in a similar way. We know, for example, that the number of epitopes on even a large autoantigen such as thyroglobulin is restricted to between 2 and 4 [17] and even this number may be halved by the symmetry of the molecule. Preliminary isoelectric focusing studies by *Lynn Nye* in our laboratory suggest that the anti-thyroglobulin response is polyclonal, although the contribution made by isotypic variation to the number of spectrotypes observed has yet to be determined. It may also be that these different clones share a relatively small number of common idiotypic specificities; if so, the chances of generating a therapeutic anti-idiotypic response would be greatly improved. The sera of patients undergoing spontaneous remissions should also be examined for anti-idiotypic specificities. Other aspects of possible future developments have been discussed elsewhere [7, 9, 15].

References

1 Adams, D. D. and Purves, H. D.: Abnormal responses in the assay of thyrotropin. Proc. Univ. Otago med. Sch. *34:* 11–12 (1956).
2 Adams, D. D.; Kennedy, T. H., and Stewart, R. D. H.: Correlation between long-acting thyroid stimulator protector level and thyroid ^{131}I uptake in thyrotoxicosis. Br. med. J. *ii:* 199–201 (1974).
3 Allison, A. C.: Self-tolerance and autoimmunity in the thyroid. New Engl. J. Med. *295:* 821–827 (1976).
4 Banga, J. P.; Anderton, B. H., and Roitt, I. M.: Separation of membrane proteins in an undenatured form by isoelectric focusing. Analyt. Biochem. *89:* 348–354 (1978).
5 Bottazzo, G. F.; Cudworth, A. G.; Moul, I. J.; Doniach, D., and Festenstein, H.: Evidence for a primary autoimmune type of diabetes mellitus (type Ib). Br. med. J. *ii:* 1253–1255 (1978).
6 Daniel, P. M.; Pratt, O. E.; Roitt, I. M., and Torrigiani, G.: The release of thyroglobulin from the thyroid gland into thyroid lymphatics; the identification of thyroglobulin in the thyroid lymph and in the blood of monkeys by physical and immunological methods and its estimation by radioimmunoassay. Immunology *12:* 489–504 (1967).
7 Doniach, D. and Marshall, N. J.: Autoantibodies to the thyrotropin (TSH) receptors on thyroid epithelium and other tissues; in Talal, Autoimmunity, pp. 621–642 (Academic Press, New York 1977).
8 Doniach, D. and Roitt, I. M.: Thyroid autoallergic disease; in Gell, Coombs and Lachman, Clinical aspects of immunology; 3rd ed., pp. 1355–1386 (Blackwell, Oxford 1975).
9 Doniach, D.; Bottazzo, G. F., and Russell, R. C. G.: Goitrous autoimmune thyroiditis (Hashimoto's disease). Clin. Endocrinol. Metabol. (in press, 1979).
10 Doniach, D.; Roitt, I. M., and Polani, P. F.: Thyroid antibodies and sex-chromosome anomalies. Proc. R. Soc. Med. *61:* 278–280 (1968).
11 Fagraeus, A. and Jonsson, J.: Distribution of organ antigens over the surface of thyroid cells as examined by immunofluorescence test. Immunology *18:* 413–416 (1970).
12 Forbes, I. J.; Roitt, I. M.; Doniach, D., and Soloman, I. L.: The thyroid cytotoxic autoantibody. J. clin. Invest. *41:* 996–1006 (1962).
13 Hall, R.; Owen, S. G., and Smart, G. A.: Evidence for genetic predisposition to formation of thyroid autoantibodies. Lancet *ii:* 187–189 (1960).
14 Rapoport, B.; Pilarisetty, R. J.; Herman, E. A.; Clark, O. H., and Congco, E. G.: Production of a non-immunoglobulin thyroid stimulator by human lymphocytes during mixed culture with human thyroid cells. J. biol. Chem. *253:* 631–640 (1978).
15 Roitt, I. M.: Future prospect for research; in Miescher, Organ-specific autoimmunity, Menarini Symposium, pp. 327–334 (Schwabe, Basel 1978).
16 Roitt, I. M. and Doniach, D.: A reassessment of studies on the aggregation of thyroid autoimmunity in families of thyroiditis patients. Clin. exp. Immunol. *2:* 727–736 (1967).
17 Roitt, I. M.; Campbell, P. N., and Doniach, D.: The nature of the thyroid auto-antibodies present in patients with Hashimoto's thyroiditis (lymphadenoid goitre). Biochem. J. *69:* 248–256 (1957).
18 Roitt, I. M.; Doniach, D.; Campbell, P. N., and Hudson, R. V.: Autoantibodies in Hashimoto's disease (lymphadenoid goitre). Lancet *ii:* 820–821 (1956).
19 Rose, N. R. and Witebsky, E.: Studies on organ specificity. V. Changes in the thyroid glands of rabbits following active immunization with rabbit thyroid extracts. J. Immun. *76:* 417–427 (1956).
20 Rose, N. R.; Bacon, L. D.; Sundick, R. S.; Kong, Y. M.; Esquivel, P., and Bigazzi, R. E.: Genetic regulation in autoimmune thyroiditis; in Talal, Autoimmunity, pp. 63–87 (Academic Press, New York 1977).
21 Stastny, P.: Association of the B-cell alloantigen DRw4 with rheumatoid arthritis. New Engl. J. Med. *298:* 869–871 (1978).
22 Werner, S. C.; Wegelius, O.; Fierer, J. A., and Hsu, K. C.: Immunoglobulins (E, M; G) and complement in the connective tissues of the thyroid in Graves' disease. New Engl. J. Med. *287:* 421–425 (1972).
23 Winand, R.; Winand-Devigne, J.; Wedeleux, P.; Etienne Decerf, J., and Kohn, L. D.: Biochemical studies on thyroid cytotoxic antibodies and interest in thyroid disease. J. clin. Endocr. Metab. (in press, 1979).

Dr. I. M. Roitt, Department of Immunology, Middlesex Hospital Medical School, Arthur Stanley House, 40–50 Tottenham Street, London WIP 9PG (England)

Immunopathology. 6th Int. Convoc. Immunol., Niagara Falls, N.Y., 1978, pp. 112–116 (Karger, Basel 1979)

Experimentally Induced Chronic Active Hepatitis in Rabbits

K.-H. Meyer zum Büschenfelde, M. Manns and U. Hopf [1]

Department of Internal Medicine, Freie Universität Berlin, Klinikum Charlottenburg, Berlin

In rabbits, it is possible to induce an autoimmune hepatitis with progression to chronic active hepatitis and cirrhosis of the liver by long-term immunization with human liver-specific proteins or allogeneic altered liver-specific proteins [6, 7, 11, 12]. The liver protein fraction used for immunization in particular contained an organ-specific membrane protein [10, 14]. The importance of the liver-specific membrane protein (LSP) in terminating the natural tolerance to autologous liver antigens has been demonstrated in several experiments [11].

In recent studies, we investigated the importance of cellular and humoral immune reactions to human and rabbit membrane proteins for the induction of liver lesions and the protective effect of rabbit LSP against the experimental induction of chronic active hepatitis. To answer our questions white New-Zealand rabbits were subdivided into 6 groups and immunized as summarized in table I.

Hemagglutinating antibodies against rabbit LSP were present in all study groups

except in the unimmunized control group. The results of the skin tests showed, in agreement with our previous studies, that the termination of the natural tolerance against autologous liver-specific antigens is possible by long-term immunization with a related but different antigen. Liver lesions could be induced in all animals of group I and group IV. After termination of the natural tolerance against rabbit LSP with human LSP, liver lesions could be induced with the allogeneic (rabbit) LSP (group II). The combined immunization with human and rabbit LSP inhibited the induction of liver lesions. The combined application of xenogeneic and allogeneic LSP seemed to have a stabilizing effect on the T cell tolerance against autologous liver antigens (group III and group V). Cellular immune reaction (skin tests) against rabbit liver specific proteins correlated with the morphological changes of the liver but not with the serum antibodies.

To study the pathogenetic importance of humoral immune reactions against the plasma membrane antigen LSP in experimentally induced chronic active hepatitis, isolated hepatocytes from rabbits (group I to group VI) were investigated for membrane-

[1] We are indebted to Miss *U. Dang* for excellent technical assistance.

Table I. Immunization of rabbits

Group I (n = 10)	HLP i.p. + CFA (20 mg protein/inj.)	41 injections over 143 weeks
Group II (n = 10)	HLP i.p. + CFA	11 injections over 18 weeks followed by RLP i.p. 30 injections over 143 weeks
Group III (n = 10)	HLP + CFA like group I RLP i.p. 1 day after HLP-inj.	
Group IV (n = 18)	HLP i.p. + CFA (5 mg protein/inj.)	25 injections over 68 weeks
Group V (n = 12)	HLP + CFA like group IV RLP i.v. (aggregate-free) 1 day prior to HLP-inj.	
GroupVI (n = 5)	CFA i.p. like group I over 143 weeks	

HLP = Human liver-specific proteins; RLP = rabbit liver-specific proteins; CFA = complete Freund's adjuvant.

fixed immunoglobulins. Furthermore, the sera were studied for circulating immune complexes by a modified Raji cell technique [4].

A good correlation between membrane-fixed IgG, circulating immune complexes and anti-rabbit LSP autoantibodies could be observed. In contrast, no correlation between liver lesions and *in vivo* fixed IgG could be detected. It is therefore suggested that the experimental chronic active hepatitis is the consequence of cellular immunity against autologous liver specific antigens. The pathogenetic importance of an antibody or immune complex-mediated lymphocytotoxicity remains open [1].

Our further studies were concentrated on the characterization of the target antigen which is believed to play an essential role in the immunopathogenesis of experimental chronic active hepatitis.

LSP of different species is a macrolipoprotein present on the surface of the liver cell membrane. LSP shows a complete organ specificity and an incomplete species specificity [3]. It was isolated from fresh human liver homogenate followed by ultracentrifugation, gel filtration on Sephadex G-100,

Sephadex G-200 or Sepharose 6B [14, 15]. Isolated LSP is unstable in most buffer systems. This has hampered the early studies with LSP since it was necessary to use freshly prepared LSP. Recently, it was demonstrated that LSP is stable in a Tris buffer containing EDTA [9]. Because of its lipoprotein nature, it is difficult to determine the molecular weight of LSP by gel filtration techniques. The finding that LSP appears in the void volume of a Sepharose 4B column suggests a molecular weight of less than 20×10^6. On the other hand, the lipoprotein was excluded from Sepharose 6B, suggesting a molecular weight between 4×10^6 and 20×10^6. Lipid and apolipoprotein moieties were partly characterized after separation on Sephadex LH 20 column chromatography [5]. A chromatography of the three Sephadex LH 20 fractions shows that LSP contains large amounts of phosphatides and triglycerides. The antigenicity of LSP is dependent on its lipid content. The delipidated apolipoprotein of LSP does not react with antisera against LSP when tested by double immunodiffusion.

LSP can be subdivided into several subcomponents when polyacrylamide gel electrophoresis is performed in the presence of sodium dodecylsulphate (SDS) [9]. Five major and several minor components can be distinguished.

Further characterization of the purified LSP has been performed by affinity chromatography and by crossed-immunoelectrophoresis. Anti-human-LSP serum prepared in a sheep is able to identify two different antigeneic determinants of the human LSP. With rabbit LSP, only one of these peaks near first dimension starting point can be identified. This peak seems to represent the non-species-specific part of the human LSP complex. It is also found when pig, rat or mouse LSP is tested against the anti-human LSP serum prepared in a sheep.

The fact that with sheep and bovine LSP no reaction could be detected against the sheep anti-LSP serum indicates that the non-species-specific fraction of LSP is not identical in all species. Absorption studies with the sheep anti-human LSP serum using LSP preparations from different species supported this hypothesis. By affinity chromatography experiments using CNBr-activated Sepharose 4B columns coupled with sheep anti-human LSP serum, it was possible to isolate and purify the species-specific fraction of the LSP complex.

To characterize further the antibodies found in sera of rabbits with experimentally induced chronic active hepatitis, human and rabbit LSP purified on Sephadex G-100 columns was tested against the rabbit serum in crossed immunoelectrophoresis. Human LSP revealed at least two different precipitin peaks with rabbit serum. When rabbit LSP was tested only, a single precipitin peak could be detected near first dimension starting point in an equivalent position where the non-species-specific moiety of LSP was demonstrated in previous experiments. This autoantibody could not be detected in sera of rabbits after short-term immunization. This

autoantibody could be absorbed by rat and rabbit LSP. In tandem-crossed immunoelectrophoresis, a pattern of nonidentity was found when compared with the species-specific fraction of human LSP. It is postulated that the autoantibody found in these animals is directed against the non-species-

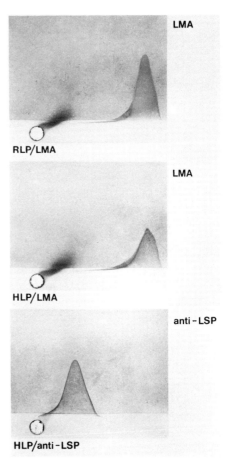

Fig. 1. Characterization of LM-Ag and LSP as two different antigens by crossed-immunoelectrophoresis. Antigens: RLP/LMA and HLP/LMA, LM-Ag purified by applying 100,000 *g* supernatants of rabbit or human liver homogenates on a LMA-coupled CNBr-activated Sepharose 4B. HLP/anti-LSP: species-specific LSP purified on anti-LSP serum coupled to CNBr-activated Sepharose 4B. Antigens were tested against the following sera, from top to bottom: LMA, LMA and anti-LSP.

specific determinant of the LSP complex [8]. These findings suggest that the break of tolerance against the non-species-specific determinant of LSP is the key reaction for the induction of experimental chronic active hepatitis.

In human autoimmune type of chronic active hepatitis, our group [2] described a liver membrane autoantibody (LMA) detected by an indirect immunofluorescence technique using isolated rabbit hepatocytes. It was of interest to study if this autoantibody has been induced in experimental chronic active hepatitis. A corresponding antigen for LMA could be purified by affinity chromatography of 100,000 g supernatants of liver homogenates on insolubilized serum of patients suffering from HB_sAg-negative, LMA-positive, chronic active hepatitis [13]. The proteins purified from human and rabbit liver homogenates, tested against γ-globulin of LMA-containing serum in crossed immunoelectrophoresis, resulted in a precipitin peak that was different from purified LSP (fig. 1). Control experiments with normal human serum and serum of patients with HB_sAg-positive, LMA-negative, chronic active hepatitis were negative. The immunological identity of the liver membrane antigen (LM-Ag) prepared from rabbit and human livers was demonstrated by tandem-crossed immunoelectrophoresis. When LM-Ag was tested against γ-globulin of rabbits with experimentally induced chronic active hepatitis, no immunoprecipitate was observed.

Summary and Conclusions

In rabbits, it is possible to induce a chronic active hepatitis by long-term immunization with human LSP. After termination of the natural tolerance against rabbit LSP with human LSP, the chronic active hepatitis can be induced by rabbit LSP. The combined immunization with human and rabbit LSP failed to induce liver lesions. As already shown in human chronic active liver diseases, membrane-fixed IgG has been detected in experimentally induced chronic active hepatitis. We conclude that experimental chronic active hepatitis is induced by the loss of tolerance to the non-species-specific determinant of the LSP complex as animals with histologically proved chronic active hepatitis show positive skin tests for rabbit LSP and bear serum autoantibodies against the non-species-specific determinant of LSP. These autoantibodies are absent in rabbit sera after short-term immunization. The liver membrane autoantibody LMA, typical for human autoimmune chronic active hepatitis, is absent in rabbit sera. Cell-mediated immunity as well as serum antibodies against the purified LSP in man are found in virus-induced and autoimmune type chronic active liver disease. Experimentally induced chronic active hepatitis more likely is a model for immune reactions found in virus-induced liver diseases of men than for chronic active hepatitis of autoimmune origin.

References

1 Hopf, U. and Meyer zum Büschenfelde, K. H.: Studies on the pathogenesis of experimental chronic active hepatitis in rabbits. II. Demonstration of immunoglobulin on isolated hepatocytes. Br. J. exp. Path. *55:* 509–513 (1974).

2 Hopf, U.; Meyer zum Büschenfelde, K. H., and Arnold, W.: Detection of a liver-membrane autoantibody in HB_sAg-negative chronic active hepatitis. New Engl. J. Med. *294:* 578–582 (1976).

3 Hopf, U.; Meyer zum Büschenfelde, K. H., and Freudenberg, J.: Liver-specific antigens of different species. II. Localization of a membrane antigen at cell surface of isolated hepatocytes. Clin. exp. Immunol. *16:* 117–124 (1974).

4 Hopf, U.; Meyer zum Büschenfelde, K. H. und Hütteroth, T. H.: Humorale Immunreaktionen an der hepatocellulären Plasmamembran bei der experimentellen chronisch-aktiven Hepatitis im Kaninchen. Klin. Wschr. *54:* 591–598 (1976).

5 Hütteroth, T. H. and Meyer zum Büschenfelde, K. H.: Clinical relevance of the liver-specific lipoprotein (LSP). Acta hepato-gastroenterol. *25:* 243–253 (1978).

6 Kössling, F. K. und Meyer zum Büschenfelde, K. H.: Zur Induktion einer aktiven chronischen Hepatitis durch heterologe lösliche Leberproteine. Virchows Arch. Abt. A Path. Anat. *345:* 365–376 (1968).

7 Kössling, F. K. und Meyer zum Büschenfelde, K. H.: Untersuchungen zur Pathogenese der aktiven chronischen Hepatitis. Z. ges. exp. Med. *153:* 150–161 (1970).

8 Manns, M.; Meyer zum Büschenfelde, K. H., and Hopf, U.: Characterization of serum-antibodies in rabbits with experimentally induced chronic active hepatitis (in preparation).

9 McFarlane, J. B.; Wojcicka, B. M.; Zucker, G. M.; Eddleston, A. L. W. F., and Williams, R.: Purification and characterization of human liver-specific membrane lipoprotein (LSP). Clin. exp. Immunol. *27:* 381–390 (1977).

10 Meyer zum Büschenfelde, K. H.: Untersuchungen über die immunbiologische Bedeutung löslicher Leberproteine. Z. ges. exp. Med. *148:* 131–163 (1968).

11 Meyer zum Büschenfelde, K. H. and Hopf, U.: Studies on the pathogenesis of experimental chronic active hepatitis in rabbits. I. Induction of the disease and protective effect of allogeneic liver specific proteins. Br. J. exp. Path. *55:* 498–508 (1974).

12 Meyer zum Büschenfelde, K. H.; Kössling, F. K., and Miescher, P. A.: Experimental chronic active hepatitis in rabbits following immunization with human liver proteins. Clin. exp. Immunol. *10:* 99–108 (1972).

13 Meyer zum Büschenfelde, K. H.; Manns, M.; Hütteroth, T. H.; Hopf, U., and Arnold, W.: LM-Ag and LSP—two different target antigens involved in the immunpathogenesis of chronic active hepatitis. Clin. exp. Immunol. (in press).

14 Meyer zum Büschenfelde, K. H. and Miescher, P. A.: Liver-specific antigens—purification and characterization. Clin. exp. Immunol. *10:* 89–102 (1972).

15 Miller, J.; Smith, M. G. M.; Mitchell, C. G.; Reed, W. O.; Eddleston, A. L. W. F., and Williams, R.: Cell-mediated immunity to a human liver-specific antigen in patients with active chronic hepatitis and primary biliary cirrhosis. Lancet *ii:* 296–297 (1972).

Dr. K.-H. Meyer zum Büschenfelde, Department of Internal Medicine, Freie Universität Berlin, Klinikum Charlottenburg, Spandauer Damm 130, D-1000 Berlin 19 (FRG)

Immunopathology. 6th Int. Convoc. Immunol., Niagara Falls, N.Y., 1978, pp. 117–122 (Karger, Basel 1979)

Immunological Renal Injury Produced by Deposition of Immune Complexes[1]

Frank J. Dixon

Research Institute of Scripps Clinic, La Jolla, Calif.

Kidney tissue is subject to injury from antibodies in several ways [2, 15]. First, antibodies specific for renal structural components can bind to their respective tissue-fixed antigens. The only target antigen of the glomerulus identified to date in man is the basement membrane, and immune responses to it can lead to a variety of anti-basement membrane diseases, including anti-glomerular basement membrane (GBM) glomerulonephritis, anti-GBM antibody-induced Goodpasture's syndrome (glomerulonephritis and pulmonary hemorrhage), and anti-tubular basement membrane (TBM) antibody-induced tubulo-interstitial nephritis. In animals, antibodies have been shown to react with the renal tubular brush border and with non-basement membrane glomerular structural elements as well. The second, more common way, in which kidneys are harmed immunologically, follows when antibodies complex with circulating nonglomerular antigens and then react adversely wherever they come to rest. For example, these circulating immune complexes can lodge in glomerular capillaries and be phagocytized by the glomerular mesangium to induce glomerulonephritis and can accumulate in tubular interstitial tissue and along the TBM to contribute to tubulo-interstitial nephritis.

The possible 'non-immunologic' initiation or perpetuation of renal disease by mediators of antibody-induced injury is an additional possibility that has attracted considerable attention. One such mediator system is complement which, in some instances, is identified in glomeruli without immunoglobulin deposits. Coagulation proteins are also thought to play a part in some forms of 'non-immune' glomerular injury associated with such conditions as systemic coagulopathies, hemolytic uremic syndrome and possibly eclampsia.

There is little reason to think that cellular immune mechanisms play an important role in glomerulonephritis, judging from histologic sampling and experimental testing. Experimental glomerulonephritis can be transferred with antibody or immune complexes alone, relegating cellular immunity to a secondary role at best. However, mononuclear leukocyte infiltration is much more prominent in tubulo-interstitial nephritis than in its glomerular analogues, and experimental studies suggest that cellular immunity may contribute to anti-TBM antibody-induced injury.

The different ways in which antibody interacts with renal tissue calls for the use of immunohistochemical (immunofluorescent, enzymatic) techniques to identify and differentiate the patterns of reactivity. Anti-basement membrane antibodies accumulate smoothly all along the basement membrane and can be shown by immunofluorescence in a characteristic linear pattern, while immune complexes which deposit irregularly from the circulation are identified in a broken, granular pattern. Methods are also available to dissociate (by elution) glomerular-bound antibodies and to identify their specificities so as to confirm the immunologic mechanisms suggested by using immunofluorescence. One can also detect anti-basement membrane antibodies and immune complexes in the circulation.

[1] Supported by United States Public Health Service Grant Al-07007 and the Elsa U. Pardee Foundation.

Experimentally Induced Immune Complex Renal Injury

Serum Sickness Models. Immune complex-induced glomerulonephritis is typified by serum sickness, and its principles have been established by study of clinical and experimental forms of this disease. Not until the 1950s were immune complexes identified as the toxic product envisioned as responsible for serum sickness by *von Pirquet* in 1911 [3–6]. To describe the course of this disease in its experimental form briefly, when a large amount of heterologous serum proteins such as bovine serum albumin (BSA) is given to a rabbit, the BSA equilibrates with the intra- and extra-vascular fluids and then circulates, disappearing slowly at its non-immune catabolic rate. Later, antibody is produced and combines with the circulating BSA to form immune complexes. As the amount of antibody increases, the immune complexes increase in size, activate complement and are eliminated rapidly from the circulation largely by fixed and circulating phagocytes. During this so-called immune elimination, small amounts of BSA in immune complex form deposit in the glomeruli (about 20 μg per total kidney weight or 4.4×10^8 molecules of antigen per glomerulus) inciting a severe but transient inflammatory response. The glomerular lesions may occur in the absence of complement and polymorphonuclear leukocytes; however, depletion of these mediators prevents the vasculitic features of acute serum sickness.

When an experimental animal's production of antibody is balanced by smaller amounts of BSA injected daily, nephrotoxic immune complexes form and can lead to widely varying forms of glomerulonephritis as judged histologically and as characterized by immune complex deposits seen in immunofluorescence and electron microscopes. Membranous glomerulonephritis, proliferative glomerulonephritis, crescent-forming glomerulonephritis, and focal mesangial proliferative glomerulonephritis all may develop in this model, but all are induced by an identical immunologic mechanism. Histology alone, then, is inadequate to identify the immunopathogenesis of a glomerulonephritic lesion. It is particularly noteworthy that the glomerular-bound immune complexes are in dynamic equilibrium with antigen and antibody from the circulation. Antigen or antibody alone binds to the glomerular-bound, immune complex. In fact, an experimentally induced antigen excess can be used to actually dissolve immune complex deposits, shortening the normal disappearance rate to less than 1 day [14]. If the immune complexes are cleared as a result of antigen excess administration before irreversible damage occurs, the nephritic process is halted and may resolve.

Various interrelated events apparently regulate glomerular deposition of immune complexes [1, 15]. For instance, large immune complexes tend to localize in the mesangium, but smaller immune complexes (around 19s) are thought to deposit along the GBM. The size of such an immune complex, and thereby its site of deposition, is governed largely by the antigen-antibody ratio and the size of the antigen. Vasoactive amines released during the immune interaction leading to immune complex formation may cause increased vascular permeability and predispose to immune complex deposition. However, the glomerular mesangium may protect the glomerular capillaries by taking up and degrading immune complexes before they can lodge in the GBM. When immune complex-induced glomerulonephritis does occur, mesangial hypertrophy and/or hyperplasia are found in the early stages. Finally, blood flow and blood pressure are among the contributors to immune complex localization. The glomerular capillary bed seems to be unique in respect to the ease with which immune complexes deposit and, in general, only when large quantities of immune complexes are available do they deposit outside the glomeruli.

Other Models of Experimental Immune Complex-Induced Glomerulonephritis. Because they resemble human immune complex-induced glomerulonephritides, several other types of immune complex-induced glomerulonephritis of animals deserve mention. Not only exogenous antigens, most often from infectious agents, but also endogenous antigens may participate in nephrotoxic immune complex formation. Viral infections, particularly when persistent, contribute to a high frequency of glomerulonephritis in animals. Mice with chronic lymphocytic choriomeningitis (LCM) virus infection can develop immune complex-induced glomerulonephritis in which anti-LCM antibody and LCM antigen complexes appear in the circulation and bound along the GBM [11]. Many other viral infections, including those with murine leukemia virus, lactic dehydrogenase virus, Aleutian disease virus, and equine infectious anemia virus, can lead to immune complex induced glomerulonephritides in which viral antigens can be identified within glomerular-bound immune complexes.

Viral infections may play a role in the systemic lupus erythematosus-like disease found in mice of the New Zealand Black (NZB) strain and of the NZB × New Zealand White (NZW) F_1 hybrid strain [8]. Mice of both strains commonly develop thymic atrophy and increased humoral antibody responses to some antigens and seem to be genetically predisposed to form antinuclear antibodies. The glomeruli, renal tubular interstitia, systemic arterioles, and choroid plexuses of these animals are involved in manifesting their immune complex disease. The immune complexes contain nuclear antigens, and the presence of native DNA-

anti-native DNA antibody-immune complexes correlates best with disease activity. In addition, viral antigens derived from C-type murine leukemia viruses have been identified in their glomeruli [16].

Endogenous antigens other than nuclear components have similarly been associated with nephritogenic immune complex formation [15]. Some examples are material in the renal tubular brush border, thyroglobulin, erythrocyte antigens and histoincompatibility antigens. The participation of renal tubular brush border antigens in immune complex-induced glomerulonephritis in rats has been described in exceptional detail. *Heymann et al.* [7] originally documented experiments in which rats repeatedly immunized with suspensions of homologous kidney eventually experienced membranous glomerulonephritis with fine granular deposits of immunoglobulin and complement along the GBM. A naturally occurring glomerulonephritis involving brush border antigens has not yet been observed in animals but has been tentatively but infrequently identified in man [9].

Immune Complex-Induced Glomerulonephritis in Man

The similarity of granular immunoglobulin deposits in humans to those in animals with experimentally induced immune complex-induced glomerulonephritis and the ever-increasing confirmation of immune complex-induced glomerulonephritis in man suggest that most, if not all, patients who are positive for granular immunoglobulin by immunofluorescence have immune complex deposits in their glomeruli. Actually, such granular deposits of immunoglobulin, usually accompanied by complement, or their electron microscopic equivalents, i.e. electron-dense deposits, are identified in upwards of 80% of glomerulonephritic kidneys. There is

Table I. Antigen-antibody systems described in human immune complex-glumerulonephritides

Exogenous antigens	Endogenous antigens	Other conditions
Iatrogenic agents	Nuclear antigens	in which antigen-
Drugs, toxoids, foreign	Thyroglobulin	antibody systems
protein	Renal tubule brush	should be identi-
Bacterial	border antigens	fiable:
Nephritogenic streptococci	Carcinoembryonic	drug-related
Staphylococcus albus	antigen	GN (prophylactic
Enterococcus	Tumor antigens	inoculations,
Salmonella typhosa	Immunoglobulin	penicillamine,
Treponema pallidum		sulfa compounds,
Diplococcus pneumoniae		trimethadione,
Parasitic		mercury, gold,
Plasmodium malariae,		heroin), bacterial
P. falciparum		endocarditis, lep-
Schistosoma mansoni		rosy, kala-azar,
Toxoplasma gondii		filarial loiasis,
Viral		dengue fever,
Hepatitis B		mumps, varicella,
Oncornavirus-related		infectious mono-
antigen		nucleosis
Measles		
Epstein-Barr virus		

no reason to assume that a single immune complex system is involved in each case. In fact, multiple antigen-antibody systems have been already identified in the complicated immune complex-induced glomerulonephritis that accompanies systemic lupus erythematosus [1]. Multiple antigen-antibody systems may be combined or appear in sequence to induce glomerular injury in individual patients.

Antigens Involved in Nephritogenic Immune Complex Formation. The causative antigens can be broadly divided into exogenous and endogenous. Exogenous antigens generally emanate from infectious agents and are the most commonly identified thus far; endogenous antigens are found in association with autoimmune disorders such as systemic lupus erythematosus or thyroiditis (table I).

Exogenous Antigens. The potential for immune complex formation lies in almost any exogenous antigenic

material such as foreign serum, toxoids, or drugs, whether therapeutic or illicit, that enters the circulation [15]. Serum sickness is, of course, the clearest example.

The aftermath of bacterial, parasitic and viral infections or infestations can be immune complex-induced glomerulonephritis, particularly when the infection is persistent. In affected individuals, antigen from the infecting agent is identifiable in glomerular immune complex deposits. Nephritogenic streptococcal infection and glomerulonephritis have a long-established association, and the latent period between infection and the onset of renal injury suggests a serum sickness type of immune response to the streptococcal infection. The results of immunofluorescence and electron microscopy used in diagnosing these patients indicate that immune complexes have deposited; moreover, streptococcal antigens have been observed in glomeruli of nephritic patients whose biopsies were obtained early in the course of the glomerulonephritis [13].

Patients are subject to immune complex-induced glomerulonephritis when an atrioventricular shunt used to treat hydrocephalus becomes infected and bacterial antigens have also been found in glomerular immune complex deposits of patients with subacute bacterial endocarditis. Pneumococcal antigens and *Salmonella typhosa* antigens have been identified in glomeruli of patients with corresponding infections. Immune complex-induced glomerulonephritides are also seen in both congenital and secondary syphilis, and immunopathologic evidence of glomerular bound anti-*Treponemal pallidum* antibody has been reported in 1 such patient. Leprosy, particularly the erythema nodosum variety, can be complicated with immune complex-induced glomerulonephritis, and there have been several reports in which circulating immune complexes have been detected. Fungal antigens have also been tentatively identified in the glomerular immune complex deposits of an individual with candidiasis.

Parasitic infections can similarly supply antigens that become part of nephritogenic immune complexes. Immune complex deposits of glomerulonephritics can contain *Plasmodium maliariae* or *Plasmodium falciparum* antigens or antibodies in patients so infected. Antigens from the infectious organism have also been identified in the congenital toxoplasmosis and in schistosomiasis of patients with immune complex-induced glomerulonephritis.

Hepatitis B antigen has been implicated both in immune complex vasculitis and glomerulonephritis, which sometimes complicates viral hepatitis. Measles antigens in glomerular immune complex deposits of patients with subacute sclerosing panencephalitis again typify the link between chronic infection and immune complex-induced glomerulonephritis. Many other viral infections are accompanied by glomerular injury, and viral antigens may be identifiable in glomerulonephritis associated with dengue fever, mumps, varicella, and infectious mononucleosis [15].

Epstein-Barr viral antigens have been identified in immune complex deposits of patients with Burkitt's lymphoma, and antibodies eluted from kidneys of these patients react with Epstein-Barr virus antigens. Recently, antigens detected by antisera reactive with feline leukemia virus have been reported in the glomerular deposits of 2 patients with acute myelocytic leukemia [12].

Endogenous Antigens. Endogenous antigens can also contribute to nephritogenic immune complex formation in man (table I). The best example is systemic lupus erythematosus, in which antibodies reactive with several nuclear components have been recovered from eluates of glomerulonephritic kidneys [1]. Nuclear antigens are seen in glomerular immune complex deposits. It has also been possible to relate quantities of circulating immune complexes with their attendant decreases in serum complement levels to the clinical course.

Another of the endogenous antigens found in human glomerulonephritis is thyroglobulin along with antithyroglobulin in immune complexes of patients with thyroiditis complicated by glomerulonephritis. In 1 such patient studied in our laboratory, two episodes of serum sickness-like glomerulonephritis occurred in conjunction with two courses of radioactive iodine therapy. This suggests that, as in experimental thyroiditis associated glomerulonephritis, radiation-induced thyroid damage can release sufficient thyroglobulin to lead to the formation of nephritogenic immune complexes.

Renal tubular antigen(s) similar to that identified as responsible for Heymann's glomerulonephritis in rats has been tentatively identified in patients with membranous glomerulonephritis in Japan and in patients with sickle cell anemia in this country [9]. Renal tubular damage due to toxic exposure or ischemia could be responsible for the induction of the immune response. A survey of several hundred patients with immune complex-induced glomerulonephritides in our laboratory has uncovered only a few questionable examples of this type of immune complex-induced glomerulonephritis.

Immune complex-induced glomerulonephritis accompanying neoplasia has now joined the list of disease states in which endogenous antigens have been identified. Carcino-embryonic antigen has been reported in glomerular immune complex deposits in 1 patient with colonic carcinoma. Anti-tumor antibodies have been eluted from immune complex deposits in neoplasm-associated glomerulonephritis. Recently, patients with renal carcinoma were reported to have immune complex-induced glomerulonephritis with renal tubular antigens in their glomeruli, and circulating cryoglobulins were found that contained a similar antigen-antibody system [10].

Detection of Circulating Immune Complexes. A new dimension in the identification and management of patients with immune complex disease is now offered by the sensitive and quantitative assays available for measuring circulating immune complexes. It is of interest that according to the methods currently being employed for this purpose, there appear to be far fewer immune complexes in the circulations of patients with primary immune complex-induced glomerulonephritis than in patients with systemic immune complex disease, such as systemic lupus erythematosus. With both Clq and Raji cell assays, most patients who have immune complex-induced glomerulonephritis that complicates systemic disease are positive, and virtually all those with active systemic lupus erythematosus show circulating immune complexes. Persons with acute primary glomerulonephritis are also frequently positive, whereas those with chronic forms of immune complex-induced glomerulonephritis such as membranous glomerulonephritis rarely have circulating immune complexes.

Little is known about possible fluctuations in levels of circulating immune complexes, but such fluctuations seem to occur and, if so, glomerulonephritis may result from recurrent brief and not easily detected bouts of immune complex deposition. The fact that many patients with primary immune complex-induced glomerulonephritis have no more reactive material detectable in their circulation than do some controls suggests that some feature of the kidney or host, possibly involving phagocytic function, may predispose to immune complex deposition in these patients. In addition to allowing one to monitor immunosuppressive therapies, quantitation of circulating immune complexes enables one to optimize the timing of transplantation so as to lessen the chances of recurrent immune complex-induced glomerulonephritis.

References

1 Cochrane, C. G. and Koffler, D.: Immune complex disease in experimental animals and man. Adv. Immunol. *16*: 185–264 (1973).
2 Dixon, F. J.: The pathogenesis of glomerulonephritis. Am. J. Med. *44*: 493–498 (1968).
3 Dixon, F. J.: The role of antigen-antibody complexes in disease. Harvey Lect. *58*: 21–52 (1963).
4 Dixon, F. J.; Feldman, J. D., and Vazquez, J.: Experimental glomerulonephritis. The pathogenesis of a laboratory model resembling the spectrum of human glomerulonephritis. J. exp. Med. *113*: 889–920 (1961).
5 Dixon, F. J.; Vazquez, J. J.; Weigle, W. O., and Cochrane, C. G.: Pathogenesis of serum sickness. Archs. Path. *65*: 18–28 (1958).
6 Germuth, F. G.: A comparative histologic and immunologic study in rabbits of induced hypersensitivity of the serum sickness type. J. exp. Med. *97*: 257–282 (1953).
7 Heymann, W.; Hackel, D. B.; Harwood, S.; Wilson, S. G. F., and Hunter, J. L. P.: Production of nephrotic syndrome in rats by Freund's adjuvants and rat kidney suspensions. Proc. Soc. exp. Biol. Med. *100*: 660–664 (1959).
8 Lambert, P. H. and Dixon, F. J.: Pathogenesis of the glomerulonephritis of NZB/W mice. J. exp. Med. *127*: 507–522 (1968).
9 Naruse, T.; Kitamura, K.; Miyakawa, Y., and Shibata, S.: Deposition of renal tubular epithelial antigen along the glomerular capillary walls of patients with membranous glomerulonephritis. J. Immun. *110*: 1163–1166 (1973).
10 Ozawa, T.; Pluss, R.; Lacher, J.; Boedecker, E.; Guggenheim, S.; Hammond, W., and McIntosh, R.: Endogenous immune complex nephropathy associated with malignancy. I. Studies on the nature and immunopathogenic significance of glomerular bound antigen and antibody, isolation and characterization of tumor specific antigen and antibody and circulating immune complexes. Q. Jl. Med. *44*: 523–541 (1975).
11 Oldstone, M. B. A. and Dixon, F. J.: Pathogenesis of chronic disease associated with persistent lymphocytic choriomeningitis viral infection. I. Relationship of antibody production to disease in neonatally infected mice. J. exp. Med. *129*: 483–505 (1969).
12 Sutherland, J. C. and Mardiney, M. R., jr.: Immune complex disease in the kidneys of lymphomaleukemia patients: the presence of an oncornavirus-related antigen. J. natn. Cancer Inst. *50*: 633–639 (1973).
13 Treser, G.; Sermar, M.; Ty, A.; Sagel, I.; Franklin, M. A., and Lange, K.: Partial characterization of antigenic streptococcal plasma membrane components in acute glomerulonephritis. J. clin. Invest. *49*: 762–768 (1970).
14 Valdes, A. J.; Senterfit, L. B.; Pollack, A. D., and Germuth, F. G.: The effect of antigen excess on chronic immune complex glomerulonephritis. Johns Hopkins med. J. *124*: 9–13 (1969).
15 Wilson, C. B. and Dixon, F. J.: Renal response to immunological injury; in Brenner and Rector, The kidney, pp. 838–940 (Saunders, Philadelphia 1976).
16 Yoshiki, T.; Mellors, R. C.; Strand, M., and August, J. T.: The viral envelope glycoprotein of murine leukemia virus and the pathogenesis of immune complex glomerulonephritis of New Zealand mice. J. exp. Med. *140*: 1011–1027 (1974).

F. J. Dixon, MD, Director, Research Institute of Scripps Clinic, La Jolla, CA 92037 (USA)

Immunopathology. 6th Int. Convoc. Immunol., Niagara Falls, N.Y., 1978, pp. 123–126 (Karger, Basel 1979)

Immunologically Mediated Tubulointerstitial Nephritis in Experimental Animals and in Man[1]

G. A. Andres, B. Albini, J. Brentjens, M. Milgrom, B. Noble, E. Ossi and C. Szymanski

Departments of Microbiology, Pathology and Medicine, School of Medicine, State University of New York at Buffalo, Buffalo, N.Y.

The possibility that there might be immunologically mediated damage directly involving renal tubles or interstitial tissue has only recently received attention. However, in the past 5 or 6 years a number of observations, made both in experimental models and human diseases, have clearly shown that such damage occurs [1, 7]. We shall briefly discuss the experimental models and present reasons for believing that similarly mediated lesions occur in man.

Tubulointerstitial (TI) Nephritis Induced by Antigen-Antibody Complexes

Experimental Models. A renal lesion that is caused predominantly by the formation of autologous immune complexes along the tubular basement membrane (TBM) has been described in rabbits injected with preparation of homologous renal tissue in adjuvant or given repeated renal allografts. Similar lesions have been recorded in rats injected with homologous kidney suspensions. The nature of the immune deposits suggests that they represent autologous immune complexes formed *in situ* between cytoplasmic antigens

released from tubular cells and antibodies coming from the circulation [6].

Recently, an experimental TI nephritis selectively involving the thick ascending limb of the loop of Henle and the distal convoluted tubules has been produced in rats by immunization with Tamm-Horsfall protein in complete Freund's adjuvant. This disease is probably induced by local formation of antigen-antibody complexes [5].

TI lesions associated with local deposition of exogenous antigen-antibody complexes may develop in the kidneys of rabbits given multiple daily injections of BSA for prolonged periods. Histologic examination shows interstitial fibrosis accumulation of mononuclear cells and neutrophils, and tubular damage. Some of the rabbits develop renal glucosuria reflecting tubular dysfunction. These TI abnormalities had not been reported in earlier studies of chronic serum sickness in rabbits. It is possible that the use of multiple daily injections, in contrast to the single daily injection given in previous experiments, may have resulted in the formation of larger amounts of complexes and/or longer persistence of critical concentration of complexes, or of different kinds of complexes with a propensity to localize in extraglomerular sites.

Human Diseases. Following descriptions in experimental models, granular TI deposits

[1] This study was supported by the United States Public Health Service Grant AI-10334 and by contract 91271 of the New York State Health Research Council.

of immunoglobulins and complement were found in man, most commonly in lupus nephritis. It appears that in about 50% of patients with lupus nephritis, tubular or interstitial deposits are present. In most of the patients, there is conspicuous interstitial fibrosis and inflammation as well as tubular cell damage, indicating that the deposits are of pathogenetic significance. Besides being found in lupus nephritis, TI deposits have been seen (although less often) in various other forms of glomerulonephritis, occasionally in renal allografts [1], and in a few patients with otherwise unexplained tubular and interstitial disease.

The functional significance of these TI lesions remains to be fully evaluated. However, several patients have been found to have renal glucosuria. Furthermore, it is highly probably that the tubular and interstitial changes can lead to renal functional impairment, as shown by the fact that in a few patients with systemic lupus erythematosus, progressive renal failure has been seen in the presence of TI lesions in the face of only mild glomerular damage. Although some of the deposits seen in man closely resemble those seen in experimental models, convincing evidence that they are, in fact, immune complexes has been obtained only in patients with lupus nephritis where the antigen (SS-DNA) has been demonstrated in deposits by immunofluorescence [3].

Interstitial deposition of Tamm-Horsfall protein has been recently reported in patients with TI nephritis. It is likely that this pathologic accumulation of Tamm-Horsfall protein results from tubular disruption with discharge of the content into the interstitium where it becomes entrapped [8]. Thus, Tamm-Horsfall protein may have pathogenetic potential and further work is needed to substantiate this hypothesis.

Accumulation of *C3* without associated IgG is occasionally found along TBM. The significance of this finding is difficult to evaluate; however, it cannot be considered as direct evidence of immune complexes. Broad, irregular deposits of C3 often are seen along proximal TBM in normal rat kidneys, and are occasionally seen in human kidneys without other compelling evidence of renal disease. One condition in which conspicuous accumulation of C3 is frequently found without associated immunoglobulins is in 'basement membrane dense deposit disease'; the nature of the deposits, however, is not known.

TI Nephritis Induced by Antibody to TBM

Experimental Models. The first form of experimentally induced antiTBM antibody disease was described by *Steblay*, who reported that guinea pigs injected with rabbit TBM preparations develop severe renal disease, characterized by linear deposits of IgG along TBM, with tubular cell damage and interstitial accumulation of mononuclear and giant cells. The evidence that the renal lesions are mediated by the anti-TBM antibodies is compelling; passive transfer of serum results not only in accumulation of immunoglobulins along TBM but in TI lesions comparable to those in actively immunized animals. Thus, despite the mononuclear nature of the interstitial infiltrate, there is no necessity to implicate delayed hypersensitivity in the damage. There is evidence that complement-dependent mechanisms are involved, but it also appears that they are not obligatory. The infiltrating leukocytes are essential since depletion of leukocytes by irradiation prior to serum transfer prevents the occurrence of the lesions. A deeper insight into the way in which these autoantibodies arise comes from recent work showing that purified anti-TBM antibody initiates the production of autoantibodies to TBM in susceptible guinea pigs which then develop severe TI nephritis

[4]. This process, that was called 'auto-immune amplification', could explain why injection of similar amounts of anti-TBM antibody into susceptible and resistant strains results in much milder disease in the latter.

Anti-TBM disease has also been induced in Brown-Norway or Lewis × Brown-Norway rats injected with suspensions of Sprague-Dawley rat kidney or with heterologous (bovine) TBM preparations. The animals develop renal disease with features similar to those of the guinea pig model. However, in some strains, the disease cannot be produced. Lewis, Wistar-Furth, and Maxx rats can produce antibodies against bovine TBM, but the antibodies do not cross-react with their own TBM, and no lesions occur. ACI, Buffalo, Wistar, and DA strains do show accumulation of anti-TBM antibodies in their kidneys, but only in minimal amounts, and they do not exhibit nephritis.

Another method of inducing the formation of anti-TBM antibodies is by transplantation of a kidney from a donor with a relevant TBM antigen (Lewis × Brown-Norway hybrid) into a strain lacking this antigen (Lewis).

Human Diseases. There is conclusive evidence that anti-TBM disease occurs in man, although only very uncommonly and almost always in association with other forms of renal disease or in allografts. One situation in which anti-TBM antibodies have been documented is in association with anti-glomerular basement membrane (GBM) antibody disease. Antibody to TBM is present in about 50% of patients with anti-GBM disease. Eluates of renal tissue have been shown to contain antibodies that react both with GBM and TBM (and sometimes with pulmonary basement membranes as well). The results of a recent study suggest that TI nephritis is most frequent and severe when both anti-GBM and anti-TBM antibodies are demonstrable and suggest that anti-TBM

antibodies contribute to the development of TI lesions [2].

Anti-TBM antibodies have been described in patients with renal allografts, and it is suggested that chronic rejection may act as a non-specific adjuvant or damages TBM so as to render it immunogenic. It was also proposed that the patients may have reacted to a foreign TBM antigen present in the allograft but not in his own kidney, as described in renal transplantation between certain strains of rats.

In the past several years, scattered reports have appeared of patients with anti-TBM antibodies and TI disease in association with what appears to be immune complex glomerular diseases. In view of the apparent rarity of anti-TBM disease, it seems that this is not a chance association, but the explanation for the phenomenon is not known. It may be appropriate to notice that antibody to GBM may develop in patients with preexisting immune complex glomerulonephritis.

Anti-TBM antibodies have also been detected in the serum of a patient with methicillin-associated interstitial nephritis [7]. A methicillin-derived antigen, as well as IgG and C3, were bound to the TBM. It was suggested that the dimethoxyphenyl-penicilloyl haptenic group, which is largely secreted by the proximal tubules, binds to the TBM and results in the formation of antibodies responsible for the disease. Lastly, of considerable interest is a patient with well docu mented anti-TBM disease without associated glomerular disease.

In summary, although lesions mediated by anti-TBM antibodies have definitely been shown to occur in man, it is obvious that this process is rare. With one known exception, anti-TBM antibodies have developed in association with other forms of renal disease. However, it is apparent that when they are formed, anti-TBM antibodies are capable of reacting with their target *in vivo* and producing TI damage.

TI Nephritis Possibly Induced by Cell-Mediated Hypersensitivity

It appears that the renal interstitium is a site where cell-mediated reaction can occur and may account for some forms of interstitial nephritis. Autologous or exogenous antigens have been implicated both in experimental animals and in man. One of the main problems in this kind of experiments is the lack of reproducibility. Recently, it has been reported that reaction with the characteristic histologic appearances of delayed reactions can be produced in the renal cortex by injection of insoluble antigens, such as heat-aggregated bovine γ-globulin, in appropriately sensitized guinea pigs [9]. Soluble antigens are generally not capable of producing such a reaction in the kidney. It has been suggested that delayed hypersensitivity plays a role in bacterial infections of the kidney or in TI nephritis developing after administration of certain drugs.

TI Nephritis Possibly Induced by Immediate Hypersensitivity of IgE-Type

Few patients with atopic diseases develop acute TI nephritis in association with manifestation of drug hypersensitivity (methicillin). Interstitial infiltration and degranulation of eosinophils are observed. Skin tests are positive. These findings are consistent with the hypothesis that immediate hypersensitivity plays a role in some forms of interstitial nephritis. Although this hypothesis is plausible, proof is lacking.

References

1 Andres, G. A. and McCluskey, R. T.: Tubular and interstitial renal disease due to immunologic mechanisms. Kidney int. *7:* 271–289 (1975).
2 Andres, G.; Brentjens, J.; Kohli, R.; Anthone, R.; Anthone, S.; Baliah, T.; Montes, M.; Mookerjee, B. K.; Prezyna, A.; Sepulveda, M.; Venuto, R., and Elwood, C.: Histologic aspects of human tubulointerstitial nephritis associated with antibodies to renal basement membranes. Kidney int. *13:* 480–491 (1978).
3 Brentjens, J. R.; Sepulveda, M.; Baliah, T.; Bentzel, C.; Erlanger, B. F.; Elwood, C.; Montes, M.; Hsu, K. C., and Andres, G. A.: Interstitial immune complex nephritis in patients with systemic lupus erythematosus. Kidney int. *7:* 342–350 (1975).
4 Hall, C. L.; Colvin, R. B.; Carey, K., and McCluskey, R. T.: Passive transfer of autoimmune disease with isologous IgG_1 and IgG_2 antibodies to the tubular basement membrane in strain XIII guinea pigs. Loss of self-tolerance induced by autoantibodies. J. exp. Med. *146:* 1246–1260 (1977).
5 Hoyer, J. R.: Autoimmune tubulointerstitial nephritis induced in rats by immunization with rat Tamm-Horsfall (TH) urinary glycoprotein (abstr.). Kidney int. *10:* 544 (1976).
6 Klassen, J.; Milgrom, F. M., and McCluskey, R. T.: Studies of the antigens involved in an immunologic renal tubular lesion in rabbits. Am. J. Path. *88:* 135–144 (1977).
7 Wilson, C. B. and Dixon, F. J.: The renal response to immunological injury; in Brenner and Rector The kidney, vol. II, p. 838–940 (Saunders, Philadelphia 1976).
8 Zager, R. A.; Cotran, R. S., and Hoyer, J. R.: Pathologic localization of Tamm-Horsfall protein in interstitial deposits in renal disease. Lab. Invest. *38:* 52–57 (1978).
9 Zwieten, M. J. van; Leber, P. D.; Bhan, A. K., and McCluskey, R. T.: Experimental cell-mediated interstitial nephritis induced with exogenous antigen. J. Immun. *118:* 589–593 (1977).

Dr. G. A. Andres, Department of Pathology, State University of New York at Buffalo, Buffalo, NY 14214 (USA)

Immunopathology. 6th Int. Convoc. Immunol., Niagara Falls, N.Y., 1978, pp. 127–131 (Karger, Basel 1979)

Immune Reactions with Antigens in or of the Glomerulus[1]

Curtis B. Wilson

Department of Immunopathology, Research Institute of Scripps Clinic, La Jolla, Calif.

Antibody deposition followed by activation of immunologic mediators (complement, polymorphonuclear leukocytes, etc.) causes most glomerulonephritides (GN) and some tubulointerstitial nephritides in man. Antibodies either react *in situ* with structural components of the kidney (or trapped foreign antigens), or they react with circulating antigens to form immune complexes (IC), which are trapped nonspecifically in the glomerulus or interstitium. Once IC deposit within the glomeruli, free antibody or antigen from the circulation may persist in interacting at these sites, continually modifying the composition of the IC. For example, one can completely dissolve glomerular IC deposits by purposely creating a state of huge antigen excess [15].

This discussion deals with the specific *in situ* immune reactions that lead to GN and tubulointerstitial nephritis [16]. Antibodies reactive with glomerular basement membrane (GBM) and tubular basement membrane (TBM) antigens are the prototype and only documented examples of such reactions in humans. Nonbasement membrane glomerular antigens and foreign antigens trapped or 'planted' in the glomerulus are identifiable in experimental animals and may have counterparts in humans.

Nephritogenic Immune Responses Involving Basement Membrane Antigens

The nephritogenicity of heterologous antikidney and anti-GBM antisera has been recognized since 1900. Such antisera given in sufficient quantities (75 μg bound/g of kidney in the rat) cause immediate GN. Smaller amounts of antibody may bind to the GBM and sensitize the host, with GN delayed until the host has produced and deposited antibodies reactive with this foreign or 'planted' antigen [11]. Heterologous anti-GBM antibodies then classically injure glomeruli by either reacting with structural antigenic determinates or by serving as 'planted' antigens.

Autoimmune responses to GBM and TBM have been induced in many species after immunization (in adjuvant) with homologous or heterologous basement membranes, or basement membrane-like materials, recovered from the urine [11, 15]. These autologous models have provided the necessary background for understanding spontane-

[1] This is publication No. 1549 from the Department of Immunopathology, Research Institute of Scripps Clinic, 10666 North Torrey Pines Road, La Jolla, California 92037. This work was supported in part by USPHS Grants AI-07007, AM-20043, AM-18626, and BRS Grant RRO-5514.

ously-occurring anti-basement membrane disease in man.

In man, anti-basement membrane antibodies cause a variety of diseases depending upon the predominant basement membrane involved [15]. GN, usually severe although sometimes mild, is generally present in these patients, about two thirds of whom have concomitant pulmonary hemorrhage with a clinical presentation of Goodpasture's syndrome. The clinical manifestations of a few patients are confined to the lung, with presentations resembling idiopathic pulmonary hemosiderosis [14]. Anti-TBM antibodies can complicate anti-GBM antibody disease or occur in association with IC-induced renal injury [15]. Anti-TBM antibodies have also developed in patients with drug toxicity, renal transplants and perhaps as a primary disease process in tubulointerstitial nephritis [15].

Anti-basement membrane antibodies produce typical linear deposits of immunoglobulin along the GBM, TBM, alveolar basement membrane (ABM), and/or occasionally choroid plexus basement membrane. Nephritis was transferred to subhuman primates with anti-GBM antibodies isolated from the sera or eluted from the kidneys [6]. Nephrotoxicity of the antibody was further demonstrated when nephritis was inadvertently transferred to renal transplants placed in patients who had residual circulating anti-GBM antibody [6, 13].

We are currently evaluating nearly 400 patients with anti-basement membrane disease identified in our laboratory since 1972. Of the first 272 patients reviewed, 65% are males and 59% developed the disease in the second and third decades of life, although patients below 10 years of age and over 70 were identified. 64% of these patients had Goodpasture's syndrome, 34% had GN alone, and the remaining few had only lung involvement. The most common presentations, either rapidly progressive GN or Good-

pasture's syndrome, often followed a preceding flu-like illness, with a few patients having arthritis as a prominant early complaint. When the presentation is Goodpasture's syndrome, the pulmonary hemorrhage and renal symptoms often begin almost simultaneously but one may precede the other by several months. Pulmonary hemorrhage is usually episodic and may be mild or severe, leading to death from hypoxia.

Diagnosis is based on classic linear deposits of IgG and less frequently IgA or IgM seen by immunofluorescence, along the basement membrane. The diagnosis is confirmed by elution study or detection of circulating anti-GBM antibody. Anti-TBM antibodies accompany anti-GBM antibodies in about 70% of patients. We have developed a radioimmunoassay for detecting circulating anti-GBM antibodies, using as an antigen the noncollagenous portion of the GBM remaining after collagenase digestion and extensive dialysis [15]. 76 of 78 patients with immunopathologic evidence of anti-GBM antibody-induced Goodpasture's syndrome, and 43 of 52 patients with anti-GBM antibody-induced nephritis alone have had detectable circulating antibodies when tested by this technique. Only 2 of 329 patients with IC nephritis were positive. Both patients developed the antibody during the course of membranous GN. Four of 56 patients with systemic lupus erythematosus had circulating anti-GBM antibody. Only 1 patient with negative renal immunofluorescence studies had anti-GBM antibodies, but this patient subsequently developed anti-GBM antibody-induced nephritis in a transplant, suggesting the inadequacy of the original immunofluorescence study.

Antibody activity estimated by percent binding of the radiolabeled antigen does not differ significantly between patients with Goodpasture's syndrome and those with GN alone. The anti-GBM antibody response is usually transient, lasting a matter of weeks or months, with only rare examples of recrudescence. No common antecedent events have been found, and only loose associations relate infectious or noxious environmental stimuli (influenza A2 infection, hydrocarbon solvent inhalation, etc.), drugs and immunologic or physical renal injury to either presentation [15]. Antigenic differences in basement membrane antigens occur between individuals. Some individuals with hereditary nephritis of the Alport's type lack the usual nephritogenic antigens in their basement membranes and may be susceptible to antibasement membrane antibody formation when transplanted with a kidney containing normal basement membrane antigens [9]. Nephrectomy has no immediate effect on levels of anti-GBM antibody activity but may hasten somewhat its eventual disappearance.

Antibodies can be found along the ABM and antibodies reactive with both ABM and GBM can be eluted from lung tissues of patients with the Goodpasture's form of the disease [5, 10]. Neither the occurrence nor severity of pulmonary hemorrhage correlates directly with the level of anti-GBM antibody detected by radio-immunoassay. In some instances, the pulmonary hemorrhage seems to be precipitated by events such as fluid overload or pulmonary or systemic infection [4]. Nephrectomy has been suggested as beneficial to patients with severe pulmonary hemorrhage of the Goodpasture's type; however, favorable responses have not been achieved uniformly [13]. Since large doses of steroids are now considered therapeutic during acute bouts of pulmonary hemorrhage, nephrectomy is considered only as a last resort.

Plasmapheresis with immunosuppression appears to enhance the disappearance of circulating anti-basement membrane antibodies [4, 7]. If treatment is instituted before irreversible renal failure occurs, beneficial effects may be noted. Plasmapheresis is also thought to have some benefit in the treatment of pulmonary hemorrhage; however, here the results are more difficult to evaluate since hermorrhages are episodic. The use of high-dose steroid therapy to control pulmonary hemorrhage coupled with improved dialysis techniques have also improved survival.

Transplantation while high levels of anti-GBM antibody persists can result in recurrent GN; however, once the anti-GBM response has subsided, clinically severe recurrence is unusual [13]. Recently, we studied a woman with Goodpasture's syndrome who received an identical twin transplant 2 years after nephrectomy and disappearance of anti-GBM antibodies. 3 months later, circulating anti-GBM antibodies reappeared with histologic and immunofluorescent evidence of recurrent anti-GBM GN. Immunosuppression and plasmapheresis reduced the quantity of antibody and retained graft function.

Other Nephritogenic Immune Responses Involving Antigens in or of the Kidney

Antigens derived from nonbasement membrane structural components of the kidney or antigens from an extra-renal source that are merely trapped or retained in various portions of the kidney can be involved in nephritogenic immune responses.

Nephritogenic Immune Responses to Nonbasement Membrane Renal Antigens. Glomerular antigens other than those of the GBM have been implicated in spontaneously occurring GN in rabbits and may be involved in human GN as well. About 5% of the New Zealand White rabbits we tested had overt GN with abnormal proteinuria; 15% more had morphologic or immunofluorescent evidence of latent GN [16, 17]. The glomerular IgG deposits are granular, with segmental confluency. Saw-tooth-like subepithelial electron-dense deposits are present but lack the typical circumscribed appearance of deposits seen in IC disease. Antibodies (circulating or eluted) from these rabbits react with nonbasement membrane glomerular constituents and the walls of small arterioles. The binding is granular as viewed by immunofluorescence, and electron microscopic studies in progress suggest interaction in the area of the epithelial cell foot processes attachment to the GBM. The reaction is not blocked by absorption using isolated GBM or actin. These observations, then indicate that non-basement membrane antigens concentrated in the walls of glomeruli and arterioles are involved in nephrotoxic immune reactions, either formed directly *in situ* or originating as circulating IC. Some human sera or eluates have rather granular reactivity with glomeruli when tested by indirect fluorescence, suggesting an immunopathogenic similarity between the spontaneous rabbit GN and some human GN. Non-basement membrane glomerular antigens have also been suggested as a cause of GN in rats given heterologous anti-renal tubular antigen antibodies [12].

Nephritogenic Immune Responses to Foreign or 'Planted' Antigens. As noted earlier, the classic example of an immune reaction involving a 'planted' antigen is the autologous phase of nephrotoxic nephritis. Anti-immunoglobulin antibodies have been identified in glomerular immune deposits in individuals with systemic lupus erythematosus, suggesting their interaction with glomerular immunoglobulin deposits [1]. *Mauer et al.* [8] described a model in which they load the glomerular mesangium with aggregated γ-globulin and then administer anti-immunoglobulin antibody. *Izui et al.* [3] suggested that DNA released by administration of bacterial lipopolysaccharide can bind to glomeruli of mice, where interaction of anti-

DNA antibody may result in *in situ* immune complex formation.

We used the lectin Concanavalin A (Con A), an extract from *Canavalia ensiformis*, to bind to the glucose and mannose of the GBM for subsequent *in situ* antibody reaction [2, 16]. Sufficient Con A was infused into the renal arteries of rats to localize $75\mu g/g$ of kidney. Rabbit anti-Con A was subsequently given intravenously. Glomerular injury ensued related to the amount of anti-Con A antibody bound (4–123 $\mu g/g$). Immunofluorescence of the perfused kidney revealed somewhat irregular but generally continuous deposits of Con A and heterologous anti-Con A antibody along the GBM accompanied by rat C3. The subsequent histologic changes included proliferative GN with polymorphonuclear leukocyte infiltration. The lesions progressed during the 5 days of observation and were accompanied by interstitial and tubular changes. Similar lesions were induced with autologous anti-Con A antibody in experiments in which rats previously sensitized to Con A had Con A perfused into their renal arteries.

The fact that material bound to the glomerular capillary wall can serve as a 'planted' antigen for *in situ* nephritogenic IC formation in rats suggests a similar potential in man. Some infectious viruses have lectin-like properties, evidenced by their ability to hemagglutinate red cells through their interaction with sialic acid. Lectin-like components have also been identified in some pathogenic bacteria.

Summary

Classically, *in situ* nephritogenic immune reactions have been considered to relate to the interaction of anti-basement membrane antibodies with their corresponding basement membrane antigens. This mechanism should now be expanded to include immune reactions with non-basement membrane glomerular antigens and 'planted' glomerular antigens as well.

References

1 Agnello, V.; Koffler, D., and Kunkel, H. G.: Immune complex systems in the nephritis of systemic lupus erythematosus. Kidney int. *3:* 90–99 (1973).

2 Golbus, S. and Wilson, C. B.: Glomerulonephritis (GN) produced by the *in situ* formation of immune complexes (IC) on the glomerular basement membrane (GBM) (abstr.). Kidney int. *12:* 513 (1977).

3 Izui, S.; Lambert, P. H., and Miescher, P. A.: *In vitro* demonstration of a particular affinity of glomerular basement membrane and collagen for DNA. A possible basis for a local formation of DNA-anti-DNA complexes in systemic lupus erythematosus. J. exp. Med. *144:* 428–443 (1976).

4 Johnson, J. P.; Whitman, W.; Briggs, W. A., and Wilson, C. B.: Plasmapheresis and immunosuppressive agents in antibasement membrane antibody-induced Goodpasture's syndrome. Am. J. Med. *65:* 354–359 (1978).

5 Koffler, D.; Sandson, J.; Carr, R., and Kunkel, H. G.: Immunologic studies concerning the pulmonary lesions in Goodpasture's syndrome. Am. J. Pathol. *54:* 293–305 (1969).

6 Lerner, R.; Glassock, R. J., and Dixon, F. J.: The role of antiglomerular basement membrane antibody in the pathogenesis of human glomerulonephritis. J. exp. Med. *126:* 989–1004 (1967).

7 Lockwood, C. M.; Rees, A. J.; Pearson, T. A.; Evans, D. J.; Peters, D. K., and Wilson, C. B.: Immunosuppression and plasma-exchange in the treatment of Goodpasture's syndrome. Lancet *i:* 711–715 (1976).

8 Mauer, S. M.; Sutherland, D. E. R.; Howard, R. J.; Fish, A. J.; Najarian, J. S., and Michael, A. F.: The glomerular mesangium. III. Acute immune mesangial injury: a new model of glomerulonephritis. J. exp. Med. *137:* 553–570 (1973).

9 McCoy, R. C.; Johnson, H. K.; Stone, W. J., and Wilson, C. B.: Variation in glomerular basement membrane antigens in hereditary nephritis (abstr.). Lab. Invest. *34:* 325–326 (1976).

10 McPhaul, J. J., jr. and Dixon, F. J.: Characterization of human antiglomerular basement membrane antibodies eluted from glomerulonephritic kidneys. J. clin. Invest. *49:* 308–317 (1970).

11 Unanue, E. R. and Dixon, F. J.: Experimental glomerulonephritis: immunologic events and pathogenetic mechanisms. Adv. Immunol. *6:* 1–90 (1967).

12 Van Damme, B. J. C.; Fleuren, G. J.; Bakker, W. W.; Vernier, R. L., and Hoedemaeker, P. J.: Experimental glomerulonephritis in the rat induced by antibodies directed against tubular antigens. V. Fixed glomerular antigens in the pathogenesis of heterologous immune complex glomerulonephritis. Lab. Invest. *38:* 502–510 (1978).

13 Wilson, C. B. and Dixon, F. J.: Anti-glomerular basement membrane antibody-induced glomerulonephritis. Kidney int. *3:* 74–89 (1973).

14 Wilson, C. B. and Dixon, F. J.: Diagnosis of immunopathologic renal disease. Editorial. Kidney int. *5:* 389–401 (1974).

15 Wilson, C. B. and Dixon, F. J.: The renal response to immunological injury; in Brenner and Rector The kidney, pp. 838–940 (Saunders, Philadelphia 1976).

16 Wilson, C. B.; Golbus, S. M.; Neale, T. J., and Woodroffe, A. J.: Nephritogenic immune responses involving antigens in or of the glomerulus. Streptococcal Diseases and the Immune Response Symp., Trinidad 1977 (Rockefeller University, New York, in press).

17 Woodroffe, A. J.; Neale, T. J., and Wilson, C. B.: Spontaneous glomerulonephritis (GN) in New Zealand White (NZW) rabbits. 7th Int. Congr. Nephrol., Montreal 1978 (abstr.).

Curtis B. Wilson, MD, Department of
Immunopathology, Research Institute of Scripps
Clinic, 10666 North Torrey Pines Road, La Jolla,
CA 92037 (USA)

Immunopathology. 6th Int. Convoc. Immunol., Niagara Falls, N.Y., 1978, pp. 132–136 (Karger, Basel 1979)

Tubular and Interstitial Renal Disease Due to Immune Complexes

J. Klassen

Departments of Medicine and Pathology, University of Calgary, Calgary, Alberta

Introduction

It is generally accepted that immune complexes can induce glomerular damage. More recently, compelling evidence has been accumulated which demonstrates that other parts of the nephron and, indeed, other organs may also be adversely affected by immune complexes [1, 13, 14]. The antigens may be of exogenous or endogenous origin as in the glomerular lesions. However, in contrast, in some forms of interstitial renal disease, the tubules also serve as the source of antigen.

Experimental Lesions Due to Locally Formed Immune Complexes

The observation that rabbits which received renal allografts developed an interstitial renal lesion in their own kidneys was the first clue suggesting that tubules could possibly be damaged by immune complexes [7]. A more reproducible lesion was then developed in rabbits by injecting them repeatedly with a suspension of homologous kidney incorporated in Freund's complete adjuvant [8]. The animals developed a progressive renal lesion characterized by extensive interstitial fibrosis, tubular degenerative changes, and sparse focal lymphocytic infiltrates and by deposition of IgG and C3 in a granular pattern along the basement membrane of proximal convoluted tubules (fig. 1). Animals with severe disease developed renal glucosuria and generalized aminoaciduria and eventually renal failure. Similar deposits could be produced *in vivo* by passive transfer of serum into normal rabbits. Further, transplantation of normal kidneys into rabbits with tubular lesions resulted in appearance of similar lesions in the graft. The immunization also induced the production of antibodies of several different specificities, including at least three kidney-specific autoantibodies. When sera from animals with the tubular lesions were layered on sections of normal rabbit kidney, binding of IgG to the cytoplasm of the proximal tubules could be demonstrated. Antibodies were eluted from kidneys with tubular lesions and labeled with fluorescein isothiocyanate [11]. The labeled eluates reacted with the corresponding antigens in the tubular deposits and also with antigens present in the cytoplasm and/or brush border of the proximal tubules (fig. 2). Similar reactions were not detected with other parts of the nephron, brain, lung, heart, liver, bowel, spleen, or muscle. The antigens appear to be soluble but may also be present in the plasma membrane but not in urine.

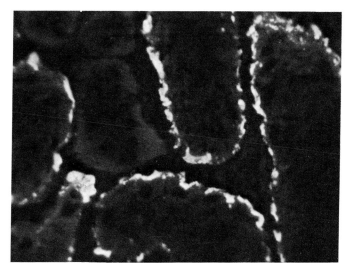

Fig. 1. Frozen section of a kidney biopsy of a rabbit with a severe tubular lesion stained with a fluorescein-labeled antiserum to IgG. Large granular deposits are seen along the basement membrane of the proximal but not of distal tubules. × 280.

The pathogenetic mechanisms of this lesion are probably as follows: as antigen 'leaks' out of the proximal tubule, it reacts with the corresponding antibody in the peritubular spaces, forming a local immune complex. It should be noted that in some animals with severe disease, the immunoreactants could no longer be detected by immunofluorescence but the lesion appeared to progress. Similar autologous immune complex tubular lesions have been produced in rats and sheep immunized with renal antigens [9].

A lesion involving the ascending thick limb of the loop of Henle, macula densa and the very earliest portion of the distal convoluted tubule has been produced in the rat by repeated injections of Tamm-Horsfall glycoprotein which is also produced by this segment of the nephron. The lesion is characterized initially by granular deposits of IgG and C3 along the basal portions of the involved tubules. Later focal tubular necrosis and marked mononuclear cell infiltration around severely involved nephrons are seen. The role of cell-mediated immunity has not been investigated.

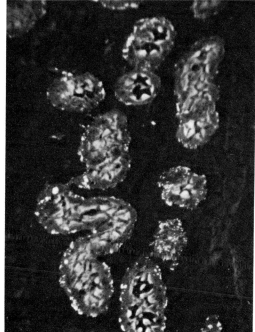

Fig. 2. Frozen section of a kidney of a rabbit with a severe tubular lesion stained with fluorescein-labeled antibodies, which had been eluted from the same kidney (fig. 1). Large granular deposits along the basement membrane of proximal tubules stain in a pattern similar to that produced with fluorescein-labeled antisera to IgG and C3. In addition, only in those tubules which have deposits, is there also staining of their brush borders. × 140.

Experimental Lesions Due to Deposition of Circulating Immune Complexes

Some rabbits, which receive multiple daily injections of bovine serum albumin, develop chronic serum sickness with deposition of circulating immune complexes in various extraglomerular sites as well as in glomeruli [3]. Deposits of IgG, C3, IgM and bovine serum albumin in Bowman's capsule, along the tubular basement membranes and around peritubular capillaries were demonstrated by immunofluorescence and corresponding electron-dense deposits were seen ultrastructurally. Accumulation of neutrophiles and mononuclear cells, interstitial fibrosis and tubular cell damage followed. There appeared to be a positive correlation between the deposits and the tubulointerstitial damage. Transient glucosuria was observed in some animals.

It is conceivable that the extraglomerular deposits occurred because the very large amounts of complexes formed saturated the usual removal mechanisms. Whether or not cell-mediated immunity played a significant pathogenetic role was not investigated. The contribution of the glomerular lesions to the interstitial and tubular damage must also be considered.

Experimental Lesions Due to Undefined Immune Mechanisms

Some rats immunized with homologous kidney incorporated in Freund's complete adjuvant develop a lesion involving the thick ascending limb of the loop of Henle and the distal convoluted tubule [9]. Staining of the basal portion of these tubules was seen. Antibodies with similar reactivity *in vitro* were present in the serum and could also be eluted from the kidney. It was hypothesized that the antigen probably was present on the cell membrane of the basal infolding of the cells, which is very marked in this segment of the nephron. A similar lesion has been seen in sheep immunized with heterologous kidney.

Human Counterparts of these Experimental Lesions

It was only after the animal models were described that similar lesions were recently observed in man. Probably in the past the deposits were overlooked or attributed to absorption droplets or to intravascular proteins. It is also possible that, as in the rabbit model of autologous immune complex disease, the immunoreactants disappear but the lesion persists or even progresses.

Tubulointerstitial deposits of immunoglobulin and complement are found in at least half of the patients with lupus nephritis [4, 10, 12]. Generally, IgG and C3 and less frequently IgM and IgA are found in granular deposits along the tubular basement membrane, and around peritubular capillaries by immunofluorescence. By electron microscopy, the deposits can be on either side of, or within, the tubular basement membrane, in the interstitium and in the walls of capillaries. The deposits may be focal, usually in the first portion of the proximal tubule, or quite widespread. In a few cases, DNA has been demonstrated in the deposits [4]. In some cases, at least, these deposits appear to make a major contribution to the interstitial fibrosis, inflammation and tubular cell damage [5]. However, in other cases with similar damage, no deposits are seen leading to the hypothesis that cell-mediated immunity may also play a role. Further, most patients also have a similar degree of glomerular involvement. Functional tubular defects have been described in some patients [17]. Cases of lupus with deposits of complexes in many organs have been described [4]. Tubulointerstitial deposits have also been infrequently seen in cases of rapidly progressive (crescentic) glomerulonephritis, membranoproliferative glomerulonephritis (especially the dense deposit disease type) membranous glomerulonephropathy and rather more commonly in glomerulonephritis associated with mixed cryoglobulins [10, 12–14].

Similar deposits have also been seen in patients who did not have glomerular lesions including several cases with idiopathic interstitial nephritis, lipoid nephrosis and Sjögren's syndrome [10, 19]. In other cases of Sjögren's syndrome, the localization of immunoglobulins appears to resemble more the lesions seen in rats, in which the basal portion of the loops of Henle and the distal convoluted tubule stain [9, 15, 16]. In many patients with Sjögren's syndrome, functional tubular defects have been described [6, 15, 16]. There is no good study of a correlation between such deposits and functional tubular defects, however. Deposits in tubular basement membranes have also been seen in renal allografts [2]. In 31 of 90 renal biopsies of renal allografts, deposits of C3 and infrequently of IgG and IgM were seen [Klassen, unpublished observations]. Deposits of Tamm-Horsfall glycoprotein [20], light chains (especially K chains) and amyloid are also seen not infrequently in the interstitium. The mechanisms whereby they induce inflammation and tubular damage have not been investigated.

As in glomerular disease due to immune complexes, in the tubulointerstitial disease only in lupus and cryoglobulinemia have the pathogenetic antigens been identified. The role of cell-mediated immunity remains to be defined. The contribution of the glomerular disease to the interstitial damage must also not be forgotten.

Since it is possible to induce an isolated immune complex-mediated lesion of the tubules, it is not surprising that similar isolated

lesions have been observed in other organs such as skin, thyroid [18] and heart and bladder [Klassen, manuscripts accepted for publication in Can. med. Ass. J. and Clin. Immunol. Immunopath.].

References

1 Andres, G. A. and McCluskey, R. T.: Tubular and interstitial renal disease due to immunologic mechanisms. Kidney int. 7: 271–289 (1975).

2 Andres, G. A.; Accinni, L.; Hsu, K. C.; Penn, I.; Porter, K. A.; Randall, J. M.; Seegal, B. C., and Starzl, T. E.: Human renal transplants. III. Immunopathologic studies. Lab. Invest. 22: 588–604 (1970).

3 Brentjens, J. R.; O'Connell, D. W.; Pawlowski, I. B., and Andres, G. A.: Extraglomerular lesions associated with deposition of circulating antigen-antibody complexes in kidneys of rabbits with chronic serum sickness. Clin. Immunol. Immunopath. 3: 112–122 (1974).

4 Brentjens, J. R.; Sepulveda, M.; Baliah, T.; Bentzel, C.; Erlanger, B. F.; Elwood, C.; Montes, M.; Hsu, K. C., and Andres, G. A.: Interstitial immune complex nephritis in patients with systemic lupus erythematosus. Kidney int. 7: 342–350 (1975).

5 Case records of the Massachusetts General Hospital case 2. New Engl. J. Med. 294: 100–105 (1976).

6 Kaltreider, H. and Talal, N.: Impaired renal acidification in Sjögren's syndrome and related disorders. Arthritis Rheum. 12: 538–547 (1969).

7 Klassen, J. and Milgrom, F.: Autoimmune concomitants of renal allografts. Transplantn Proc. 1: 605–608 (1969).

8 Klassen, J.; McCluskey, R. T., and Milgrom, F.: Nonglomerular renal disease produced in rabbits by immunization with homologous kidney. Am. J. Path. 63: 333–358 (1971).

9 Klassen, J.; Sugisaki, T.; Milgrom, F., and McCluskey, R. T.: Studies on multiple renal lesions in Heymann nephritis. Lab. Invest. 35: 577–585 (1971).

10 Klassen, J.; Andres, G. A.; Brennan, J. C., and McCluskey, R. T.: An immunologic renal tubular lesion in man. Clin. Immunol. Immunopath. 1: 69–83 (1972).

11 Klassen, J.; Milgrom, F., and McCluskey, R. T.: Studies of the antigens involved in an immunologic renal tubular lesion in rabbits. Am. J. Path. 88: 135–144 (1977).

12 Lehman, D. H.; Wilson, C. B., and Dixon, F. J.: Extraglomerular immunoglobulin deposits in human nephritis. Am. J. Med. *58:* 765–786 (1975).

13 McCluskey, R. T. and Klassen, J.: Immunologically mediated glomerular, tubular and interstitial renal disease. New Engl. J. Med. *288:* 564–570 (1973).

14 McCluskey, R. T. and Colvin, R. B.: Immunological aspects of renal tubular and interstitial diseases. Annu. Rev. Med. *29:* 191–203 (1978)

15 Pasternak, A. and Linder, E.: Renal tubular acidosis: an immunopathological study on four patients. Clin. exp. Immunol. *7:* 115–120 (1970).

16 Talal, N.; Zisman, E., and Schur, P. H.: Renal tubular acidosis, glomerulonephritis, and immunological factors in Sjögren's syndrome. Arthritis Rheum. *11:* 774–779 (1968).

17 Tu, W. H. and Shearn, M. A.: Systemic lupus erythematosus and latent renal tubular dysfunction. Ann. intern. Med. *67:* 100–107 (1967).

18 Werner, S. C.; Wegelius, O.; Fierer, J. A., and Hsu, K. C.: Immunoglobulins (E, M, G) and complement in connective tissues of the thyroid in Grave's disease. New Engl. J. Med. *287:* 421–429 (1972).

19 Winer, R. L.; Cohen, A. H.; Sawhney, A. S., and Gorman, J. T.: Sjögren's syndrome with immune-complex tubulointerstitial renal disease. Clin. Immunol. Immunopath. *8:* 494–503 (1977).

20 Zager, R. A.; Cotran, R. S., and Hoyer, J. R.: Pathologic localization of Tamm-Horsfall protein in interstitial deposits in renal disease. Lab. Invest. *38:* 52–57 (1978).

Dr. J. Klassen, Department of Laboratories, Foothills Hospital, Calgary, Alberta T2N 2T9 (Canada)

Immunopathology. 6th Int. Convoc. Immunol., Niagara Falls, N.Y., 1978, pp. 137–141 (Karger, Basel 1979)

Pathophysiology of Pemphigus[1]

Beno Michel and John R. Schiltz[2]

Division of Dermatology, Department of Medicine, Case Western Reserve University and University Hospitals of Cleveland, Cleveland, Ohio

Pemphigus is a dermatologic condition characterized by blisters which occur on a non-inflammatory base on skin and mucous membranes. Histologically, an intraepidermal split develops through the stratum granulosum in *p. foliaceus* or above the basal cell layer in *p. vulgaris* and isolated keratinocytes known as acantholytic cells are present in the blister cavity. In 1964, *Beutner and Jordan* [2] demonstrated the presence of circulating antibodies to the intercellular cement substance (ICS) of stratified squamous epithelia in the sera of pemphigus patients, and subsequently *Beutner et al.* [3] demonstrated the presence of tissue-fixed immunoglobulins to the ICS of the epidermis of these patients. Since their observations, studies have attempted to determine whether these antibodies are responsible for producing the lesions of pemphigus [8, 14, 20]. In this review, we will summarize our results from experiments in which normal human skin or epidermal cells were cultured with whole pemphigus serum or purified pemphigus IgG (PIgG).

Organ Culture Studies

Michel and Ko [12, 13] demonstrated that the histologic changes of pemphigus could be produced in normal human skin culture in the presence of whole pemphigus serum. *Schiltz and Michel* [15] later demonstrated that it was the IgG fraction from the pemphigus serum that was responsible for the tissue injury, and that complement was not required.

Light-Microscopic Observations [4, 12, 13, 15]. When normal skin was grown in normal serum or in F-10 medium containing normal IgG (NIgG) no changes were observed during the first 24 h. After 72 h, a layer of loose keratin and a new parakeratotic layer were noted (fig. 1a). Similar changes were present at 120 h, but at no time was acantholysis seen in these controls. When normal skin was grown in the presence of pemphigus serum or F-10 medium plus pemphigus IgG (PIgG) a reproducible series of events occurred. At 24 h, the ICS began to widen and a split developed above the basal cell layer. After 40 h, acantholytic cells were seen with characteristic small pyknotic nuclei surrounded by a 'halo' and an eosinophilic cytoplasm. Extensive acantholysis was present at 72 h (fig. 1b) and, at a later stage, marked epidermal necrosis was noted. These changes were shown to be antibody-concentration-dependent, and pemphigus antibody with a minimum titer of 80 was required for the histological changes to develop. This provided strong evidence for a pathogenetic role of the pemphigus antibody. Similar observations have been made by *Deng et al.* [4] using monkey skin cultured in whole pemphigus serum.

Direct Immunofluorescence Observations [4, 12, 13, 15]. Direct immunofluorescence studies using fluorescein-labelled goat anti-human immunoglobulin antibodies demonstrated the presence of tissue-fixed IgG to the ICS of normal skin cultured with PIgG, whereas IgA,

[1] Supported by National Institutes of Health Grant AM-19115.

[2] The authors gratefully acknowledge the expert technical assistance of Mr. *Robert Papay* and Mrs. *Patricia Bronson.*

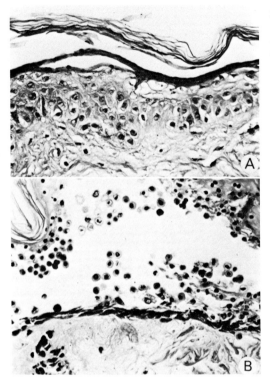

Fig. 1. Photomicrographs of normal human skin explants which had been cultured 72 h in F-10 medium containing 32 mg of normal IgG/ml (A) or 32 mg of pemphigus IgG/ml (B), the latter at an anti-ICS titer of 200. HE. × 180.

IgM, and C3 were absent. The IgG became fixed to the ICS *before* acantholysis occurred and the most intense staining was seen between 6 and 24 h. As acantholysis progressed, the fluorescence gradually decreased and at 72–120 h only residual peripheral fluorescence was seen and this was confined to the surface of the acantholytic cells.

RNA and Protein Metabolism in Pemphigus 'Lesions' [15]. Skin explants grown in F-10 + PigG or F-10 + NIgG were removed at specific intervals and pulsed for 2-hour periods (without antibodies) with ³H-uridine or ³H-amino acids, and autoradiographs were prepared to assess RNA and protein synthesis. The extent of accumulation of these radioactive macromolecules by the basal cells and *stratum Malpighii* and *stratum granulosum* cells were evaluated by counting average grains per cell. These studies demonstrated that pemphigus IgG caused a markedly reduced incorporation by the

non-basal cells by 43 h. The reduction was to less than 10% of normal IgG controls. At 67 h, a time when acantholysis was extensive, the basal cells were unaffected whereas the cells above the basal cell layer were devoid of activity. Thus, in the presence of pemphigus antibody, the suprabasilar 'target cells' gradually lost the capacity to accumulate RNA and protein and the definitive acantholytic cells were completely devoid of such activity.

Electromicroscopic Observations [1, 7, 9]. Ultrastructural studies of explants of human skin grown in PIgG [9] demonstrated that the sequence of histologic changes were identical to those which occur in the pemphigus patient. Similar observations have been reported by *Barnett et al.* [1] using monkey skin. As shown for spontaneous pemphigus [7], acantholysis began as a dissolution of the ICS in non-desmosomal areas. In later stages, the desmosomal attachments were destroyed and the tonofilaments retracted and clumped in a perinuclear position. The hemidesmosomes, which function to anchor the basal cells to the underlying basal lamina, were unaffected, leaving what is referred to as a 'row of tombstones'.

Studies Using Human Epidermal Cells in Suspension Culture [16–18]

As an alternate approach to studying the interaction of pemphigus antibodies with epidermal cells, cell suspensions were prepared by trypsinization and incubated with normal or pemphigus IgG. During 18-hour periods, PIgG became bound to individual cells (immunofluorescence) and caused the killing of 75% of the cells (trypan blue exclusion) as compared to only 14% in NIgG control cultures. Radioactive tracer studies were employed to evaluate the effects of NIgG or PIgG on the ability of epidermal cells to accumulate newly synthesized proteins. Following incubation with mixtures of ³H-amino acids, a simple fractionation scheme was devised which separated the labelled proteins into 3 fractions: (1) the medium fraction, as prepared by centrifugation; (2) the intracellular, water-soluble, fraction as prepared by several cycles of freezing/thawing of the cell pellet, and (3) the remaining water-insoluble fraction. Using this system it was demonstrated that relative to the NIgG controls, PIgG inhibited the accumulation of newly synthesized proteins by nearly 60%. Furthermore, PIgG caused a shift in the distribution of the newly-synthesized proteins from the insoluble cellular fraction to the medium. In the normal IgG-treated cultures 44% of the labelled proteins were recovered in the insoluble fraction and 42% in the medium. In the PIgG-treated cultures, 14% were recovered in the insoluble fraction and 76% in the medium. Since no significant changes occurred in the intracellular, water-soluble fraction, we assumed that the increased radioactivity in the medium of PIgG-treated cells was derived from the cell-associated insoluble fraction. It was further shown that the inhibition of protein accumulation and the shift in partitioning from an insoluble to soluble fraction was dependent upon antibody concentration. Maximal effects occurred at a pemphigus antibody titer of 150, and no effects were seen at titers below 50.

K inetic experiments demonstrated that in the presence of NIgG, proteins continued to accumulate during a 4-hour incubation period. The cell-associated, insoluble fraction accumulated linearly until it accounted for about 33% of the total proteins at 2 h. However, in the presence of PIgG (antibody titer of 150) protein accumulation ceased after $1\frac{1}{2}$ h and at 2 h the cell-associated, insoluble fraction was similar to the controls (approximately 38%). Beginning at 2 h, however, a rapid loss of insoluble labelled protein began to occur in the PIgG-treated cultures and in 1 h 70% of this preformed material was lost into the medium. These data suggested that the solubilization resulted from enzymatic digestion in the pemphigus antibody-treated cultures.

Enzyme Hydrolase Studies [17, 18]

We reasoned that if the solubilization of the insoluble material which occurred in the presence of PIgG was due to enzymes released by the keratinocytes, these enzymes might be recovered in the medium. Consequently, we assayed the medium for standard lysosomal hydrolases (β-glucuronidase, aryl sulfatase, and acid phosphatase) and for the non-lysosomal cytoplasmic enzyme leucine aminopeptidase. We could not detect such activity due to lack of sensitivity of the assays. Therefore, a more sensitive assay was developed which was based on the ability of enzyme hydrolases to solubilize a ^{3}H-labelled substrate prepared from epidermal cells. The assay was developed using the enzymes extracted from the normal human epidermis. These enzymes had broad pH optima between 4.5 and 6.5, the activity could be destroyed by boiling 15 min and nearly 70% of the solubilized radioactive material was dialyzable. Using this approach, the medium from epidermal cell suspensions or whole epidermis which had been cultured with NIgG or PIgG were assayed for enzyme activity at various pH values. The results demonstrated that in the medium of epidermal cultures containing PIgG, a large peak of enzyme activity occurred between pH 6 and 6.5 (fig. 2). This activity was not present in

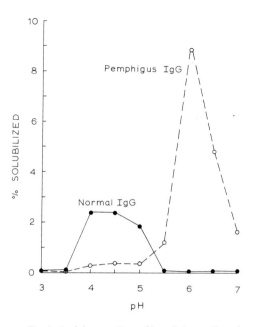

Fig. 2. Activity-vs-pH profiles of the medium from whole epidermis which had been incubated for 48 h with normal IgG or pemphigus IgG (24 mg/ml antibody protein, pemphigus anti-ICS, titer 160). The ordinate represents the percent of a ^{3}H-labeled protein substrate which was solubilized during the assay.

the medium of epidermis cultured with NIgG. Furthermore, the intracellular enzymes had lower pH optima (presumably of lysosomal origin) and the pH profiles were similar for both cultures. We interpreted these results to suggest that PIgG caused the release, synthesis or activation of an enzyme(s) with pH optimum of 6–6.5. We propose that it is this enzyme(s) which is responsible for the observed solubilization of labelled epidermal cell material.

Discussion

The demonstration that patients with pemphigus have tissue-fixed and circulating antibodies to epidermis represented a major advance in the diagnosis and understanding of this disease. To ascribe pathogenicity to these antibodies, it was necessary to determine that they could produce the histologic changes of pemphigus. Organ culture studies have provided this evidence. Pemphigus IgG became bound to the 'target cells' in the epidermis and typical acantholytic changes developed. Furthermore, the damage occurred in the absence of complement. In view of the well documented observations by *Jordan et al.* [10, 11] that products of complement activation can be found in the blister fluid from pemphigus patients and that C3, C1q, C3PA, and properdin are deposited in the area of blister formation, the exact role of complement in pemphigus *in vivo* remains to be established. Autoradiographic studies showed that RNA and protein accumulation in the keratinocytes above the basal cells was inhibited and ultrastructural studies confirmed that the changes produced in culture are identical to those observed in the spontaneous disease. Cell suspension studies further demonstrated that PIgG-inhibited protein accumulation and caused a shift from cell-associated insoluble proteins to soluble proteins and that the effect was antibody concentration and time-dependent.

Evidence has been presented that in the presence of PIgG, keratinocytes release, or activiate an enzyme(s) capable of solubilizing labelled insoluble epidermal material. This is not a new concept since several earlier studies suggested a possible role for enzymes in pemphigus [18]. More recently, *Farb et al.* [5, 6] using cultured monolayers of mouse epidermal cells, showed that pemphigus serum caused these cells to become less adherent to the culture dish. Since the effect was prevented by soybean trypsin inhibitor (STI), they postulated that this effect, as well as pemphigus acantholysis, was caused by the pemphigus antibody-induced release of a neutral proteinase. However, in recent experiments, we tested STI to determine whether this compound would prevent antibody-induced acantholysis in organ cultured skin, and found that the acantholysis was entirely unaffected [19].

Based on organ culture and cell suspension studies, we propose the following hypothesis to account for the pathogenesis of pemphigus acantholysis. According to this hypothesis, the pemphigus antibody plays a pivotal role. The antibody binds to the epidermal cell surface, produces a loss of integrity of the cell surface, and leads to a cessation of RNA and protein synthesis. This results in cell death, and during the process, the cells respond by a release or activation of hydrolytic enzymes. This process of autolysis results in the production of the characteristic histologic changes of pemphigus and the acantholytic cell.

References

1 Barnett, L. M.; Beutner, E. H., and Chorzelski, T.P.: Organ culture studies of pemphigus antibodies. 2. Ultrastructural comparison between acantholytic changes *in vitro* and human pemphigus lesions. J. invest. Derm. *68:* 265–271 (1977).
2 Beutner, E. and Jordon, R.: Demonstration of skin antibodies in sera of pemphigus vulgaris patients by indirect immunofluorescent staining. Proc. Soc. exp. Biol. Med. *117:* 505–510 (1964).
3 Beutner, E.; Lever, W.; Witebsky, E.; Jordan, R., and Chertock, B.: Autoantibodies in pemphigus vulgaris: response to an intercellular substance of epidermis. J. Am. med. Ass. *192:* 682–688 (1965).
4 Deng, J. S.; Beutner, E. H., and Shu, S.: Organ culture studies of pemphigus antibodies. 1. Studies of antigen stability in explants of normal monkey skin and kinetics of acantholytic changes. Archs Derm. *113:* 923–926 (1977).
5 Farb, R.; Fountain, E.; Yost, F., and Lazarus, G.: Molecular model for the induction of acantholysis in pemphigus vulgaris (abstr.). Clin. Res. *25:* 281A (1977).
6 Farb, M. R.; Dykes, R., and Lazarus, G. S.: Anti-epidermal-cell-surface pemphigus antibody detaches viable epidermal cells from culture plates by activation of proteinase. Proc. natn. Acad. Sci. USA *76:* 459–463 (1978).
7 Hashimoto, K. and Lever, W.: An electron microscopic study of pemphigus vulgaris of the mouth and the skin with special reference to the intercellular cement. J. invest. Derm. *48:* 540–552 (1967).

8 Holubar, K.; Chorzelski, T. P.; Gauto, M., and Beutner, E. H.: Studies in immunodermatology. 3. Induction of intraepithelial lesions in monkey by intramucosal injection of pemphigus antibodies. Int. Archs Allergy appl. Immun. *44:* 631–643 (1973).

9 Hu, C. H.; Schiltz, J. R., and Michel B.: Pemphigus autoantibody-induced *in vitro* suprabasilar acantholysis: a unique phenomenon of epidermal injury. Am. J. Path. *90:* 345–362 (1978).

10 Jordon, R. E.; Day, N. K.; Luckasen, J. R., and Good, R. A.: Complement activation in pemphigus vulgaris blister fluid. Clin. exp. Immunol. *115:* 53–56 (1973).

11 Jordon, R. E.; Schroeder, A. L.; Rogers, R. S., II, and Perry, H. O.: Classical and alternate pathway activation of complement in pemphigus vulgaris lesions. J. invest. Derm. *63:* 256–259 (1974).

12 Michel, B. and Ko, C. S.: Effect of pemphigus and bullous pemphigoid sera and leukocytes on normal skin in organ culture: an *in vitro* model for the study of bullous diseases (abstr.). J. invest. Derm. *62:* 541 (1974).

13 Michel, B. and Ko, C. S.: An organ culture model for the study of pemphigus acantholysis. Br. J. Derm. *96:* 295–302 (1977).

14 Sams, W. M., jr. and Jordon, R. E.: Pemphigus antibodies: their role in disease. J. invest. Derm. *56:* 474–479 (1971).

15 Schiltz, J. R. and Michel, B.: Production of epidermal acantholysis in human skin *in vitro* by the IgG fraction from pemphigus serum. J. invest. Derm. *67:* 254–260 (1976).

16 Schiltz, J. R. and Michel, B.: Effect of pemphigus autoantibodies on human epidermal cells in organ or suspension culture (abstr.). J. invest. Derm. *66:* 279 (1976).

17 Schiltz, J. R. and Michel B.: Pemphigus autoantibody interaction with human epidermal cells in culture. A proposed mechanism for pemphigus acantholysis (abstr.). J. invest. Derm. *70:* 212 (1978).

18 Schiltz, J. R. and Michel, B.: Effects of the pemphigus autoantibody on human epidermal cells in suspension culture; a proposed mechanism for pemphigus acantholysis. J. clin. Invest. *62:* 772–788 (1978).

19 Schiltz, J. R.; Hu, C. H., and Michel, B.: Steroids, aurothioglucose and soybean trypsin inhibitor do not prevent pemphigus-induced acantholysis *in vitro.* Br. J. Derm. (in press, 1979).

20 Wood, J. W.; Beutner, E. H., and Chorzelski, T. P.: Studies in immunodermatology. II. Production of pemphigus-like lesions by epidermal injection of monkeys with Brazilian pemphigus foliaceus serum. Int. Archs Allergy appl. Immun. *42:* 556–564 (1972).

Dr. B. Michel, Division of Dermatology, Department of Medicine, Case Western Reserve University, and University Hospitals of Cleveland, Cleveland, OH 44106 (USA)

Immunopathology. 6th Int. Convoc. Immunol., Niagara Falls, N.Y., 1978, pp. 142–147 (Karger, Basel 1979)

A Unified Concept of Autoimmunity and the Nature of Stratum Corneum Antigen (SCAg) Conversion Phenomenon[1]

Ernst H. Beutner, Stefania Jablonska, Tadeusz P. Chorzelski and Walter L. Binder

Departments of Microbiology and Dermatology, State University of New York at Buffalo, Medical and Dental Schools, Buffalo, New York, and Department of Dermatology, Warsaw School of Medicine, Warsaw

Introduction

The three major areas of research on the nature and cause of psoriasis that have appeared in the literature are: (a) histopathologic studies on the skin lesions; (b) epidemiologic and genetic studies on predisposing factors (including HLA typing), and (c) biochemical studies on the hyperproliferative responses which characterize psoriatic lesions. This report as well as the following one deal with a fourth area of research, notably the immunopathology of the disease as it relates to reactions of stratum corneum antibodies (SCAb). The *in vivo* reactions of SCAb relate to the above-mentioned three areas of research as follows: (a) They may, to some extent, be determined by the epidemiologic and genetic factors which predispose to psoriasis. (b) They appear to precede the hyperproliferative responses and the changes in biochemical activities. (c) They are consistent with the types of histopathologic changes which are stressed in many of the current studies of the subject. In brief, SCAb are a group of physiologic autoantibodies whose *in vivo* reaction results from alterations in the stratum corneum (SC).

[1] Supported by grants from the Summerhill Foundation and the Polish Academy of Science (10.5) and by fellowships from the National Psoriasis Foundation and from a NIH Training Grant (501580E).

The Nature of Autoimmunity: a Unified Concept

The ambient concepts of autoimmunity deal with it either as a pathologic or a physiologic process. None but a unified concept deal adequately with both extremes. It may be stated simply as follows. If one considers all forms of autoimmunity from the viewpoint of their effects on their producer, they can be classified into a spectrum ranging from purely physiologic, to intermediate, and to unequivocally pathologic responses. These effects of autoimmune responses depend, in large part, on the accessibility of their antigens to *in vivo* reactions. In part, they also depend on the nature and effects of the *in vivo* reaction on the producer of autoimmunity. Three groups of etiologic factors can be distinguished [2]: (a) the etiology of the *in vivo* reactions of 'physiologic' autoantibodies entails a normal immune response and the appearance of an altered or abnormal self. The etiology of 'pathologic' autoimmunity may be attributable either to (b) abnormal T and B cell function (including T suppressor cell function), or to (c) abnormal antigenic stimuli interacting with a normal immune system. Various combinations of these three etiologic mechanisms come into play in various forms of autoimmunity. A clear distinction between these three etiologic mechanisms aids greatly in clarifying such major medical problems as the role of altered antigens in eliciting rheumatoid factor production [18].

Physiologic autoimmune responses are directed to antigens which are normally absent (novel antigens) or hidden by molecules on their surface or by their anatomical location or by some combination of these factors. These autoimmune responses are common or universal events. According to the 'transporteur' theory of *Grabar* [12], they aid in the removal of damaged, altered, senescent or novel tissue antigens which are not adequately degraded by autolytic enzymes. It is of little value to gaining an understanding of pathologic auto-immunity, and there is, at present, little hard evidence that common physiologic autoimmune responses actually do play a protective role. From the viewpoint of the unified concept, responses identified as being of the physiologic type need to be studied primarily in terms of the nature of and natural occurrence of the auto-antigens since the autoantibody production is a normal response.

Pathologic autoimmune responses tend to be directed to antigens which, in *normal* tissue, are present in forms which are, at least in part, accessible to the actors of immune response. These autoimmune responses tend to be rare events, presumably in consequence of antigenic suppression of the T cell (low dose) and B cell (high dose) function. According to the *horror autotoxicus* concept of *Ehrlich* [10] and its various latter-day variants, notably *Burnet*'s [8] 'forbidden clone theory', and present-day concepts on losses of T suppressor cell functions, auto-immunity should be regarded as an abnormal and therefore pathologic process. These concepts are of interest in studies of autoimmunity in pemphigus and certain other diseases considered in this book. They focus attention on possible etiologies of the autoimmune responses. They tend to be misleading in considering universal autoimmune responses such as those to SCAb which entail a different set of etiologic mechanisms [2].

Methods and Materials

Direct and indirect immunofluorescent (IF) studies, if carried out under defined conditions, can yield findings that are reproducible. The reproducibility of the authors' IF findings is borne out by subsequent reports on IF studies on SCAb [3, 4]. IF findings correlate with the earlier and more extensive studies of SCAb reaction by red cell labeling methods [15]. However, it has not as yet been possible to reproduce the latter methods. Direct IF tests reveal Ig, C and fibrin deposits in lesions.

Indirect IF (IIF) and complement IIF tests, using normal human skin as antigenic substrate, serve to detect circulating SCAb.

Results

Studies on SCAb. Indirect IF staining tests as well as complement IIF staining with normal human sera containing SCAb performed on sections of normal, non-volar skin show reactions in the stratum granulosum

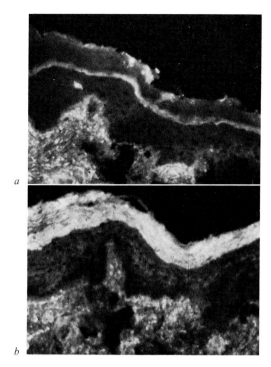

Fig. 1. a Frozen section of normal human skin (4μm) treated with phosphate-buffered saline (PBS) followed by ⅛ U/ml of an anti-human IgG conjugate with a molar F/P ratio of 2.9. Note negative reaction in SC and nonspecific staining of stratum granulosum. The latter is due to the high F/P ratio of the conjugate. × 300. *b* Skin section as above, treated with a 1 : 10 dilution of a normal human human serum with a SCAb titer of 40 followed by the same conjugate as above. Note strongly positive (3 +) IF staining throughout the SC. × 300.

and SC (fig. 1a, b) [3]. A comparable distribution of complement-fixing SCAb had been demonstrated in original immune adherence studies of *Krogh and Tönder* [16] and in the extensive studies carried out in this and other red cell labeling studies which had been reported by this group prior to the initiation of our IF studies of this system.

The results obtained variously by red blood cell (RBC) labeling and IF labeling methods of studying SCAb may be summarized as follows:

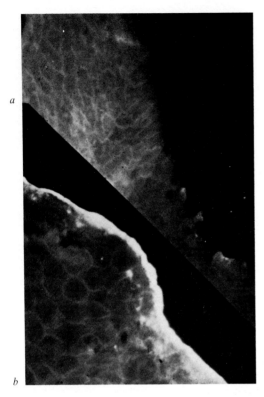

Fig. 2. a Frozen section of normal human callus (4μm) soaked for 24 h in a 1: 16 dilution of normal human serum (SCAb titer of 20) that had been *absorbed* with homogenized callus. The callus was sectioned and stained by direct IF with ¼ U/ml of an anti-human IgG conjugate with a molar F/P ratio of 1.2. Note negative IF reaction at the cut edge. × 600. b Section of a callus comparable to the one above, soaked for 24 h in a 1: 16 dilution of the same normal human serum that was unabsorbed. The callus was rinsed, sectioned and stained as above. Note the strongly positive IF stain (3+) at the cut edge of the callus. × 600.

(1) SCAb fulfill the definition of true autoantibodies (RBC and IF methods) [3, 16].

(2) SCAb are of the IgG and/or IgM class (RBC and IF methods) [3, 16].

(3) SCAb occur in virtually all human sera (RBC and IF methods) [3, 16].

(4) The SCAg include proteins (RBC and

IF methods) [3, 16] and polysaccharides (RBC methods) [16]. The latter appear to include an α6-linked glucose determinant.

(5) Though SCAb are true autoantibodies they fail to bind *in vivo* or in organ cultures of skin to normal SC (IF methods) (fig. 1a, b) [5].

(6) Mechanical trauma of the SC converts the SC antigens from a non-reactive form to a form which is reactive both *in vivo* and in culture (IF methods) (fig. 2a, b).

(7) SCAb appear to react *in vivo* with the SC of virtually all psoriatic lesions and in some but not all lesions of other dermatoses (RBC and IF methods) [3, 16].

While the indirect IF staining and other *in vitro* serologic tests with SCAb (points 1 and 2 above) give reactions comparable to those of pemphigus antibodies and certain other disease-specific autoantibodies to the skin, the properties of SCAb listed as points 3 and 4 above serve to identify them as physiologic autoimmune responses. In contrast to the SCAb, pemphigus antibodies react with their antigens in normal skin *in vivo* [1] and as indicated by one of the papers in this symposium [17] also in culture. This, together with the other properties of pemphigus antibodies [2] serve to identify it as a pathologic autoimmune response. This and the following report afford, respectively, indirect and direct evidence which indicates that the *in vivo* reactions of SCAb occur not only under certain 'normal' conditions but also that more extensive binding of SCAb precedes the development of the earliest detectible histologic or clinical signs which are characteristic of psoriasis. This report stresses the observations which lead to the conclusion that trauma converts SC antigens from a non-reactive to a reactive form and the relation of this '*SCAg conversion phenomenon*' to the events which precede and appear to lead up to the earliest detectible changes of typical psoriatic lesions.

Experimental Evidence for the Existence of the SCAg Conversion Phenomenon. Three lines of evidence indicate that trauma of the SC caused by cutting, scratching, or scraping changes it from its normal, non-reactive form to a form which can bind SCAb either *in vivo* or in culture. Preliminary studies with proteolytic enzymes suggest that they can enhance this conversion phenomenon. The following five lines of evidence point to the existence of the SCAg conversion phenomenon.

(1) The failure of normal, intact SCAg to react *in vivo* is apparent not only from the negative IF reactions obtained in staining frozen sections of normal skin for bound IgG but also from the fact that free circulating SCAb coexist with intact SC.

(2) Tissue culture studies of normal skin explants reveal that SCAb fail to bind to SCAg even if the explants are bathed in serum containing elevated SCAb titers (i.e. 40–80) while explants grown in sera with comparable titers of pemphigus antibodies bind them in 4–24 h. The presence of SCAg in the explants is demonstrable by cutting frozen sections of them and performing indirect IF staining reactions with the same serum in which the explants are grown.

(3) Cuts or scratches of explants convert the SCAg to a form which does bind SCAb in culture.

(4) SCAg of volar SC does not react with SCAb of most sera in indirect IF staining technique. However, binding does occur at cut edges of the volar SC in tests of sera with elevated titers of SCAb. The immunologic specificity of this IF staining for SCAb is borne out by absorption with callus homogenates (fig. 2a, b).

(5) Soaking pieces of callus in trypsin (1 mg/ml) for varying periods of time and then testing for indirect IF staining of the cut edges with SCAb revealed that 4 h of the enzyme treatment markedly increased the intensity of the reaction while 24 h of this treatment decreased or abolished the SCAb reactivity.

Three mechanisms may be implicated in the failure of SCAb to bind *in vivo* with intact SCAg: (1) biochemical sequestration; (2) physical blocking by lipids, and (3) anatomical sequestration.

Evidence for a Role of the SCAg Conversion Phenomenon in the Koebner Phenomenon. The following six observations lend support to the interpretation that abnormally extensive SCAg conversion triggers the development of psoriatic lesions.

(1) *Krogh and Tönder* [16] reported a decrease in SCAb titers during active phases of psoriasis.

(2) *Farber et al.* [11] observed that patients in whom the Koebner phenomenon (or the 'isomorphic reaction' as they call it) is provoked by a cut parallel to the skin surface develop psoriasis at the site of *entry* of the knife into the skin. *Bizzozero* [7] reported similar findings. *Jablonska* [unpublished results] finds that 'stripping' of the SC provokes psoriasis at the edge of the stripped area.

(3) *Comaish et al.* [9] reported that treatment of scratches with paraffin oil inhibits the development of Koebner reactions in patients with active psoriasis. *Binder* [6] found that treatment of skin explants with paraffin oil after scratching inhibits the SCAg conversion.

(4) Organ specificity studies of SCAb reveal that SCAg-like substances occur not only in the skin but also in various mucous membranes, including those of the oral cavity, the esophagus, and the conjunctiva.

(5) If indeed SCAb play the suggested role in the development of psoriasis, then patients with hypo- (or a-) gammaglobulinemia should be free of psoriasis. Surveys of four centers which specialize in studies of such patients have failed to reveal a single case of psoriasis [6].

(6) One report has appeared on a set of twins in Sweden both of whom had hypogammaglobulinemia and psoriasis [6]. *Binder et al.* [5] showed that direct IF studies of a psoriatic lesion of one of these patients yielded typical IgG and C deposits on the SCAg sites and that the serum contained detectable SCAb.

These six observations suggest that an abnormally strong SCAg conversion phenomenon leads to the clinical manifestations of the Koebner phenomenon.

Studies on Autoreactive Cell-mediated Immune Responses in Psoriasis. Several reports deal with the suppression of T cells in active psoriasis [13, 19]. The relation of this response to humoral factor(s) is detailed in the following report [14].

If we define an autoreactive cell-mediated immune (CMI) response as immunologically specific reactions with autologous antigens demonstrable by accepted *in vitro* and/or *in vivo* tests for CMI, then none such have as yet been reported to be associated with psoriasis. Until and unless such reports appear, the role of autoreactive CMI in this disease lies in the realm of science fiction.

The available data suggest that the observed suppression of T cells is a secondary phenomenon and that it is not associated with autoreactive CMI.

Summary

The unified concept of autoimmunity distinguishes between the pathologic and physiologic types on the basis of the effects of the immune responses on their producer. Three distinct etiologies of *in vivo* reactions are differentiated. *In vivo* reactions of physiologic forms of autoimmunity are caused by alterations in autologous antigens. The *in vivo* reactions of pathologic forms of autoimmunity which are directed to normal tissue components are caused by the abnormal immune responses. These may be due either to abnormal antigenic stimuli or the abnormal function of T and B cells or a combination of the two.

Stratum corneum (SC) antibodies are an example of a physiologic autoimmune response. Trauma converts the SC from a non-reactive to a reactive form that permits SC antibodies to bind *in vivo*, fix complement and attract leucocytes. It is postulated that their normal function is to aid in the removal of damaged SC components. The observations reviewed suggest that abnormally reactive SC antigens may be the underlying cause of psoriasis.

References

1 Beutner, E. H. and Chorzelski, T. P.: Studies on etiologic factors in pemphigus. J. cutan. Path. *3:* 67–74 (1976).

2 Beutner, E. H.; Chorzelski, T. P., and Binder, W. L.: Nature of autoimmunity: pathologic versus physiologic responses and a unifying concept; in Beutner, Chorzelski and Bean Immunopathology of the skin; 2nd ed., pp. 147–180 (Wiley & Sons, New York 1979).

3 Beutner, E. H.; Chorzelski, T. P., and Jablonska, S.: Autoimmunity in psoriasis. I. Studies on the possible significance of the universal stratum corneum antibodies in the pathogenesis of psoriasis; in Farber and Cox Psoriasis: Proc. 2nd Int. Symp. (Yorke Medical Books, New York 1977).

4 Beutner, E. H.; Jablonska, S.; Bean, S.; Shu, S., and Saikia, N.: Autoimmunity in psoriasis: an extended four compartment test with complement immunofluorescence (abstr.). J. invest. Derm. *64:* 298 (1975).

5 Binder, W. L.; Beutner, E. H., and Jablonska, S.: Comparisons of sites of psoriatic lesions, tissue distribution of stratum corneum (SC) and the relation of Koebner phenomenon to the conversion of SC antigens from hidden to reactive form by scratching (abstr.). Fed. Proc. Fed. Am. Socs. exp. Biol. *37:* 1487 (1978).

6 Binder, W. L. and Beutner, E. H.: Studies in immunodermatology. VIII. Immunofluorescence studies of stratum corneum antibodies. Int. Archs Allergy appl. Immun. (in press).

7 Bizzozero, E.: Experiences sur le signe de Köbner dans le psoriasis. Bull. Soc. fr. Derm. Syph. *38:* 1047–1049 (1931).

8 Burnet, M.: Autoimmune disease as a breakdown in immunological homeostasis; in Cellular immunology (Cambridge University Press, Cambridge 1970).

9 Comaish, J. S. and Greener, J. S.: The inhibiting effect of soft paraffin on the Koebner response in psoriasis. Br. J. Derm. *94:* 195–200 (1976).

10 Ehrlich, P. und Morgenroth, J.: Über Haemolysine. 3. Mitteilung. Berl. klin. Wschr. *37:* 453–458 (1900).
11 Farber, E. M.; Roth, R. J.; Aschehim, E.; Eddy, D., and Epinette, W. W.: Role of trauma in isomorphic response in psoriasis. Archs Derm. *91:* 246–251 (1965).
12 Grabar, P.: Hypothesis. Auto-antibodies and immunological theories: an analytical review. Clin. Immun. Immunopath. *4:* 453–466 (1975).
13 Guilhou, J. J. and Meynadier, J.: Immunological aspects of psoriasis. II. Associated impairment of thymus dependent lymphocytes Br. J. Derm. *95:* 295–301 (1976).
14 Jablonska, S.; Beutner, E. H.; Jarzabek-Chorzelska, M.; Maciewjowska, E.; Rzesa, G.; Chowzniec, O., and Chorzelski, T. P.: Clinical significance of autoimmunity in psoriasis; in Milgrom and Albini, Immunopathology, pp. 148–153 (Karger, Basel 1979).
15 Krogh, H. K.: Antibodies to stratum corneum in man; in Beutner, Chorzelski, Bean and Jordon Immunopathology of the skin: labeled antibody studies; 1st ed. (Dowden, Hutchinson & Ross, Stroudsburg 1973).
16 Krogh, H. K. and Tönder, O.; Stratum corneum antigens and antibodies; in Beutner, Chorzelski and Bean Immunopathology of the skin; 2nd ed., pp. 413–425 (Wiley & Sons, New York 1979).
17 Michel, B. and Schiltz, J.: Pathophysiology of pemphigus; in Milgrom and Albini, Immunopathology, pp. 137–141 (Karger, Basel 1979).
18 Milgrom, F.: Antibodies to altered autologous antigens; in Milgrom and Albini, Immunopathology, pp. 56–61 (Karger, Basel 1979).
19 Obalek, S.; Haftek, M., and Glinski, W.: Immunological studies in psoriasis. The quantitative evaluation of cell mediated immunity in patients with psoriasis by experimental sensitization to 2, 4-dinitrochlorobenzene. Dermatologica *155:* 13–23 (1977).

Dr. E. H. Beutner, Departments of Microbiology and Dermatology, State University of New York at Buffalo, Medical and Dental Schools, Buffalo, NY 14214 (USA)

Immunopathology. 6th Int. Convoc. Immunol., Niagara Falls, N.Y., 1978, pp. 148–153 (Karger, Basel 1979)

Clinical Significance of Autoimmunity in Psoriasis[1]

S. Jablonska, E. H. Beutner, M. Jarzabek-Chorzelska, E. Maciejowska, G. Rzesa, O. Chowaniec and T. P. Chorzelski

Department of Dermatology, Warsaw School of Medicine, Warsaw, and Departments of Microbiology and Dermatology, State University of New York at Buffalo, Medical and Dental Schools, Buffalo, N.Y.

Introduction

Psoriasis is a common proliferative disease of epidermis. Genetic predisposition plays a role, although the mode of inheritance is not clear [7]. Clinical features vary from common psoriasis to severe pustular, arthropatic and erythrodermic varieties.

Psoriatic arthritis is analogous to the rheumatoid arthritis (RA) which is considered to be an immunologic disorder. Rheumatoid factor (RF), which is generally absent from the circulation in psoriasis, may be detected by a rosette test on the surface of lymphocytes [12].

As in RA, IgM and IgG immunoglobulins and fibrinogen have been found in synovial tissue [8].

In spite of the proliferative character of the fully developed lesion, a very early event is penetration of the white cells into the epidermis with damage of the basal cells. The important feature is exocytosis and exoserosis with accumulation of polymorphs in the stratum corneum (Munro micro-abscesses). The penetration of white cells through elongated dermal papillae into the epidermis has been described by *Pinkus and*

Mehregan [11] as a 'squirting papilla'. This phenomenon has not been understood until recently. The possible explanation is provided by our studies which point to the significance of autoimmune mechanisms.

Because no valid animal model of psoriasis is available, we have studied the Koebner phenomenon to evaluate the sequence of immunologic and histologic events in the development of psoriatic lesions.

Material and Methods

Studies on immune deposits have been performed in over 300 cases of psoriasis and in 120 control cases (30 healthy people and 90 cases of various skin diseases).

The Koebner phenomenon, which is an inducement of psoriatic lesions by traumatization of the skin, was provoked mainly by scratching. Psoriatic lesions develop in about 7–20 days at the site of the scratch if a positive Koebner reaction is obtained. The Koebner phenomenon has been studied in 152 patients with psoriasis and in 19 healthy controls.

Direct and indirect immunofluorescence (IF) studies were carried out using anti-IgG and anti C3 and/or C4 conjugates with molar F/P ratios in the range of 1.9–2.9 diluted to $\frac{1}{4}$–$\frac{1}{8}$ unit/ml. The same conjugates absorbed with normal human sera served as control for non-specific staining, according to the method described by *Beutner et al.* [3]. Comparisons between the indirect (IIF) and direct (DIF) give some insight into the saturation of the antigenic sites of the stratum corneum by the *in vivo* deposited immunoglobulins, presumably stratum

[1] Supported by grants from the Polish Academy of Sciences (10.5), the National Psoriasis Foundation and by an NIH Training Grant (501580E).

Table I. Relation of the activity of psoriasis of selected types to the development of the Koebner reaction

Activity of psoriasis and types of lesions	Koebner reactions	
	positive/ total	percent positive
Receding lesions (with partially cleared centers) under topical treatment[1]	0/48	0
Stationary lesions under topical treatment[1]	2/32	6
Single stationary, untreated lesions	0/4	0
Rapidly spreading plaques with central clearing	2/5	40
Active guttate psoriasis	8/16	50
Active spreading plaques or guttate psoriasis, topical treatment[1]	15/32	47
Chronic active psoriasis (psoriasis inveterata)	6/6	100

[1] The scratch sites were untreated; they were protected by a watch glass from the topical agents used for treatment.

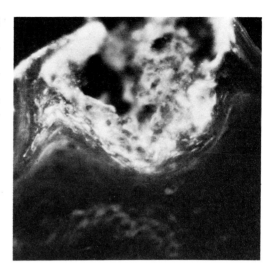

Fig. 1. Koebner phenomenon 72 h after scratch. DIF staining for IgG. Diffuse staining of the crust and some immune deposits in the SC at the SCAg sites at the edge of the crust (intercellular staining visible at the lower right margin of stained crust). This IF pattern is the same in psoriatics and controls. × 335.

corneum antibodies (Sc Ab). Additional binding in the IIF method would point to the presence of free antigenic determinants. Failure to obtain additional binding would point to saturation of the stratum corneum antigen sites.

Histological (routine H + E staining) and immunological (DIF and IIF) studies were carried out in various time intervals from 2 h to 7 days (4, 24, 48, 72, 96 h, and 5, 7 and 11 days).

Results

In essentially all active lesions of psoriasis, DIF showed immunoglobulins in stratum corneum deposited in a characteristic psoriatic pattern (intercellular and cytoplasmic), and in a majority of cases also complement was demonstrable at the same location [2].

The Koebner phenomenon was induced in 49% of the active untreated cases of psoriasis (16/31). The results were negative in patients with single small psoriatic plaques (table I). However, in patients treated topically for psoriasis except for the test site, which was protected by a watch glass, the results were negative if the lesions were receding and partially cleared in the central area. If the lesions were still progressing and were spreading peripherally, the Koebner phenomenon developed in about 47% of the cases, very much like in untreated active cases (table I). In healthy controls, the scratched areas healed in 3–4 days with no visible traces. The histological picture within 3–4 days did not differ in psoriatics and controls. In both

Table II. Koebner's phenomenon. IF changes induced by scratching in patients with psoriasis and normal control subjects

Time of biopsy after scratch, days	Number of cases biopsied	Number of cases with IgG deposits in stratum corneum at edge of crust	Number of cases with psoriatic pattern of IF stain in the stratum corneum		Number of cases with negative stain for IF deposits and histological features of psoriasis	Koebner-positive	
			histology with no features of psoriasis	histology with features of psoriasis		number of cases	days after scratching
Patients with psoriasis							
2	4	2	4	0	none	3	8–11
3	7	5	6	1	none	3	10–14
4	14	3	13	1	none	6	6–14
5	15	6	14	1	none	5	9–17
6	2	0	2	1	none	1	17
7	11	1	5	5	none	6	10–20
8–11	3	0	2	1	none	3	8–12
Totals	56	17	46	10	none	27	
Normal subjects							
2	4	4	none	none	none	none	
3	3	3	none	none	none	none	
4	6	1	none	none	none	none	
5	Since only normal skin was present in the scratch no further biopsies were taken						

groups, 2 h after the scratch, there was extensive inflammatory reaction composed almost exclusively of polymorphonuclear leukocytes (PMN) mainly around the blood vessels. The PMN appeared in the epidermis and accumulated at the site of the scratch where a crust was formed. At 12–72 h, there were still no detectable differences between scratches of active psoriatics and controls. Even at 96 h, some proliferation of the epidermis around the crust was observed in both groups (fig. 1).

The main difference was noticeable after 4 days. In controls, there was a complete healing, whereas in cases of psoriasis with a positive Koebner phenomenon there was a massive penetration of PMN into the epider-

mis, resulting in destruction of the basal cells. Thereafter, characteristic histological features of psoriasis started to develop [10].

DIF staining of an early Koebner phenomenon (12–96 h) showed in both groups binding of immunoglobulins in a limited area around the crust in a pattern characteristic of SCAb. In patients with active psoriasis, 4 days after the scratch, deposits became more widespread, progressively spreading throughout the stratum corneum in the next several days (table II; fig. 2, 3).

Histologic and immunohistologic studies of uninvolved skin in cases with active psoriasis revealed accumulation of PMN deep in the corium, often around hair follicles and sweat ducts.

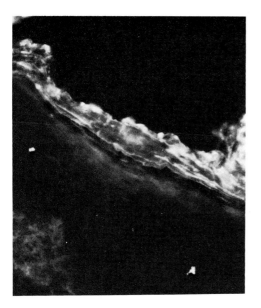

Fig. 2. Koebner phenomenon 96 h after scratch in a patient with psoriasis. DIF staining for IgG. Immune deposits appear in the stratum corneum beyond the edge of the crust (the crust is to the right side of the picture). These SC deposits tend to become more widespread than in controls. × 335.

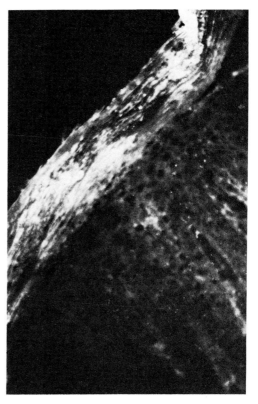

Fig. 3. Koebner phenomenon 7 days after scratch in a patient with active psoriasis. Early development of psoriatic IF pattern as seen by direct staining for IgG is followed by the appearance of histologic features of psoriasis. × 335.

In the earliest erythematous 'pre-pinpoint lesions' without clinical and histological features of psoriasis, there were widespread PMN infiltrates also in the upper dermis with some tendency to invade the basal cell layer but still not penetrating into the stratum corneum. DIF studies did not show immune deposits in the stratum corneum either in seemingly uninvolved skin or in 'pre-pinpoint lesions'.

Discussion

Our studies indicate that the depositions of immunoglobulins, presumably *in vivo* bound SCAb with concomitant binding of complement in the stratum corneum may be a part of the autoimmune mechanism of psoriasis. This mechanism seems to be responsible for the release of chemotactic factor(s) inducing the so-called squirting papilla and formation of Munro micro-abscesses in the stratum corneum. Indeed, a chemotactic factor has been isolated from the psoriatic scales by *Tagami and Ofuji* [13, 14].

Studies on the Koebner phenomenon have shown that epidermal trauma may induce psoriatic lesions 7–20 days after a scratch, that the earliest events are the same in psoriatics and normal controls and are probably related to the normal repair mechanism operating in wound healing [1, 9]. This mechanism is switched off after clearing of immune complexes within 4 days in normals in contrast to psoriatics in whom depositions of immunoglobulins and complement in the stratum corneum are progressively enlarged with continuous attraction of PMN resulting in a self-perpetuating disease process. The earliest event seems to be deposition of immunoglobulins and complement in the stratum corneum, followed by histologic and clinical changes of psoriasis.

The role of some blood-borne factors participating in the development of psoriatic lesions is indicated by constant finding of negative Koebner reactions in patients with lesions receding either spontaneously or after external treatment (even if the site of the scratch is not treated). Also, favorable results of hemo- and peritoneal dialysis. especially those of continuous peritoneal dialysis, point to the existence of such factors. Since the continuous peritoneal dialysis is associated with the removal of a great number of PMN, it is possible that these cells may be involved in some part of the mechanism of psoriasis.

The studies of the uninvolved skin of active psoriatics show the presence of PMN in the dermis; there are especially extensive infiltrates in the 'pre-pinpoint lesions'. This provides further circumstantial evidence of the significance of PMN in the disease process. *Braun-Falco and Christophers* [4, 5], studying the earliest psoriatic lesions of pinpoint type, found mainly lymphocytic infiltrates, which according to *Cormane et al.* [6] is evidence of the role of cell-mediated immunity in psoriasis. We also could confirm predominantly lymphocytic infiltrations in the fully developed psoriatic plaques; however, our studies of the lesions which have not yet developed (the prelesional changes) point rather to the involvement of PMN in the earliest stages of their formation.

The specific mechanism seems to be associated with the conversion of stratum corneum antigen to its reactive form and the binding of SCAb and complement.

Summary

The immunofluorescence studies of psoriatic plaques using direct and indirect methods have shown deposits of immunoglobulins and in a majority of cases also deposits of complement. The resulting release of chemotactic factors seems to be responsible for an accumulation of PMN in the stratum corneum (Munro micro-abscesses).

The studies on Koebner phenomenon in psoriatics and normal controls have shown within 4 days similar deposits of immunoglobulins localized around the scratch in both groups. In contrast to normals, immunoglobulins in psoriatics are progressively deposited during the next several days until the characteristic IF pattern of psoriasis is developed. These immune deposits seem to precede the histologic and clinical appearance of psoriatic lesions.

References

1 Beutner, E. H.; Chorzelski, T. P., and Binder, W. L.: Nature of autoimmunity. Pathologic versus physiologic responses and a unifying concept; in Beutner, Chorzelski and Bean Immunopathology of the skin, 2nd ed., pp. 147–180 (Wiley & Sons, New York 1979).
2 Beutner, E. H.; Jarzabek-Chorzelska, M.; Jablonska, S.; Chorzelski, T. P., and Rzesa, G.: Autoimmunity in psoriasis. A complement immunofluorescence study. Archs Derm. Res. *261:* 123–134 (1978).
3 Beutner, E. H.; Jablonska, S.; Jarzabek-Chorzelska, M.; Maciejowska, E.; Rzesa, G., and Chorzelski, T. P.: Studies in immunodermatology. VI. IF studies of autoantibodies to the stratum corneum and of *in vivo* fixed IgG in stratum corneum of psoriatic scales. Int. Archs Allergy appl. Immun. *48:* 301–323 (1975).
4 Braun-Falco, O. and Christophers, E.: Structural aspects of initial psoriatic lesions. Arch. Derm. Forsch. *251:* 95–110 (1974).

5 Braun-Falco, O. and Christophers, E.: The dermal inflammatory reaction in initial psoriatic lesions. Archs Derm. Res. *258:* 9 (1977).

6 Cormane, R. H.; Hunyadi, J. et Hammerlinck, F.: Mecanismes immunologiques du psoriasis. Annls Derm. Syph. *103:* 567 (1976).

7 Farber, E. M.; Nall, M. L.; Morhenn, V., and Kaye, J.: Unanswered questions about psoriasis; in Farber and Cox Psoriasis. Proc. 2nd Int. Symp., Stanford (Yorke Medical Books, New York 1977).

8 Fyrand, O.; Mellbye, O. J., and Natvig, J. B.: Direct immunofluorescence studies on immunoglobulins and complement (C3) in synovial joint membranes in psoriatic arthritis; in Farber and Cox Psoriasis. Proc. 2nd Int. Symp., Stanford (Yorke Medical Books, New York 1977).

9 Grabar, P.: Hypothesis. Autoantibodies and immunological theories. An analytical review. Clin. Immunol. Immunopath. *4:* 453–466 (1975).

10 Jablonska, S.; Chorzelski, T. P.; Beutner, E. H.; Maciejowski, E.; Jarzabek-Chorzelska, M., and Rzesa, G.: Autoimmunity in psoriasis. Relation of disease activity and forms of psoriasis to immunofluorescence findings. Archs Derm. Res. *261:* 135–146 (1978).

11 Pinkus, H. and Mehregan, A. H.: The primary histologic lesion of seborrheic dermatitis and psoriasis. J. invest. Derm. *46:* 109–116 (1966).

12 Rimbaud, P.; Meynadier, J.; Guilhou, J. J., and Clot, J.: Anti-IgG activity on peripheral blood lymphocytes in psoriasis. Archs Derm. *108:* 371–373 (1973).

13 Tagami, H. and Ofuji, S.: Leukotactic properties of soluble substances in psoriasis scale. Br. J. Derm. *95:* 1–8 (1976).

14 Tagami, H. and Ofuji, S.: Characterization of a leukotactic factor derived from psoriatic scale. Br. J. Derm. *97:* 509–518 (1977).

Dr. S. Jablonska, Department of Dermatology, Warsaw School of Medicine, Koszykowa 82a, PL-02-008 Warsaw (Poland)

Immunopathology. 6th Int. Convoc. Immunol., Niagara Falls, N.Y., 1978, pp. 154–160 (Karger, Basel 1979)

Clinical Significance of Autoimmunity in Pemphigus[1]

Tadeusz P. Chorzelski, Ernst H. Beutner and Stefania Jablonska

Department of Dermatology, Warsaw School of Medicine, Warsaw, and Departments of Microbiology and Dermatology, State University of New York at Buffalo, Medical and Dental Schools, Buffalo, N.Y.

Introduction

Pemphigus, one of the most severe skin disorders, is characterized by bullae due to loss of intercellular cohesions of keratinocytes (acantholysis). Clinical features may be variable and four main varieties are recognized:

(1) Pemphigus vulgaris is the most severe form. It was usually fatal before treatment with corticosteroids and immunosuppressants was introduced. In the vast majority of cases cutaneous lesions are preceded by bullous changes and erosions in the oral mucosa.

(2) Pemphigus vegetans is a form of pemphigus vulgaris presenting vegetating lesions, localized mainly in the intertriginous areas and in the buccal mucosa.

(3) Pemphigus erythematosus is a form which combines facial lesions resembling lupus erythematosus and changes on the trunk suggestive of seborrheic dermatitis (pemphigus seborrhoicus).

(4) Pemphigus foliaceus is characterized by flaccid bullae which disrupt easily with a tendency to spread and cover large areas of the skin (erythroderma of the type of exfoliative dermatitis).

[1] Supported in part by grants from the Summerhill Foundation and from the Polish Academy of Sciences (10.5).

Although the recognition of four main clinical types of pemphigus is fully justified there are some cases which combine features of the different types.

In pemphigus vulgaris and vegetans acantholytic bullae are formed suprabasally (fig. 1), in the other forms acantholysis is superficial (subcorneal acantholytic bullae). Characteristic acantholytic cells are clearly demonstrable also in cytological smears (Tzank test).

Immunologic Phenomena in Pemphigus

The mechanism of formation of acantholytic bulla was an enigma until 1964. The breakthrough was the discovery by *Beutner and Jordon* [1] by means of immunofluorescence technique (IF) of specific antibodies reactive with intercellular structures at the sites where acantholysis begins (fig. 2). At the ultra-structural level pemphigus antibodies bind to surface antigens of the keratinocytes. This appears to lead to the development of acantholysis [4]. The biochemical nature of the pemphigus antigen varies in the different mammalian species examined, man, rabbit, ox and guinea pig [4]. The human pemphigus antigen is a labile protein with a slow gamma mobility, a molecular weight of about 70,000 and little or no carbohydrate or lipid.

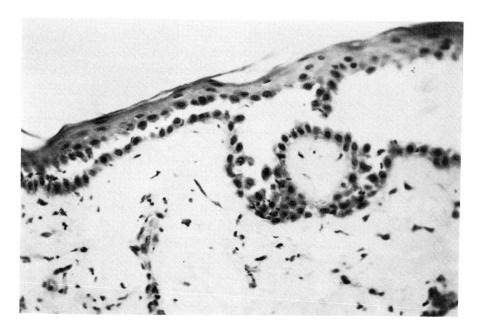

Fig. 1. Pemphigus vulgaris. Note suprabasal bulla with numerous acantholytic cells. HE. ×200.

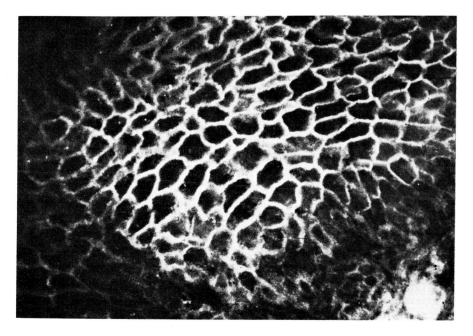

Fig. 2. Indirect immunofluorescence staining with anti-IgG conjugate on section of monkey esophagus. (Conjugate characteristics: goat anti-human IgG molar F/P 4.9; 4 U/ml, dilution 1/16.) Note specific fluorescence of the intercellular area of the epithelium. ×500.

The wide use of direct and indirect IF methods in clinical practice made it possible to recognize forms of pemphigus, which previously could not have been diagnosed. IF tests for pemphigus antibodies became the most important diagnostic criterion; it is of greater significance than histology, since acantholysis may not be detectable in some early cases of pemphigus and on the other hand it may occur in some other diseases.

Pemphigus antibodies are autoantibodies, belong to IgG class and may occur in all four subclasses. They are found in essentially all active cases at least during some phases of the disease. However, some exceptional cases of pemphigus have no demonstrable pemphigus antibodies in the circulation. One of the reasons that the sera may be negative is that in some cases pemphigus antibodies

exhibit a limited species or organ specificity but this may change to a broad reactivity during the course of the disease. Such changes in specificity are associated with corresponding changes in the distribution of lesions in some, but not all cases. In a few cases the sera of patients yield *in vitro* reactivity of pemphigus antibodies with the patients' own skin but not with the normal skin of other individuals [7].

It is to be presumed that in some cases the antibodies have a high affinity to epidermal intercellular antigens and are therefore absorbed out *in vivo* (positive *in vivo* binding) and antibodies reactive *in vitro* with mucous membranes are left in circulation.

The apparent transient negative findings may also occur in cases with acute exacerbation due to the blocking of antibodies by the

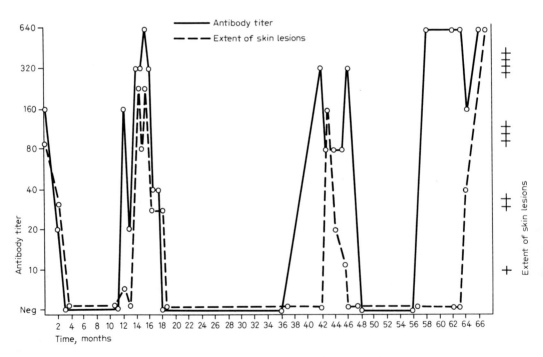

Fig. 3. Fluctuation of pemphigus antibody titers as compared to the severity of the disease over a 5-year period.

pemphigus antigens resulting in the formation of immune complexes in circulation. The antibodies might become detectable after inactivation of the thermolabile antigen by heating the serum [3].

The titers of pemphigus antibodies in general parallel the clinical state of the disease, i.e. the activity and extent of bullous lesions [9] (fig. 3). This is evident only in systematically repeated examinations under standard conditions with defined conjugates, the same substrates and controlled test conditions. Accidental detection of pemphigus antibodies in patients without clinical evidence of pemphigus at the time of sampling has shown that pemphigus antibodies may precede the appearance of skin and/or mucosal lesions.

Treatment either with high doses of corticosteroids or with corticosteroids in combination with immunosuppressants produces a gradual fall in the titer of pemphigus antibodies to undetectable levels. A rise of titer or persistence of high titer, in spite of subsidence of the lesions upon treatment, is suggestive of an impending relapse.

Regardless of the *in vitro* reactivity of patients' sera in tests for circulating antibodies, the *in vivo* fixation of IgG to the intercellular areas is a constant finding within the lesion and surrounding, apparently normal skin [4].

Complement Reactions in Pemphigus

There is general agreement that pemphigus antibodies do not bind complement *in vitro* though they are of the subclasses IgG1 and IgG3. An exception is a recent report by *Nishikawa et al.* [18] who found some complement fixing pemphigus sera. This may be due to the coexistence of pemphigus-like antibodies which are known to fix complement. Since it is well recognized that burns,

bullous pemphigoid, dermatitis herpetiformis and other forms of epidermal damage can elicit the formation of pemphigus-like antibodies it should not be surprising that pemphigus bullae can also elicit them [10].

Intercellular binding of complement occurs in some pemphigus lesions, particularly in untreated cases [12] but not in the adjacent normal skin. The question arises why complement can be fixed *in vivo* whereas the pemphigus antibodies are incapable of fixing it *in vitro*. Apparently *in vivo* complement fixation does not depend on pemphigus antibodies themselves but on secondary immunological phenomena, such as the binding of pemphigus-like antibodies or rheumatoid factor. This remains to be proven.

Pathogenic Significance of Pemphigus Antibodies

Several lines of indirect evidence point to an autoimmune pathogenesis of pemphigus. One is the coexistence of this disease with other autoimmune syndromes such as myasthenia gravis, thymoma and lupus erythematosus [5], Addisonian pernicious anemia [15] and bullus pemphigoid [11]. Occurrence of pemphigus with such diseases as myasthenia gravis, thymoma and SLE with suppressed T cells may be due to a loss of inhibitory function of the thymus resulting in the formation of various types of auto-antibodies. Pemphigus associated with Hodgkin's disease or lymphoma might also suggest that T cell suppression could play an etiologic role in the development of pemphigus antibodies [14].

One important set of observations relevant to the etiology of autoimmune responses in pemphigus derives from studies of Brazilian pemphigus foliaceus. This disease affects all ethnic groups which live in the narrowly circumscribed endemic regions in South-

Central Brazil [2]. One endemic region, for example, includes the suburbs around the water reservoir of Sao Paulo, Brazil, but not other districts of the same metropolitan area. Such observations clearly indicate that the etiology of this form of pemphigus is some unusual antigenic stimulus, possibly some local arbovirus. The reactive antigen differs from those of nonendemic pemphigus [23].

Familial incidence of pemphigus and other immune disturbances is not restricted to relatives living in the same area thus suggesting a genetic predisposition to autoimmune responses, at least in some cases. On the other hand, the increased occurrence of pemphigus antibodies in relatives of patients with pemphigus foliaceus is restricted to family members (and neighbors) living in the same endemic area [6].

The pathogenic role of the pemphigus antibodies is now documented by three types of direct evidence, notably the passive induction of acantholysis by transfer of pemphigus antibodies into animals [4, 8], the passive induction of acantholysis by growth of skin explants in pemphigus antibody-containing sera [16, 21] and the passive transfer of pemphigus from mother to newborn child [19].

Although passive transfer of pemphigus by transfusion has been a failure [20], work begun earlier [8] was continued with the view towards demonstrating the pathogenicity of the antibodies by intradermal or intramucosal injection of pemphigus sera to rabbit and monkeys [4]. The experiments proved that repeated injections at the same site are not only followed by in vivo binding of the antibodies but may give rise to acantholytic lesions resembling those of true pemphigus.

Cultures of skin in sera or IgG fractions containing pemphigus antibodies showed that these sera are indeed capable of inducing acantholysis [16, 21]. This, in addition, shed

new light on the much argued problem of the role of complement, which appeared to be unnecessary for the cytopathogenic effect as reported by Michel and Schiltz [17] in this volume.

Recently we performed tissue culture studies of the skin of patients with pemphigus both in the acute stage of their disease (with in vivo bound intercellular IgG) and in the remission phase (without detectable immunoglobulins in the intercellular spaces of the epidermis). After 24–48 h, skin of the patients with active disease cultured in normal serum showed formation of acantholytic clefts, whereas skin of the same patients in remission did not differ from the control. It is noteworthy that during the active disease no lesions developed in the area of the biopsy in contrast to the intraepidermal changes in the skin explant. This points, on the one hand, to the pathogenic potential of pemphigus antibodies and on the other hand to some additional mechanisms operating in vivo which may prevent the formation of acantholytic bulla. Interestingly, explants of normal skin biopsy specimens from a patient with pemphigus foliaceus developed suprabasal clefts in tissue culture as in pemphigus vulgaris while the patient had typical subcorneal acantholytic lesions. These apparent discrepancies shed light on the mechanism of action of the pemphigus antibodies. The pathogenic effects of pemphigus antibodies are also indicated by the beneficial responses of patients to plasmapheresis [19]. Also, the development of transient acantholytic blisters with in vivo bound pemphigus antibodies in a newborn child of a mother afflicted with pemphigus points to pathogenic potential of these antibodies [19].

Provoking Factors in Pemphigus

Some factors appear to provoke the development of pemphigus antibodies while others appear to precipitate the development of lesions in patients who already have the antibodies. The presence of pemphigus-like antibodies in burns has been repeatedly reported [22]. They are detectable as a rule during the second week after a burn and disappear some weeks later. Their pathogenic role is doubtful because of their inability to bind *in vivo*. The formation of pemphigus-like antibodies is undoubtedly a secondary and transient phenomenon, caused by the release of epidermal antigens altered by thermal injury or other forms of trauma. In some cases, however, true pemphigus antibodies rather than pemphigus-like antibodies are produced. In such situations the antibodies acquire properties of *in vivo* fixation and result in the development of true pemphigus. Indeed, some postburn pemphigus cases have been described [10].

Drugs may also be one of the factors which evoke pemphigus. Especially striking is the incidence of pemphigus induced by prolonged penicillamine therapy which is used primarily for the treatment of rheumatoid arthritis, scleroderma and Wilson's disease [13]. The mechanism of action of penicillamine remains to be determined.

UV testing in patients with active pemphigus and circulating antibodies may precipitate a formation of bullae with characteristic histologic and immunologic features. Sunlight may play a similar role particularly in precipitating pemphigus erythematosus and pemphigus foliaceus [4].

In conclusion, clinical observations as well as experimental studies have convincingly shown the role of autoimmunity in the pathogenesis of pemphigus. The direct evidence for the pathogenic potential of pemphigus antibodies is described by *Michel and Schiltz* [17] in their report on the cytopathic effect of pemphigus antibodies in tissue culture.

Summary

The well-established diagnostic and prognostic value of the detection of pemphigus antibodies by indirect immunofluorescence and their apparent *in vivo* binding by direct immunofluorescence becomes understandable now in the light of their pathogenic significance. The pathogenic potential of pemphigus antibodies is well documented by experimental and natural passive transfer of the disease as well as by their capacity to produce typical acantholytic 'lesions' in tissue cultures of skin. These findings afford a firm foundation for studies on different etiologic mechanisms, e.g. in pemphigus associated with thymomas versus Brazilian pemphigus. They also afford a basis for analytic studies on the mechanism of action of pemphigus antibodies, e.g. by comparisons of the *in vivo* and *in vitro* effects of pemphigus antibodies.

References

1 Beutner, E. H. and Jordon, R. E.: Demonstration of skin antibodies in sera of pemphigus vulgaris patients by indirect immunofluorescent staining. Proc. Soc. exp. Biol. Med. *117:* 505–510 (1964).

2 Beutner, E. H.; Chorzelski, T. P., and Jordon, R. E.: Autosensitization in pemphigus and bullous pemphigoid (Thomas, Springfield 1970).

3 Beutner, E. H.; Sporer, R., and Chorzelski, T. P.: Pemphigus antigens in human sera (abstr.). J. invest. Derm. *62:* 342 (1974).

4 Beutner, E. H.; Chorzelski, T. P.; Bean, S. F., and Jordon, R. E. (eds.): Immunopathology of the skin: labeled antibody studies (Dowden, Hutchinson & Ross, Stroudsburg 1973).

5 Beutner, E. H.; Chorzelski, T. P.; Hale, W. L., and Hausmanowa-Petrusewicz, I.: Auto-immunity in concurrent myasthenia gravis and pemphigus erythematosus. J. Am. med. Ass. *203:* 845–849 (1968).

6 Castro, R. M.; Chorzelski, T. P.; Jablonska, S., and Marquart, A., jr.: Anti-epithelial antibodies in healthy people living in an endemic area of South American pemphigus foliaceus (fogo selvagem). Preliminary report. Castellania *4:* 111–112 (1976).

7 Chorzelski, T. P. and Beutner, E. H.: Autoantibodies in some bullous diseases. Ann. N.Y. Acad. Sci. *177:* 224–226 (1971).

8 Chorzelski, T. P.; Beutner, E. H., and Jarzabek, M.: Passive transfer of pemphigus in experimental animals (abstr.). Int. Archs Allergy appl. Immun. *39:* 106 (1970).

9 Chorzelski, T. P.; Weiss, J. F. von, and Lever, W. F.: Clinical significance of autoantibodies in pemphigus. Archs Derm. *93:* 570–576 (1966).

10 Chorzelski, T. P.; Jablonska, S.; Beutner, E. H., and Kowalski, M.: Can pemphigus be provoked by a burn? Br. J. Derm. *85:* 320–325 (1971).

11 Chorzelski, T. P.; Maciejowska, E.; Jablonska, S.; De Mento, F. J.; Grover, R. W.; Holubar, K., and Beutner, E. H.: Coexistence of pemphigus and bullous pemphigoid. Archs Derm. *109:* 849–853 (1974).

12 Cormane, R. H. and Chorzelski, T. P.: 'Bound' complement in the epidermis of patients with pemphigus vulgaris. Dermatologica *134:* 463–466 (1967).

13 Degos, R.; Touraine, R.; Belaich, S., and Revuz, J.: Pemphigus chez un malade traité par pénicillamine pour maladie de Wilson. Bull. Soc. fr. Derm. Syph. *76:* 751–753 (1969).

14 DeGuerra, H. A.; Reis, A. P., and Guerra, M. V. N.: T and B lymphocytes in South American pemphigus foliaceus. Clin. exp. Immunol. *23:* 477–480 (1976).

15 Mackie, R. M.; Saikia, N. K., and Moreley, W. N.: A case of pemphigus vulgaris in association with addisonian pernicious anaemia. Br. J. Derm. *88:* 139–143 (1973).

16 Michel, B. and Ko, C. S.: An organ culture model for the study of pemphigus acantholysis. Br. J. Derm. *96:* 295–302 (1977).

17 Michel, B. and Schiltz, J.: Pathophysiology of pemphigus; in Milgrom and Albini Immunopathology, pp. 137–141 (Karger, Basel 1979).

18 Nishikawa, T.; Kurihara, S.; Harada, T.; Sugawara, M., and Hatano, H.: Capability of complement fixation of pemphigus antibodies *in vitro*. Archs Derm. Res. *260:* 1–6 (1977).

19 Ruocco, V.; Rossi, A.; Argenziano, G.; Astarita, C.; Alviggi, L.; Farzati, B., and Papaleo, G.: Pathogenicity of the intercellular antibodies of pemphigus and their periodic removal from the circulation by plasmapheresis. Br. J. Derm. *98:* 237–241 (1978).

20 Sams, W. M., jr. and Jordon, R. E.: Pemphigus antibodies: their role in disease. J. invest. Derm. *56:* 474–479 (1971).

21 Schiltz, J. R. and Michel, B.: Production of epidermal acantholysis in normal human skin *in vitro* by the IgG fraction from pemphigus serum. J. invest. Derm. *67:* 254–260 (1976).

22 Thivolet, J. et Beyvin, A. J.: Recherches par immunofluorescence d'autoanticorps sériques vis-à-vis des constituants de l'épiderme chez les brûlés. Experientia *24:* 945–946 (1968).

23 Wood, G. W. and Beutner, E. H.: Blocking immunofluorescence studies on the specificity of pemphigus autoantibodies. Clin. Immunol. Immunopath. *7:* 168–175 (1977).

Prof. Dr. T. P. Chorzelski, Department of Dermatology, Warsaw School of Medicine, Koszykowa 82a, PL-02-008 Warsaw (Poland)

Immunopathology. 6th Int. Convoc. Immunol., Niagara Falls, N.Y., 1978, pp. 161–166 (Karger, Basel 1979)

Immunological Considerations in Thermal Injury[1]

Felix T. Rapaport, Radoslav J. Bachvaroff, Kyoichi Kano and *Felix Milgrom*

Department of Surgery, State University of New York at Stony Brook, Health Sciences Center, Stony Brook, N.Y., and the Department of Microbiology, State University of New York at Buffalo, Buffalo, N.Y.

Continued progress in the management of the early post-burn shock phase and in the topical therapy of the burn wound [27] have contributed significantly to improve burn therapy. The recent revival of techniques of early excision and resurfacing of the burn wound [16] and use of hyperalimentation [38] constitute other important landmarks in the treatment of burns. The main effect of such advances appears, however, to be limited to moderate reductions in the mortality of severe burns involving 40–60% body surface area. The injured patients are now less toxic, and their wounds are generally cleaner. The leading cause of death continues to be sepsis, however, involving a continually changing microbial flora, and the overall mortality of severe burns has shifted to a later phase, termed 'burn disease' [21], associated with extensive metabolic derangements. This discussion highlights evidence supporting the concept that severe thermal injury is also associated with profound alterations in host mechanisms of immunological responsiveness, and proposes the thesis that a better understanding of such changes may be of usefulness in further decreasing mortality of burn disease.

[1] Supported by Grant GM 24481, National Institute of General Medical Sciences, Bethesda, Md.

Immunological Sequelae of Thermal Injury

Cellular Studies. The first suggestive evidence of an effect of thermal injury upon cellular mechanisms of immune responsiveness was provided by the demonstration that severe burns can produce prolongations in skin allograft survival [33]. The potential bearing of this observation upon therapy is supported by the demonstration that HLA serological typing techniques can produce even further skin allograft survival in burned patients [8]. Further attempts to assess parameters of delayed hypersensitivity in burns have resulted in the demonstration of the ability of thermal injury to inhibit manifestations of tuberculin hypersensitivity in burned guinea pigs and in man [34], with a direct relationship between the severity of the injury and the degree of inhibition of cutaneous hypersensitivity responses. Thermal injury has also been shown to produce marked decreases in the output of thoracic duct lymphocytes, in a fashion similar to that resulting from total body irradiation [10].

Humoral Studies. Significant decreases in circulating immunoglobulin levels have been documented in the first 48 h after severe burns, in parallel with a fall in the total serum protein values. The IgG and IgA components are most severely affected, but IgM values appear to show relatively little change [20]. The fall in immunoglobulins is generally followed with a gradual return to normal and occasionally elevated levels. *Arturson and Fjellström* [5] and others have documented falls in the factors of complement, with return to normal or elevated levels within 7–10 days, and *Decoulx et al.* [12] have reported similar falls in serum properdin levels. $F(ab')_2$-like fragments of immunoglobulin similar to those produced by *in vitro* papain digestion have also been detected in the serum of burned patients [14].

The recent introduction of polyacrylamide gel electrophoresis in continuous molecular sieve gradient techniques has provided a further opportunity to identify changes in serum protein contents following severe thermal injury. This technique, which can recognize as many as 40 well-defined protein bands of known molecular weights in normal mammalian sera has been applied in this laboratory to compare serum components in normal and burned mice at serial intervals after injury [32]. There is an immediate fall in albumin (69,000 d) after injury, with return to normal by 9 days; transferrin levels (90,000 d) rise at 24 h, reaching a peak at 9 days and returning to normal at 30 days. Haptoglobulins (100,000 d) behave similarly; IgG (150,000 d) and IgA (160,000 d) decrease until the 15th day, but return to normal by 20 days. C1 complement activator (104,000 d) fluctuates during the first 2 weeks, but C1q (400,000 d) levels are sharply depressed during the first 2 weeks. A particularly prominent finding in these studies was the *de novo* appearance of a thick lipoprotein band of large molecular size $(1-1.5 \times 10^6$ d) within 48 h after thermal injury, with persistence until the 15th day. Further isolation and characterization of this lipoprotein may be of usefulness in gaining a better understanding of the mechanisms implicated in triggering changes in immunological function in thermal injury.

Attempts to relate these observations to the ability of burned subjects to initiate and maintain humoral responses have yielded contradictory results. Normal serum antibody responses have been documented in burned patients and experimental animals. *Alexander and Moncrief* [3], however, have noted decreases in the humoral response of burned subjects to primary antigenic challenge, with no evidence of interference with secondary responses.

Recent progress in cellular immunology has been of usefulness in providing further insight into this important question. In the course of these studies, severe thermal injury has been shown to have the capacity to increase the rate of generation of antibody-forming cells in mice [31]. The intensity of stimulation was proportional to the extent of injury, and the effect was observed in animals burned within one hour before or after sensitization with test antigens; the effect persisted for as long as 14 days after injury, thereafter waning and disappearing by the 21st day. Responses to T-cell dependent antigen, such as sheep erythrocytes, or sheep erythrocytes coupled to TNP, and to antigens not requiring T and B cell cooperation, such as DNP-Ficoll, appeared to be equally affected. Although the mechanisms underlying this form of enhanced antibody responses were not clear, the results were consistent with the possibility that the burn wound releases factors capable of enhancing immunological responsiveness in the injured animal. Such factors were shown not to be endotoxins [31].

Altered Tissue Antigenicity as a Consequence of Thermal Injury

An impressive array of data has accumulated to support the notion that thermal injury can trigger autoimmune-like manifestations in the burned host. Two principal mechanisms have been invoked for such responses. The first is formation of altered tissue constituents as a consequence of burning; the second is release into the host of normally intracellular antigen(s) to which the individual—by virtue of the sequestered nature of such antigens—has not had an opportunity to develop tolerance. Exposure to such antigens in the course of injury may then stimulate an immunological response directed against a particular target organ [26]. The altered tissue constituent and/or toxin hypothesis has been studied extensively by *Rosenthal* and his associates [36], *Allgöwer et al.* [4] and many others.

The careful studies of *Newton et al.* [28], *Matter et al.* [25] and *Hilder and Jogan* [15], have failed, however, to confirm the production of such antigenic material(s) in burned skin, and *Fox et al.* [13] could only detect the appearance of thromboplastic extracts in burned mouse skin.

Experiments in this laboratory have provided further data regarding this question. In the course of these studies [18], rabbits were immunized with extracts of normal guinea pig skin and of burned skin obtained at serial intervals after injury. After absorption with normal and burned skin extracts and with pooled guinea pig serum and plasma, the resulting antisera were used to study the antigenic properties of burned skin. Double diffusion gel precipitation tests and immunoelectrophoretic studies of normal skin and of burned skin specimens obtained at various intervals after injury provided clear-cut evidence of the presence in burned skin of an antigenic component which was not detectable in normal skin. However, detection of this component required continued contact of the skin with the host after injury; burning of the skin *in vitro*, after its removal from the donor animal failed to produce the 'new' antigen(s). More detailed study of this material demonstrated its identity with fibrinogen. These studies would appear to weaken the suggestion that thermal injury can produce *de novo* antigenic or toxic products. Rather, as has been suggested by *Ablin* [1] and by *Hilder and Jogan* [15], the autoimmune manifestations of thermal injury may be a consequence of the release of normally intracellular components which have not been recognized as self by the host [26].

With regard to the second possibility, the original evidence implicating autoimmune mechanisms in severe thermal injury was provided by *Atherton et al.* [6] in 1960, in their demonstration of a correlation between burns mortality in rats and the appearance of a strongly positive direct Coombs' test at 48–96 h after injury. A number of other humoral responses of the autoimmune category have been reported in burned individuals. These include cytotoxic leukocyte autoantibodies [29], rheumatoid factor and antinuclear antibody [30] and anticollagen antibodies [9]. Studies in this laboratory have, in addition, isolated an IgG hemagglutinating autoantibody specific for syngeneic erythrocytes in the thoracic duct lymph of burned rats. This antibody can be detected on the surface of erythrocytes from burned rats, and its presence has been implicated in postburn anemia states [7, 19]. Additional studies in this laboratory have characterized a number of other antibodies whose appearance supports the existence of an ongoing autoimmune type of altered tissue reactivity as a consequence of thermal injury. These include heterophile antibodies, as well as rheumatoid factor, in the sera of burned patients, rabbits and guinea pigs [17]. The observation that autoantibodies similar to those documented in patients with pemphigus—an autoimmune disease of skin—can occur in severely burned patients has provided additional support of

the possibility that skin-specific antigens released in the course of thermal injury trigger
an autoimmune type of tissue-specific response in the injuried host. Such antibodies, which combine with the intracellular
matrix of stratified squamous epithelium,
have been described in this laboratory by
Ablin et al. [2], and by a number of other
investigators [30].

Evidence to support the possibility that
thermal injury can induce immunologically
mediated organ-specific damage has been
provided by studies designed to produce
classical autoimmune-like tissue damage by
thermal injury. Studies in this laboratory [35]
have shown that unilateral burns of guinea
pig testis with an electrode yielding a temperature of 220 °C at the burn site produces
autoimmune responses similar to those produced by immunization of the host with
testicular tissue in Freund's adjuvant. The
burned animals formed organ-specific antibodies and developed characteristic pathological changes in the germinal components
of the contralateral unburned testis. These
results, which have been confirmed recently
by other investigators [11, 23], are in keeping
with the concept that immunological responses triggered by the release into the host
of normally sequestered antigen(s) may be
implicated in the burn disease syndrome.

Recent studies in this laboratory designed
to decrease the lethal effects of severe burns
may also be of relevance to this consideration.
These experiments were based upon the observation that repetitive exposure to trauma,
such as the Noble-Collip drum technique,
or production of intestinal ischemia or massive hemorrhage, may increase host tolerance
to progressively more severe injury, with
some evidence of cross-resistance between
various different forms of trauma. In an
attempt to ascertain whether a conditioning
regimen might also be of usefulness in decreasing burns mortality, groups of mice

were subjected to six consecutive full-thick-
ness 1.5 % body surface area skin burns, given
at 21-day intervals, with complete healing of
each preceding injury before application of
the next challenge. Three weeks after com-
pletion of conditioning, all mice received a
30 % body surface area burn. Contrary to
the anticipated results, the 21-day mortality
of such 30 % body-surface area burns was
34 % in mice conditioned with consecutive
small burns, in contrast with a much lower
mortality of 9 % in concurrent controls given
similar injury without preparation [37]. It
would therefore appear that such small burns,
which were not sufficient to cause any marked
physiological changes in the animals, did
have a deleterious effect upon the host's
resistance to thermal injury. The possibility
that this increases susceptibility might be
related to some form of autoimmune-like
mechanisms is currently under investigation.

Conclusions

It is evident that this very brief overview
has not done full justice to the important
question of immunological consequences of
thermal injury. The fragmentary data that
could be presented would appear, however,
to be consistent with the conclusion that
severe thermal injury can indeed cause profound alterations in the host's mechanisms
of immunological responsiveness, and that
better understanding of these changes may
contribute to improvements in the current
mortality of this type of tissue damage. Progress in the management of the physiological
derangements associated with early burns
and in the treatment of the burn wound have
led to the survival of increasing numbers
of extensively burned patients into a later
period, 'burn disease', during which septice-
mia continues to be the principal cause of
death. Burn sepsis was first recognized as a

life-threatening problem in association with infections by group A hemolytic streptococci [22]. The subsequent widespread use of penicillin in order to prevent this complication then produced a shift from Gram-positive to Gram-negative organisms—and particularly *Pseudomonas aeruginosa* [24]—as the predominant microorganisms. Viral and mycotic infections have recently begun to pose an additional ominous threat to burn patients. The relationship of this problem to immunological mechanisms is evident in view of the extensive literature demonstrating marked impairments in host resistance to a variety of microorganisms (especially *Pseudomonas aeruginosa*) after thermal injury.

Taken together, the experimental and clinical data support the notion that improved understanding of the mechanisms of host immunological responsiveness which are specifically affected by thermal injury may contribute to further progress in treatment, with decreases in morbidity and mortality. It is equally clear, however, that much additional knowledge is required before such data can be transposed from the laboratory bench to the bedside. Another aspect of this problem which may be worthy of further consideration is the evidence that controlled unilateral burns of paired organs can trigger a sequence of responses leading to immunologically mediated organ-specific damage. This observation would appear to point to the potential usefulness of the thermal modality in providing experimental models for further study of disease states in which autoimmune types of altered tissue reactivity have been implicated.

References

1 Ablin, R. J.: Autoallergy in burns. Plast. reconstr. Surg. *48:* 170 (1971).
2 Ablin, R. J.; Milgrom, F.; Kano, J.; Rapaport, F. T.,

and Beutner, E. H.: Pemphigus-like antibodies in patients with skin burns. Vox Sang. *16:* 73–75 (1969).
3 Alexander, J. W. and Moncrief, J. A.: Immunologic phenomena in burn injuries. J. Am. med. Ass. *199:* 257–260 (1967).
4 Allgöwer, M.; Burri, C.; Cueni, L.; Engley, F.; Fleisch, H.; Gruber, U. F.; Harder, F., and Russell, R. G. G.: Study of burn toxins. Ann. N.Y. Acad. Sci. *150:* 807–815 (1968).
5 Arturson, G. and Fjellström, K. E.: Alteration of serum complement factors following burn trauma (abstr.). Trans. 3rd Int. Congr. Plastic Surg., Washington 1963, p. 99.
6 Atherton, S.; Merrill, N., and McCarthy, M. D.: Evidence for a lethal autoimmune response in severely burned rats (abstr.). Fed. Proc. Fed. Am. Socs exp. Biol. *19:* 195 (1960).
7 Bachvaroff, R.; Browne, L. R., and Rapaport, F. T.: Erythrocyte changes in severe thermal injury. Surg. Forum *23:* 501–503 (1972).
8 Batchelor, J. R. and Hackett, M.: HL-A matching in treatment of burned patients with skin allografts. Lancet *ii:* 581–583 (1970).
9 Bray, J. P.; Estess, F., and Bass, J. A.: Anticollagen antibodies following thermal trauma. Proc. Soc. exp. Biol. Med. *130:* 394–398 (1969).
10 Casson, P.; Gesner, B. M.; Converse, J. M., and Rapaport, F. T.: Immunosuppressive sequelae of thermal injury. Surg. Forum *19:* 509–511 (1968).
11 Collazo, E. F.; Thierer, E., and Mancini, R. E.: Immunologic and testicular response in guinea pigs after unilateral thermal injury. J. Allergy clin. Immunol. *49:* 167–173 (1972).
12 Decoulx, P.; Amoudru, C.; Claeys, C.; Hamon, G. et Monot, G.: Les moyens de défense anti-bacteriens chez les brulés. Intérêt du dosage de la properdine. Presse méd. *72:* 257–260 (1964).
13 Foy, C. J. jr.; Holder, I. A., and Malin, L. L.: Toxic thromboplastic extracts of skin. J. Am. med. Ass. *187:* 655–658 (1964).
14 Goldberg, C. B. and Whitehouse, F., jr.: F(ab')$_2$-like fragments from severely burned patients provide a new serum immunoglobulin component. Nature, Lond. *228:* 160–162 (1970).
15 Holder, I. A. and Jogan, M.: Antigenic components of normal and burned mouse skin. Experientia *26:* 1363–1365 (1970).
16 Jackson, D. MacG.: Burns as a special problem in trauma. J. Trauma *10:* 991–996 (1970).
17 Kano, K.; Milgrom, F., and Rapaport, F. T.: Immunologic studies in thermal injury: heterophile antibodies. Proc. Soc. exp. Biol. Med. *125:* 142–146 (1967).
18 Kano, K.; Milgrom, F., and Rapaport, F. T.: Im-

munologic studies in thermal injury: antigenic properties of burned guinea pig skin. Proc. Soc. exp. Biol. Med. *128:* 1165–1168 (1968).

19 Kano, K.; Milgrom, F.; Witebsky, E., and Rapaport, F. T.: Immunologic studies in thermal injury: hemagglutinating factor in the lymph of burned rats. Proc. Soc. exp. Biol. Med. *123:* 930–935 (1966).

20 Kohn, J.: Abnormal immune response in burns. Post-grad. med. J. *48:* 335–337 (1972).

21 Koslowki, L.: Die Pathophysiologie der Verbrennungs-Krankheit in Lichte neuer Forschungsergebnisse. Arch. Klin. Chir. *329:* 880–888 (1971).

22 Liedberg, N. C. F.; Kuhn, L. R.; Barnes, B. A.; Reiss, E., and Amspacher, W. A.: Infection in burns. II. The pathogenicity of streptococci. Surgery Gynec. Obstet. *98:* 693–699 (1954).

23 Mancini, R. E.; Mazzolli, A., and Thierer, E.: Immunological and testicular response of guinea pigs sensitized with homogenate from homologous thermal injured testis. Proc. Soc. exp. Biol. Med. *139:* 991–996 (1972).

24 Markley, K.; Gurmendi, G.; Mori-Chavez, P., and Bazan, A.: Fatal pseudomonas septicemias in burned patients. Ann. Surg. *145:* 175–181 (1957).

25 Matter, P.; Chambler, K.; Bailey, B.; Lewis, S. R.; Blocker, T. G., and Blacker, V.: Experimental studies with reference to antigen-antibody phenomena following severe extensive burns. Ann. Surg. *157:* 725–736 (1963).

26 Milgrom, F.: When does self-recognition fail? Ser. Hemat. *9:* 17–25 (1965).

27 Moncrief, J. A.: Burns. New Engl. J. Med. *288:* 444–454 (1973).

28 Newton, W. T.; Fuji, K., and Moyer, C. A.: Immune specificity of burn toxin. Arch. Surg., Lond. *85:* 912 (1962).

29 Price, W. R.; Wood, M., and Childers, D.: Presence of leukocyte antibodies in major thermal burns. Am. J. Surg. *118:* 871–873 (1969).

30 Quismorio, F. P.; Bland, S. L., and Friou, G. J.: Autoimmunity in thermal injury: occurrence of rheumatoid factors, antinuclear antibodies and anti-epithelial antibodies. Clin. exp. Immunol. *8:* 701–711 (1971).

31 Rapaport, F. T. and Bachvaroff, R. J.: Kinetics of humoral responsiveness in severe thermal injury. Ann. Surg. *184:* 51–59 (1976).

32 Rapaport, F. T. and Bachvaroff, R. J.: *De novo* appearance of a high molecular weight serum lipoprotein in severely burned mice (abstr.). Fed. Proc. Fed. Am. Socs exp. Biol. *37:* 1600 (1978).

33 Rapaport, F. T.; Converse, J. M.; Horn, L.; Ballantyne, D. L., and Mulholland, J. H.: Altered reactivity to skin homografts in severe thermal injury. Ann. Surg. *159:* 390–395 (1964).

34 Rapaport, F. T.; Milgrom, F.; Kano, K.; Gesner, B.; Solowey, A. C.; Casson, P.; Silverman, H. I., and Converse, J. M.: Immunologic sequelae of thermal injury. Ann. N.Y. Acad. Sci. *150:* 1004–1008 (1968).

35 Rapaport, F. T.; Sampath, A.; Kano, K.; McCluskey, R. T., and Milgrom, F.: Immunological effects of thermal injury. I. Inhibition of spermatogenesis in guinea pigs. J. exp. Med. *130:* 1411–1425 (1969).

36 Rosenthal, S. R.: Substances released from the skin following thermal injury: 'burn toxin'. Surgery, St Louis *46:* 932–947 (1959).

37 Ball, S.; Bachvaroff, R. J., and Rapaport, F. T.: Effects of multiple repeated small burns upon host resistance to severe thermal injury (abstr.). Fed. Proc. Fed. Am. Socs exp. Biol. *37:* 622 (1978).

38 Wilmore, D. W.; Curreri, P. W., and Spitzer, K. W.: Supranormal dietary intake in thermally injured hypermetabolic patients. Surgery Gynec. Obstet. *132:* 881–886 (1971).

Dr. F. T. Rapaport, Department of Surgery, State University of New York at Stony Brook, Health Sciences Center, Stony Brook, NY 11794 (USA)

Immunopathology. 6th Int. Convoc. Immunol., Niagara Falls, N.Y., 1978, pp. 167–172 (Karger, Basel 1979)

Hemolytic Anemia with Autoantibodies[1]

H. Hugh Fudenberg[2]

Department of Basic and Clinical Immunology and Microbiology, Medical University of South Carolina, Charleston, S.C.

The discovery of Coombs' antiglobulin reagent in 1945 [3] led to the demonstration in the late 1940s that most cases of hemolytic anemia which were not due to intrinsic red blood cell (RBC) defects (e.g. abnormal hemoglobin or defective or inactive enzymes) were associated with a positive direct Coombs' test, implying autoimmunity to RBC [8, 19]. Furthermore, the eluates from patients' RBC contained 'incomplete' antibody to human RBC. Within 8 years, the discovery of corticoids [5, 7] was followed by the demonstration that such patients in the main responded dramatically to these drugs.

At just about the same time, agammaglobulinemia was described by *Bruton* [1] and by *Janeway and Gitlin* [18]. These two syndromes (agammaglobulinemia and 'autoantibody hemolytic anemia'), very different in both clinical manifestations and type of therapy, provided the basis for early clinical applications of immunologic theory and the beginning of clinical immunology as a separate discipline in medicine. Autoantibody hemolytic anemia was the first disease generally accepted in humans as being 'autoimmune'. Before that, there was a great controversy as to whether 'autoimmunity' even existed [17]. This was also the first disease in which IgM antibodies were identified (i.e. chronic cold agglutinin hemolytic anemia), and it was a disease which for some time caused a controversy as to how 'autoantibodies' should be defined. The less restrictive nomenclature defined autoantibodies as any antibody which was provoked by native or denatured material and which reacted with host material. However, these particular antierythrocyte antibodies react better with human RBC than with the RBC of other species, and they react better with RBC from the same individual or individuals with RBC antigens of the same genetic type than with other human RBC [6]. Therefore, a 'restrictive' definition of autoimmunity was proposed [9], for disease associated with autoantibodies which react with cells or tissues from the same species and react better (or at least as well) with the patient's own cells or tissues than with tissues from individuals of different genetic type [11]. Thus, anti-RBC antibodies conform to the restrictive definition of autoantibody. Another point of interest is that these were the first human antibodies that were shown to be destructive for the target cell involved (e.g. cold agglutinin hemolysis).

It was also shown subsequently by a number of workers that the amount of antibody on the cells in warm antibody hemolytic anemia (WAHA) was related to the severity of the disease [12]. It is worth mentioning that cold agglutinin hemolytic anemia shows some relationship between the fine structure of antigenic determinants and the chemical nature of the antibodies produced. Table I demonstrates some aspects of cold antibody hemolytic anemia and WAHA. In the latter, usually IgG, sometimes both IgG and complement, or sometimes complement alone may be detected on the RBC (about half of the cases are associated with underlying disease, such as lymphoma or systemic lupus erythematosus, SLE). IgG alone is usually present in idiopathic WAHA, as opposed to IgG plus complement

[1] This is Publication No. 242 from the Department of Basic and Clinical Immunology and Microbiology, Medical University of South Carolina. Research supported in part by USPHS Grant AI-13484.

[2] I thank *Charles L. Smith* and *Michelle R. DiMaria* for assistance in preparing the manuscript.

Table I. Autoantibody hemolytic anemia

	Specificity	Destruction site	Response to steroids
Warm			
γ (usually γ_1 and γ_3)	anti-U (15%) anti-nl, anti-pdl, anti-dl (85%)	RES	$++++$
$\gamma + C_3d$	anti-nl, anti-pdl, anti-dl	RES	$+++$
C_3d	?	RES	$++$
Cold			
IgMκ_{ii} (90%)	anti-I	intravascular	$0-+$
IgMκ	anti-I	intravascular	$0-+$
IgAκ_{iv}	anti-Pr$_1$	intravascular	?
IgMκ_{iv}	anti-Pr$_2$	intravascular	?

in SLE. The destruction site of these antibody-coated cells is not within the bloodstream, and with positive direct Coombs' tests, complement fixation does not occur because the antibodies bind to the RBC. Macrophages and monocytes in peripheral blood have receptors for the Fc fragment of IgG [15] and for complement [16], and these macrophages remove the coated cells.

About 85% of these antibodies have specificity for one or another antigen of the Rh system, either a 'complete' or an 'incomplete' antigen. About 15% of the cases have specificity for the U antigen, which is present in 99.9% of the population. The response to steroids in WAHA with IgG is almost always dramatic, more than 95%, with IgG and complement about 75%, and with complement alone about 25%. The response of high-titer cold agglutinin hemolytic anemia to steroids is practically zero. The severity of the latter depends more on the thermal amplitude (the temperature range at which the antibody reacts) than on the titer [4]. Hence, the incidence of this disease is much higher in, e.g. Buffalo, N.Y. than in Charleston, S.C. (There is also a high incidence of this disease in Southern California during the spring, when air conditioning is turned on and outdoor swimming pools are first used [*Fudenberg,* unpubl. observations].)

The destruction of coated RBC in cold agglutinin hemolytic anemia is an immunological reaction type II, the lysis being complement-dependent. As mentioned above, steroids rarely are of help. Most of the antibodies are directed toward the I antigen [28], which is present on the RBC of 99.9% of the human population; a few are directed toward i [20], and some others are directed toward other antigens on the RBC, termed Pr$_1$, Pr$_2$, etc. [23]. (Pr$_1$ is further subdivided into Pr$_{1d}$ and Pr$_{1h}$ [16].)

Titers of the anti-I and anti-i antibodies increase when the cells are pretreated with proteolytic enzymes, whereas the titers of anti-Pr (Pr$_1$, Pr$_2$, etc.) decrease. The anti-I and anti-i antibodies are almost always (in 8 out of 8 cases we studied) IgM κ subclass II, variable-region (V$_H$) subclass I; this also appears to be true for the constant and variable regions of the heavy chains of anti-i. In the Pr antibodies, we have found IgA or IgM constant regions and a special kind of κ chain, type IV [14]. Indeed, type IV was discovered during our studies of cold agglutinins [27]. The anti-Pr antibodies have variable-region heavy chains other than type I (i.e. V$_H$II or V$_H$III).

In 1957, Dr. *Kunkel* and I [11] used starch-block electrophoresis to separate the serum from patients with anti-I high-titer cold agglutinin anemia into fractions of different mobility. The cold agglutinins were all found in the fast γ area on electrophoresis and confined to the 19S fraction in density gradient centrifugation [10]. They were later shown to be IgM by electrophoresis [*Fudenberg and Kunkel,* unpubl. observations]. This was the first demonstration of 19S IgM autoantibody. Table II suggests that differences in fine

Table II. Autoantibodies in acquired hemolytic anemia and their serologic reactivity for selected RBC

	Anti-nl	Anti-pdl	Anti-dl	Suggested antigenic make-up of RBC
'Normal' cells CDe/CDe, cDE/cDE, etc.	+	+	+	nl, pdl, dl
'Partially deleted' cells –D–/–D– or cD–/cD–	–	+	+	pdl, dl
'Fully deleted' cells –––/––– (Rh$_{null}$)	–	–	+	dl

antigenic structure exist between the I and Pr antigens, as shown by amino acid composition of the antibodies. (The Pr antigen, as mentioned above, is subdivided into Pr$_1$, Pr$_2$, Pr$_3$, and Pr$_4$, and Pr$_1$ is further subdivided as are Pr$_2$, etc.; presumably, these are more similar to one another than to the I and i antigens.) Table II also shows that the heavy chain variable regions of all the IgM high-titer cold agglutinins with anti-I and anti-i specificity were IgM with μ type constant regions and were light chain κ type II. So this very fine difference in antigenic specificities is accompanied by preferential selection of one or another subclass of heavy and light chains, a point meriting comment in regard to the current controversy regarding generation of antibody diversity.

In terms of IgG WAHA antibodies, the specificities can be described in several ways. To oversimplify, normal RBC have the antigens C or c, D or d, and E or e, although anti-d has never been found. In conventional terminology, these are called 'nl' (normal). In some humans, the RBC lack both C and c or both E and e; these are designated 'partially deleted' (pdl) cells. In the absence of E and e, C and c, and D and d as well, the cells are designated –––/––– or 'Rh$_{null}$' (or 'completely deleted' [dl] cells). There are nonhuman sera that react with pdl cells, and all three types of antisera can be obtained by absorption of anti-Rh with the appropriate RBC. One can define the specificity of the absorbed antisera by testing against nl, pdl, and dl cells [24]. Obviously, nl will react with all three antisera. If the cells do not react, they lack the antigenic determinants concerned.

By performing a checkerboard of serologic tests with antisera absorbed with each of these three cell types, in 85% of the cases the eluates can be shown to react with anti-nl, anti-pdl, or anti-dl. Normal cells react with all three antisera. In the event that the given RBC do not react with the anti-nl serum, they lack antigenic determinants characteristic of nl but react with the rare RBC having partial or full deletions [25]. The antibodies of WAHA, after appropriate absorption, show specificity in 85% of the cases toward one of these three antigenic types.

Proof of autoimmunity was provided in 1 case studied by *Mohn et al.* [21], who described a patient positive for the E antigen who later developed RBC eluates with anti-E antibodies. We have observed similar findings in several patients of type CDe/cDe who developed hemolytic anemia with anti-e in the eluate [*Fudenberg*, unpubl. observations]. Data derived from such studies argue against the clonal selection hypothesis of *Burnet* [2], which is incorrect for other reasons as well.

In our studies, WAHA was idiopathic in about half the cases and in the other half was associated with chronic lymphatic leukemia, lymphoma, SLE and also, in a very small percentage of cases, with other disorders. The survival time of the RBC in terms of apparent half-life varies from 5 to 21 days, and the γ-globulin detectable by micro-Kjeldahl precipitin test, using rabbit antihuman IgG against eluates obtained from washed stromata of 200 ml of RBC from each patient, was small, ranging from 1.80 μg/ml protein nitrogen down to undetectable levels. However, the RBC survival was inversely related to the amount of IgG detectable in the precipitin test, especially for given patients in whom serial studies were performed during stable stages before therapy, during mild therapy, and after remission [12].

Table III shows the reactions of eluates with a panel of RBC of various Rh antigen compositions as well as of the pdl type and of the 'Rh$_{null}$' type. In our studies of 55 patients, 64% had eluates with a single specificity within the Rh system; 36% had multiple specificities (10% had anti-U or other specificity as well) [25, 26]. The vast majority of cases had only IgG antibodies, and a few had only IgM. The demonstration of serum complement components on the RBC seemed to be associated with autoantibodies of multiple immunoglobulin classes or multiple RBC specificities (table IV). The fixation of complement on the RBC of patients with acquired hemolytic anemia together with the progressive formation of multiple RBC antibodies may represent the natural evolution of the disease [22].

The variability encountered in multiple antibodies may reflect continuous differences in the antigenic stimulus, resulting from al-

tered configuration of RBC antigenic determinants. Assuming that trapping and processing of antigen are prerequisites for the induction of antibody response, it may be postulated that an adequate concentration of anti-nl on the RBC antigen site inhibits further synthesis of this antibody but not necessarily the enhancement of antibody synthesis for other unbound antigens on the immunizing RBC (anti-pdl and anti-dl). The suggestion that multiple antibody and im-

Table III. Distribution of 'anti-nl', 'anti-pdl' and 'anti-dl' in 55 RBC eluates

Autoantibody specificity	Number observed	Percentage	
Anti-nl	24[1]	44	
Anti-pdl	5	9	64%
Anti-dl	6	11	
Anti-nl plus pdl	4[2]	7	
Anti-nl plus pdl plus dl	14	26	36%
Anti-pdl plus dl	2	3	
Total	55		

[1] Two RBC eluates in this group disclosed antibody activity for well-defined Rh antigens, one anti-e and one anti-C.
[2] One RBC eluate in this group possessed anti-e in addition to anti-nl and anti-pdl.

Table IV. Indirect antiglobulin reactivity of various autoantibodies for specific preparations of anti-IgG, anti-IgM, anti-IgA and anti-complement

Immunoglobulin pattern of observed autoantibodies	Anti- 'nl'	Anti- 'pdl'	Anti- 'dl'	Anti- 'nl + pdl'	Anti- 'nl + pdl + dl'	Anti- 'pdl + dl'
IgG	18	4	2	–	–	–
IgM	4	1	3	–	–	–
IgG + IgM	2	–	1	1	–	–
IgG + IgA	–	–	–	–	1	–
IgG + IgM + C	–	–	–	3	8	2
IgG + IgM + IgA + C	–	–	–	–	3	–
IgG + IgA + C	–	–	–	–	2	–
Totals	24	5	6	4	14	2

munoglobulin formation follows a predetermined sequence of development as a consequence of variability in antigen presentation is not in agreement with the idea that the disease results primarily from an aberration of the normal humoral immune mechanism. The findings suggest instead that the initial development of autoantibodies (anti-nl, anti-pdl, and anti-dl) results from a defect in the structural composition of the Rh antigen, which is thereafter rejected by a normal immune mechanism. The subsequent development of additional specificities to other RBC antigens involving multiple immunoglobulin classes does not necessarily indicate the establishment of an aberrant immune apparatus, as would be expected by *Burnet*'s theory, but is comparable with 'broadening' of antibody specificities as observed elsewhere [13].

References

1 Bruton, O. C.: Agammaglobulinemia. Pediatrics *9:* 722–728 (1952).
2 Burnet, F. M.: The clonal selection theory of acquired immunity (Cambridge University Press, Cambridge 1959).
3 Coombs, R. A.; Mourant, A. E., and Race, R. R.: A new test for the detection of weak and 'incomplete' Rh agglutinins. Br. J. exp. Path. *26:* 255–266 (1945).
4 Dacie, J. V.: The haemolytic anaemias. Congenital and acquired (Grune & Stratton, New York 1954).
5 Dacie, J. V.: The auto-immune haemolytic anaemias. Am. J. Med. *18:* 810–821 (1955).
6 Dacie, J. V. and Cutbush, M.: Specificity of autoantibodies in acquired haemolytic anaemia. J. clin. Path. *7:* 18–21 (1954).
7 Dameshek, W.: Haematological application of ACTH and cortisone. Br. med. J. *ii:* 612 (1952).
8 Dameshek, W.: Hemolytic anemia. Distinct and indirect indications, pathogenetic mechanisms and classifications. Am. J. Med. *18:* 315–325 (1955).
9 Fudenberg, H. H.: Are autoimmune diseases immunologic deficiency states? Hosp. Pract. *3:* 43–53 (1968).
10 Fudenberg, H. H. and Franklin, E. C. Rheumatoid factors and the etiology of rheumatoid arthritis. Ann. N.Y. Acad. Sci. *124:* 884–895 (1965).
11 Fudenberg, H. H. and Kunkel, H. G.: Physical properties of the red cell agglutinins in acquired hemolytic anemia. J. exp. Med. *106:* 689–702 (1957).
12 Fudenberg, H. H.; Barry, I., and Dameshek, W.: The erythrocyte-coating substance in autoimmune hemolytic disease: its nature and significance. Blood *3:* 201–215 (1958).
13 Fudenberg, H. H.; Rosenfield, R. E., and Wasserman, L. R.: Unusual specificity of auto-antibody in auto-immune hemolytic disease. J. Mt Sinai Hosp. *25:* 324–329 (1958).
14 Gergely, J.; Wang, A. C., and Fudenberg, H. H.: Chemical analysis of variable regions of heavy and light chains of cold agglutinins. Vox Sang. *24:* 432–440 (1973).
15 Huber, H. and Fudenberg, H. H.: Receptor sites of human monocytes for IgG. Int. Archs Allergy appl. Immun. *34:* 19–31 (1968).
16 Huber, H.; Polley, M. J.; Linscott, W. D.; Fudenberg, H. H., and Müller-Eberhardt, H. J.: Human monocytes: distinct receptor sites for the third component of complement and for immunoglobulin G. Science *162:* 1281–1283 (1968).
17 Jandl, J. H. and Simmons, R. L.: The agglutination and sensitization of red cells by metallic cations: interactions between multivalent metals and the red-cell membrane. Br. J. Haemat. *3:* 19–38 (1957).
18 Janeway, C. A. and Gitlin, D.: Gamma globulins. Adv. Pediat. *9:* 65–136 (1957).
19 Kidd, P.: Elution of an incomplete type of antibody from the erythrocytes in acquired haemolytic anaemia. J. clin. Path. *2:* 103–108 (1949).
20 Marsh, W. L. and Jenkins, W. J.: Haematology. Anti-i: a new cold antibody. Nature, Lond. *188:* 753 (1960).
21 Mohn, J. F.; Lambert, R. M.; Bowman, H. S., and Brason, F. W.: Experimental production in man of autoantibodies with Rh specificity. Ann. N.Y. Acad. Sci. *124:* 477–483 (1965).
22 Roelcke, D.: Serological studies on the Pr_1/Pr_2 antigens using dog erythrocytes. Vox Sang. *24:* 354–361 (1973).
23 Roelcke, D.; Ebert, W.; Metz, J., and Weicker, H.: I-, MN- and Pr_1/Pr_2-activity of human erythrocyte glycoprotein fractions obtained by Ficin treatment. Vox Sang. *21:* 352–361 (1971).
24 Vos, G. H.; Petz, L., and Fudenberg, H. H.: Specificity of acquired haemolytic anaemia autoantibodies and their serological characteristics. Br. J. Haemat. *19:* 57–66 (1970).
25 Vos, G. H.; Petz, L. D., and Fudenberg, H. H.: Specificity and immunoglobulin characteristics of autoantibodies in acquired hemolytic anemia. J. Immun. *106:* 1172–1176 (1971).

26 Vos, G. H.; Petz, L. D.; Garratty, G., and Fudenberg, H. H.: Autoantibodies in acquired hemolytic anemia with special reference to the LW system. Blood *42:* 445–454 (1973).

27 Wang, A. C.; Fudenberg, H. H.; Wells, J. V., and Roelcke, D.: A new subgroup of the kappa chain variable region associated with anti-Pr cold agglutinins. Nature new Biol. *243:* 126–128 (1973).

28 Wiener, A. S.; Unger, L. J.; Cohen, L., and Feldman, J.: Type-specific cold auto-antibodies as a cause of acquired hemolytic anemia and hemolytic transfusion reactions: biological test with bovine red cells. Ann. intern. Med. *44:* 221–240 (1956).

Dr. H. H. Fudenberg, Department of Basic and Clinical Immunology and Microbiology, Medical University of South Carolina, Charleston, SC 29403 (USA)

A Postscript to Dr. Fudenberg's Lecture

Dr. Philip Levine (Sloan-Kettering Institute, New York and Ortho Diagnostics, Raritan, N. J.): In the course of hearing Dr. *Fudenberg* delivering his paper on 'Hemolytic Anemia with Antibodies', it occurred to me that the several types of this disease—the cold and the warm varieties—could be explained on the basis of the biochemical structure of the ABO, P, MN, and Rh blood group systems and their reaction with their respective antibodies. The ABO, P, and I antigens on the red cell membrane are glycosphingolipids whose structures and genetic synthetic pathways are in large measure understood. It has long been known that antibodies to these antigens (including those for M and N glycopeptides) are maximally reactive at low temperature. These observations have been firmly established by *Lalezari* in his studies of these antibodies in the autoanalyzer where the tests could be carried out at controlled temperatures of 10, 20, and 37 °C.

These findings allow for a clear distinction between antibodies specific for the ABO, P (glycosphingolipids), and MNSs (glycopeptides), which react best at 10 °C and minimally at 37 °C, from antibodies specific for Rh and Duffy which react maximally at 37 °C and only weakly at 10 °C. In contrast to the ABO and P glycosphingolipids and the MNSs glycopeptides in which the terminal determinant is a very small, low-molecular-weight substance, the Rh antigen—structurally a very large high-molecular-weight lipoprotein—was shown by myself to be an integral component of the structural membrane itself. This followed from my attempt to explain the fully compensated hemolytic anemia in all Rh$_{null}$ individuals tested.

It has long been suspected that autoimmune hemolytic anemia of the warm variety is induced by viruses or drugs which attach to the membrane and thus conform to the self-nonself concept.

Lesions resulting from deposition in selected tissues of immune complexes of 20–22 S (Svedberg) units are characteristic of cancer, rheumatoid arthritis, lupus erythematosus etc. There is now increasing evidence to indicate that Coombs' positive hemolytic anemia of the warm variety also falls in this general group of the self-nonself concept of diseases.

Finally, I suggest that the terms 'autoimmune' and 'autoimmunization' should be deleted from the medical literature. It is becoming increasingly clear that the diseases previously associated with these terms conform to the self-concept with recognition of the nonself as a foreign antigen which stimulates the production of specific antibodies.

Immunologically Mediated Systemic Diseases

Immunopathology. 6th Int. Convoc. Immunol., Niagara Falls, N.Y., 1978, pp. 173–177 (Karger, Basel 1979)

Systemic Lupus Erythematosus[1]

P. A. *Miescher*

Hôpital Cantonal, University of Geneva, Geneva

This paper summarizes the main clinical and immunopathologic aspects of systemic lupus erythematosus (SLE) as a baseline for the subsequent contributions on a number of more specific immunopathological questions.

It might be appropriate to mention the early discovery of the LE cell phenomenon being due to the action of antinuclear antibodies on damaged neutrophils [6]. Soon thereafter it became possible to analyze further antinuclear antibodies and to define those directed against nucleoprotein [7], DNA [1, 3, 8, 12] and histone [5]. After those early discoveries, a multitude of immune phenomena have been discovered, making SLE one of the 'richest' autoimmune conditions.

Definition

SLE has become the prototype of autoimmune pathology. Most clinicians accept the following definition of this disease: an inflammatory, noninfectious, self-perpetuating, multi-systemic disease with a predominantly vascular immunopathology and with antinuclear antibodies during disease activity,

[1] This work was supported by the Dubois-Ferrière/Dinu Lipatti Foundation and the K. and M. Arnold Fund.

as well as other autoimmune phenomena. If one included patients suffering from lupus-like conditions, but not exhibiting antinuclear antibody activity during the active stage of the disease, one would create more problems rather than simplify the lupus concept.

As in a number of other autoimmune conditions, one has to distinguish between the idiopathic type, which is probably genetically based, and the drug-induced type. Drug-induced SLE is a drug-specific and limited lupus-like condition which disappears upon discontinuation of the offending drug.

Symptoms and Signs

It is interesting to note the initial symptoms which cause patients to consult a physician (table I). In 9 SLE patients referred to us with a diagnosis other than SLE, 2 were thought to have rheumatoid arthritis, 2 multiple sclerosis, 1 epilepsy, 1 hemolytic anemia, 1 Schoenlein-Henoch's purpura, and 1 rheumatic fever. Table II summarizes the main clinical and laboratory findings of our Geneva and New York series (265 patients).

Table III summarizes the final diagnoses of 127 patients who were referred with an original diagnosis of SLE.

Table I. Initial symptoms of 122 SLE consecutive cases

Symptom	Percent
Arthritis	51.0
Skin rash	38.5
Fever	6.4
Neurological features	2.5
Hemolytic anemia	0.8
Purpura	0.8

Table II. Main clinical and laboratory findings of 265 consecutive cases

Findings	Percent
Fever	97
Skin rash	72
Joint involvement	81
Kidney involvement	
Biology	61
Biopsy	99
Heart involvement	51
Serous membrane	56
Pulmonary involvement	15
GI involvement	25
Peripheral vessel involvement	24
CNS involvement	40
Peripheral NS involvement	14
Eye involvement	25

Table III. Final diagnosis of 127 patients referred with a diagnosis of SLE

Final diagnosis	Number of patients
SLE	113
Rheumatoid arthritis	3
Systemic scleroderma	3
Mixed connective tissue disease	2
Malignancy	1
Periodic fever	1
Degenrative muscle disease	1
No final diagnosis	3

While the diagnosis of SLE has become very easy in typical cases, there still remain a number of patients who pose great differential diagnostic problems. Depending on the definition of SLE, some of the undiagnosed patients may be labelled by some authors as suffering from SLE. However, the example of Venocuran®-induced 'pseudo-LE' [2] warrants caution with the diagnosis of SLE. Indeed, patients taking this drug developed antibodies to mitochondria in very high titers, and gradually developed a lupus-like clinical picture which disappeared upon discontinuation of the medication. Before the finding that Venocuran® was the etiologic agent of this condition, it has been thought to be a disease related to SLE.

Etiology and Pathogenesis

There has been much dispute about the *etiology* of SLE. Besides the drug-induced variety, viruses have been implicated. However, evidence is increasing that SLE is a disorder which has a polygenic genetic basis. Exogenous factors, such as viruses, may act as triggers in the realization of a genetically based disease.

The *vascular immunopathology* represents a basic pathogenic mechanism while cytotoxic autoimmune phenomena occur in a minority of patients. Three different types of vascular immunopathology may be differentiated. Figure 1 illustrates the immune complex type of vascular damage in which a preformed antigen-antibody complex becomes deposited on the endothelial part of the vessel with an inflammatory reaction triggered by the biological activity of the immune complexes. The second antibody-induced vascular immunopathology may be called the 'passive agglutination' type of vascular damage (fig. 2). As in the well-known passive hemagglutination reaction, the anti-

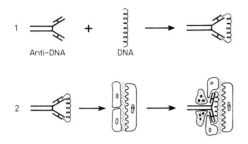

Fig. 1. Immune complex-type glomerular damage.

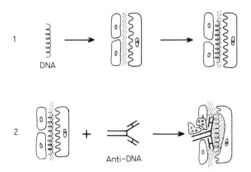

Fig. 2. Passive agglutination-type glomerular damage.

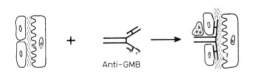

Fig. 3. Autoimmune-type glomerular damage.

genic determinant becomes first coated on the target organ, which suffers from the subsequent interaction of the fixed antigen with the corresponding antibody. *Izui et al.* [4] have demonstrated this pathway in the experimentally induced DNA-anti-DNA immune complex nephritis of the mouse. This is probably the prevalent mechanism respon-

sible for the glomerular damage in patients with SLE. Indeed, with the high affinity of DNA for basement membrane type of structures, one understands the exceedingly high incidence of glomerular damage in SLE, an incidence which is much higher than in any other immune complex disease. The third mechanism of antibody-induced vascular damage is mediated by autoantibodies (fig. 3). In SLE, antibodies against the glomerular basement membrane have been demonstrated with respective lesions within the glomeruli. More recently, antibodies against tubular basement membrane have also been shown. Their pathogenic significance is still uncertain.

With regard to blood cell damage, we may recognize again three different mechanisms. The first involves preformed immune complexes which may produce thrombocytopenia and/or leukopenia by coating the respective cells which are subsequently eliminated from the blood circulation (serum sickness-type lesion [9–11]). The second mechanism again involves the passive agglutination-type damage in which blood cells first become coated with the antigen and then with the antibody. DNA appears to have a high affinity for blood platelets, which may account for the frequent thrombocytopenia in patients with SLE. The third mechanism of antibody-induced blood cell damage involves autoantibodies against respective cells, in particular against red cells and platelets. With regard to thrombocytopenia, patients exhibiting a moderate reduction of the number of circulating platelets accompanying a high disease activity probably represent the immune complex type or the passive agglutination-type of thrombocytopenia. On the other hand, patients with no apparent disease activity and, in particular, with no circulating immune complexes, exhibiting thrombocytopenic purpura with a platelet count below 20,000 per mm^3, probably represent autoimmune thrombocytopenia.

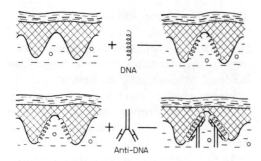

Fig. 4. Mechanism of DNA-mediated dermal immunopathology.

With regard to the skin lesions, we are probably dealing with a passive agglutination type of tissue damage with DNA coating the dermal collagen and with the antibodies locally triggering the immune complex type of inflammation (fig. 4).

Course of Disease

The course of the disease varies greatly from patient to patient. While a number of exacerbations can be related to exogenous factors, such as sunburn or wasp stings, in some patients no apparent cause can be found for either a particularly violent or mild course of the disease. Genetic factors probably are relevant for the disease manifestations in individual patients. This is particularly well illustrated by 4 of our patients who suffered from what may be called the equivalent of the NZB mouse disease, i.e. immune hemolytic anemia with or without thrombocytopenia and a lupus-like pathology, including antibodies to DNA and to coagulation Factor X complex in 2 patients. Three of the patients were males. The disease duration varied between 15 and 25 years without any change in the disease pattern other than varying degrees of immune hemolytic anemia or thrombocytopenia. A kidney biopsy performed in order to clarify this

disease condition showed, in all 4 patients, minimal lesions with subendothelial deposits but with no impairment of the renal function and with no proteinuria or pathological urinary sediment.

Treatment

Treatment of SLE has been a matter of much controversy. The disease does not lend itself easily to well-controlled studies. Indeed, treatment appears only successful if it is constantly adjusted to the disease activity of the patient, an arrangement which makes scientific studies very difficult. Yet, it appears that we have achieved a great deal with the development of treatment during the past 30 years. At the present time, we have a number of drugs at our disposal. Steroids still represent the basis of treatment, in particular in patients with kidney involvement. Other anti-inflammatory drugs are useful although only in combination with steroids. Immunosuppressive drugs may not be crucial in terms of survival in patients with kidney involvement. However, they are very much appreciated by the patients who cannot be treated with steroids alone without suffering severe side reactions which are particularly awkward for females. Antimalarial drugs were also appreciated before the introduction of immune suppressants for their steroid-sparing effect. However, they are of limited use because of the ocular side reactions which, once established, tend to increase despite discontinuation of the drug. Yet, if applied under control of electroretinograms, these drugs can be useful, but must be discontinued at the first sign of eye toxicity. Colchicine has been proved beneficial in patients suffering from immune hemolytic anemia in permitting reduction of steroid administration. Colchicine reacting with microfilamentous structures also reacts with the basic protein structures of the red cell membrane which contain the Rh 'antigenic matrix', i.e. the substrate against which autoantibodies of the warm type are usually directed. Plasmapheresis has proved useful in some acute cases in removing immune complexes and 'harmful' antibodies. Oral anticoagulants may become life-saving in patients with venous thrombosis as one of the main disease manifestations.

Cause of Death

The mortality of patients with SLE was very high some 20 years ago. Today, it has become a rather rare event for a SLE clinic to lose a patient. In part, this development is due to the fact that mild forms of SLE which were missed in the past are diagnosed today. However, prognosis has undoubtedly also changed for severe cases. The majority of our patients initially had a very high disease activity. Yet in the past 10 years, we only lost 9 out of 127 patients: 4 patients died in renal failure after a disease duration of 2, 3, 5, and 7 years, respectively; 2 patients with severe kidney involvement died of infection; 2 patients committed suicide, and 1 patient died of lethal complications during surgery (lobectomy for advanced tuberculosis). In the 6 patients with severe kidney involvement who died, treatment was started rather late, at a time when irreversible azotemia had already been established. It appears to us that improvement of treatment during the past 20 years plays a major role in the decreased mortality of patients with SLE. Furthermore, it has been our experience that the earlier patients with severe SLE are effectively treated, the better their prognosis.

References

1 Cepellini, R.; Polli, E., and Celada, F. A.: DNA-reacting factor in serum of a patient with lupus erythematosus diffusus. Proc. Soc. exp. Biol. Med. 96: 572–575 (1957).
2 Grob, P. J.; Müller-Schoop, J.; Häcki, M. A., and Joller-Jemelka, H. I.: Drug-induced pseudolupus. Lancet ii: 144–146 (1975).
3 Holman, H. R. and Deicher, H.: The reaction of the lupus erythematosus cell factor with deoxyribonucleoprotein of the cell nucleus. J. clin. Invest. 38: 2059–2064 (1959).
4 Izui, S.; Lambert, P. H., and Miescher, P. A.: Endotoxin and lupus-like syndrome; in Miescher, Proc. 7th Int. Symp. Immunopathology, pp. 191–204 (Schwabe, Basel 1977).
5 Kunkel, H. G.; Holman, H. R., and Deicher, H. R.: Multiple 'autoantibodies' to cell constituents in systemic lupus erythematosus. Ciba Found. Symp. on Cellular Aspects of Immunity, pp. 429–435 (Churchill, London 1960).
6 Miescher, P. A. et Fauconnet, M.: Les constituants antigéniques du leucocyte polynucléaire. Schweiz. med. Wschr. 84: 1036–1038 (1954).
7 Miescher, P. A. et Fauconnet, M.: L'absorption du facteur LE par des noyaux cellulaires isolés. Experientia 10: 252–254 (1954).
8 Miescher, P. A. and Straessle, R.: New serological methods for the detection of the LE factor. Vox Sang. 2: 283–287 (1957).
9 Miescher, P. A. und Miescher, A.: Die Sedormid-Anaphylaxie. Schweiz. med. Wschr. 82: 1279–1282 (1952).
10 Miescher, P. A.; Straessle, R. et Miescher, A.: Etude expérimentale du mécanisme des cytopénies anaphylactiques. Sang 26: 76–82 (1955).
11 Miescher, P. A. and Miescher, A.: Immunologic drug-induced blood dyscrasias. Klin. Wschr. 56: 1–5 (1978).
12 Seligmann, M.: Etudes immunologiques sur le lupus erythémateux disséminé et les anticorps anti-acide desoxyribonucléiques; in Grabar and Miescher, 1st Int. Symp. on Immunopathology, pp. 402–415 (Schwabe, Basel 1959).

Dr. P. A. Miescher, Hôpital Cantonal, Université de Genève, CH-1200 Genève (Switzerland)

Immunopathology. 6th Int. Convoc. Immunol., Niagara Falls, N.Y., 1978, pp. 178–181 (Karger, Basel 1979)

Clinical Significance of Immune Response to the Cytoplasmic Antigen Ro in Patients with Systemic Lupus Erythematosus[1]

Morris Reichlin and Peter J. Maddison

Departments of Medicine and Biochemistry, Veterans Administration Hospital, State University of New York at Buffalo, School of Medicine, Buffalo, N.Y.

Introduction

One of the serological hallmarks of patients with systemic lupus erythematosus (SLE) is the presence of antibodies to nuclear constituents. Characterized nuclear antigens reactive with the sera of SLE patients include native DNA, single-stranded DNA, nuclear RNA protein, DNA-histone, and Sm. The latter antigen does not contain nucleic acid and is thought to be an acidic glycoprotein [7]. SLE patients also frequently produce antibodies to cytoplasmic constituents, such as ribosomes, single-stranded RNA, and Ro. Antibodies to Ro, also thought to be an acidic glycoprotein, were found primarily in the sera of patients with SLE and Sjögren's syndrome [1]. The prototype serum first used to characterize the Ro system was from a patient who had many features of SLE and satisfied at least four of the preliminary criteria of the ARA [2] but at no time were serum globulins found that would stain the nuclei of mouse liver cells. Over the years, we have been evaluating retrospectively the incidence of antibodies to Ro in various diseases and have been struck by a number of

phenomena which are the basis of this paper. The most interesting thing to emerge from these studies is that a sizable number of patients exist who resemble our original patient. Such patients have clinical features which suggest SLE and yet lack antinuclear antibodies (ANA). It is common to find antibodies to Ro in this clinical setting and yet in about 1/3 to 1/2 of these patients antibodies to Ro are not present but antibodies of other specificities (which do not stain nuclei) are found. We designate these patients as having ANA negative SLE, an appellation which has recently appeared in the literature based on clinical observations alone [3].

The second thing that we report in this paper is the diagnostic specificity of antibodies to the Ro antigen based on a retrospective clinical analysis and finally data are presented comparing ANA-positive SLE patients with antibodies to Ro with ANA-positive SLE patients possessing antibodies of other specificities.

Results

Diagnostic Specificity of Anti-Ro. Antibodies to Ro are detected by a precipitin reaction in agarose gel utilizing a partially purified extract of human liver or spleen

[1] Work cited in this paper supported by USPHS Grant AM 10428 and funds from the Veterans Administration.

Table I. Diagnosis made in 72 patients whose sera contain antibodies to Ro

	Patients	
	n	%
Systemic lupus erythematosus	58[1]	81
Sjögren's syndrome	4[2]	6
Rheumatoid arthritis	2	3
Progressive systemic sclerosis	1	1
Cutaneous vasculitis	1	1
Non-rheumatic disease	6	8

[1] 45 patients (63 %) fulfilled preliminary criteria of the ARA for SLE.
[2] Two patients had polymyositis; one had rheumatoid arthritis.

Table II. Clinical findings in patients fulfilling ARA criteria for SLE with antibodies to the cytoplasmic antigen Ro; a comparison with patients with different antibody specificities

Clinical feature	Patients with precipitating antibodies		No precipitating antibodies
	Ro (n = 38)	nRNP (n = 30)	(n = 26)
	n	%	n	%	n	%
Facial rash	25	66	16	53	18	69
Discoid	7	18	2	7	4	15
Raynaud's syndrome	6	16	18	60	3	12
Photosensitivity	16	42	5	17	4	15
Polyarthritis	32	84	28	93	17	65
Pleurisy/pericarditis	16	42	17	57	11	42
Renal disease[1]	16	42	4	13	14	54
Neuropsychiatric	6	16	4	13	5	19
Cytopenia	26	68	20	67	19	73
Positive anti-ssDNA	16	42	4	13	18	69
Positive RA latex	27	71	8	26	3	12
Sjögren's syndrome	6	16	0		0	

[1] RBC > 5 per MPF and/or casts in urine sediment and/or proteinuria > 500 mg/24 h and/or deteriorating creatine clearance.

which has been subjected to $(NH_4)_2SO_4$ fractionation and DE_{52} chromatography. Identification of antibodies to Ro is confirmed by demonstration of a reaction of identity between the serum in question and a prototype serum monospecific for the Ro antigen with the antigen preparation employed [1].

Utilizing the precipitin technique, we have found 72 patients whose sera contained antibodies to the cytoplasmic antigen Ro. Table I lists the diagnoses of these patients. The disease which provided the major number of positive reactions was SLE (58 cases) while Sjögren's syndrome, rheumatoid arthritis (RA), scleroderma and cutaneous vasculitis provided 4, 2, 1 and 1 cases, respectively. The incidence of positive reactions for anti Ro among large numbers of RA patients is low, the 2 patients listed coming from a group of 73, an incidence of 3%. Similarly, the scleroderma patient with anti-Ro comes from a group of 20, an incidence of 5%. Thus, the only two diseases with a substantial incidence of antibodies to Ro are SLE and Sjögren's syndrome. Finally, six instances of antibodies to Ro were found among 5,000 sera screened from hospital patients with nonrheumatic diseases. This represents a 'false positive' incidence of about 1/1,000. Interestingly, 5 of these 6 patients were quite elderly, ranging in age from 60 to 80 years.

Clinical Features of Patients with Anti-Ro. We have done a retrospective clinical analysis of SLE patients with antibodies to Ro and contrasted them with two other groups of SLE patients: those with antibodies to nRNP and those with no precipitating antibodies, all of whom however were ANA-positive with the majority having complement-fixing antibodies to DNA. The clinical and serological data are listed in table II. The sizes of the three patient groups were 38, 30 and 26 patients, respectively. All of these patients fulfilled the preliminary criteria of the ARA for

SLE. As has been previously reported, the group possessing antibodies to nRNP is notable for two features: a high incidence of Raynaud's phenomenon and a low incidence of complement-fixing antibodies to ssDNA and serious renal diseases. The patients with antibodies to Ro are distinguishable from the other two groups by two features. These are the high incidence of photosensitivity and positive latex fixation reactions for rheumatoid factors in the anti-Ro group. Photosensitivity occurred in 42% of the anti-Ro patients but only in 17 and 15% of the anti-nRNP patients and the group with no precipitins, respectively. Even more dramatic is the 71% incidence of latex reactivity among the anti-Ro patients as compared to an incidence of 26 and 12%, respectively, in the other two groups. These two features are even more dramatically characteristic of the ANA-negative SLE patients with antibodies to the Ro antigen. It is notable that these patients have the expected frequency of renal involvement and unlike the anti-nRNP group are not protected from the development of serious renal disease [4]. Seven patients in the anti-Ro group have died and in 6 cases death was directly related to lupus nephritis. In 2 cases, study of the postmortem kidneys demonstrated considerable enrichment of anti-Ro in the glomerular eluates suggesting specific deposition of Ro-anti-Ro immune complexes [5].

ANA Negative SLE Patients. We have collected a total of 27 patients who have the clinical picture of SLE but lack demonstrable antinuclear antibodies on the conventional mouse liver substrate. Of these, 17 have antibodies to Ro and in the remainder antibodies to ssDNA were demonstrable by a double antibody radioimmunoassay in 4 patients' sera. No antibodies to nDNA were demonstrable in any of these patients by the *Crithidia lucilia* assay. In only 6 patients, no antibodies of any specificity were found. In table III are

Table III. Clinical findings in 27 patients with 'ANA-negative SLE': comparison between those with and without anti-cytoplasmic antibodies

Clinical feature	With anti-cytoplasmic antibodies (n = 17)		No anti-cytoplasmic antibodies (n = 10)	
	n	%	n	%
Malar rash	8	47	9	90
Discoid rash	6	35	0	
Photosensitivity	11	65	8	80
Polyarthritis	10	59	5	50
Pleurisy or pericarditis	8	47	4	40
Hematologic disease	10	59	1	10
Renal disease	3	18	3	30
Positive RA latex test	15	88	0	

listed the clinical features of the ANA-negative patients with and without antibodies to Ro antigen. It is notable that photosensitivity is very high in both groups but that only the anti-Ro group has a high incidence of latex reactivity. Indeed, 15 of the 17 patients with anti-Ro had positive latex fixation reactions. These data show that photosensitivity is not tightly linked to the presence of anti-Ro but that the presence of rheumatoid factors and anti-Ro are very tightly linked in this subgroup of ANA-negative patients. We have previously reported that patients who present with striking photosensitive lupus dermatitis who possess anti-Ro in their serum are at an apparently higher risk for the development of systemic disease [6].

Conclusions

Antibodies to Ro occur frequently in only SLE and Sjögren's syndrome. They occur in a low incidence (less than 5%) in other connective tissue diseases, such as RA and scleroderma. Although the vast majority of untreated active SLE patients produce some type of antinuclear antibody, a small fraction of otherwise typical SLE patients have no demonstrable ANA on the conventional liver and kidney substrates in their sera. We estimate that this represents about 5% of SLE patients and at least half of these can be serologically linked to other SLE patients by the presence of antibody to the cytoplasmic macromolecule Ro. Thus, these antibodies help to serologically define a group of patients with clinical features of SLE who lack ANA. The other features of SLE patients which are distinctively associated with the presence of anti-Ro are a high incidence of photosensitive rashes and an extraordinary incidence of rheumatoid factors. This latter feature, while unexplained, has a clinical corollary in the fact that these antibodies also occur frequently in the sera of patients with Sjögren's syndrome.

References

1 Clark, G. M.; Reichlin, M., and Tomasi, T. B.: Characterization of a soluble cytoplasmic antigen reactive with sera from patients with systemic lupus erythematosus. J. Immun. *102:* 117–122 (1968).

2 Cohen, A. S.; Reynolds, W. E.; Franklin, E. C.; Kulka, J. P.; Ropes, M. W.; Shulman, L. E., and Wallace, S. L.: Preliminary criteria for the classification of systemic lupus erythematosus. Bull. rheum. Dis. *21:* 643–648 (1971).

3 Fessel, W. J.: ANA-negative systemic lupus erythematosus. Am. J. Med. *64:* 80–86 (1978).

4 Maddison, P. J.; Mogavero, H., and Reichlin, M.: Patterns of clinical disease associated with antibodies to nuclear ribonucleoprotein. J. Rheum. (in press).

5 Maddison, P. J. and Reichlin, M.: The participation of antibodies to a soluble cytoplasmic antigen in the nephritis of systemic lupus erythematosus (abstr.). Clin. Res. *24:* 576 (1976).

6 Provost, T. T.; Ahmed, R. R.; Maddison, P. J., and Reichlin, M.: Antibodies to cytoplasmic antigens in lupus erythematosus: serological marker for systemic disease. Arthritis Rheum. *20:* 1457–1463 (1977).

7 Tan, E. M. and Kunkel, H. G.: Characteristics of a soluble nuclear antigen precipitating with sera of patients with systemic lupus erythematosus. J. Immun. *96:* 464–471 (1966).

Dr. M. Reichlin, Veterans Administration Hospital, 3495 Bailey Avenue, Buffalo, NY 14215 (USA)

Immunopathology. 6th Int. Convoc. Immunol., Niagara Falls, N.Y., 1978, pp. 182–184 (Karger, Basel 1979)

Defective Suppressor T Cells and Autologous Mixed Lymphocyte Reactions in Patients with Systemic Lupus Erythematosus

I. Green, T. Sakane and A. D. Steinberg

The Laboratory of Immunology, National Institute of Allergy and Infectious Diseases, and The Arthritis and Rheumatism Branch, National Institute of Arthritis, Metabolism and Digestive Diseases, National Institutes of Health, Bethesda, Md.

Systemic lupus erythematosus (SLE) is an autoimmune disease of unknown cause. Patients with SLE produce a wide variety of antibodies to tissue components [5]; it is these autoantibodies which lead to circulating immune complex formation and the disease manifestation [2]. Among the several possibilities which may explain this increased B cell autoreactivity is a relative loss of suppressor T lymphocytes [1, 3, 4, 10, 13, 14]. In this paper, we will demonstrate that this is indeed the case. Moreover, in the course of the studies concerning suppressor T cells, we made a most interesting accidental observation, that is, the autologous mixed lymphocyte reaction failed to occur.

To investigate suppressor T cells in patients with SLE, we used a modification [9] of the two-stage culture system as originally described by *Shou et al.* [12]. In the first culture, highly purified T cells are exposed to concanavalin A (Con A) to generate suppressor cells. Three days later, these cells were added to a second culture of responder cells. The responder cells were stimulated with either mitogens or allogeneic cells. The suppressor cells and the responder cells were from the same individual in most cases. In some experiments, the suppressor cells of one individual were mixed with responder cells from another individual.

In our total experience, Con A-activated lymphocytes from all 20 normal subjects studied generated suppressor T cells for mitogenic responses of both T cells and B cells. Lymphocytes from 18 of these 20 normals were also able to generate suppressor T cell activity for the T cell response to allogeneic cells. In contrast, T lymphocytes from most SLE patients failed to manifest such suppressor T cell activity for the T cell response to allogeneic cells, the T cell response to Con A and the B cell response to PWM. However, no significant impairment in generation of suppressor T cells was observed for the PHA response of T cells [10].

To determine whether the defect in the suppression phenomena observed in the lymphocytes of patients with SLE represents a defect in the development of suppressor cells, or a defect in ability of their cells to respond to suppressor cell signals, cell mixing experiments were performed. Responder cells from either normal individuals or patients with SLE could be suppressed equally by normal T cells activated by Con A. Thus, the suppressor defect in SLE was not a result of failure to respond to suppressor signals. However, when SLE cells were used as the source of the suppressor cells, there was impaired suppression. That is, the Con A-activated T cells from SLE patients produced significantly less suppression of responder cells from either normals or SLE patients. These cell mixing studies, therefore, suggest that lymphocytes from patients with SLE fail to generate adequate suppressor T cell function, but still retain the capacity to respond to normal suppressor T cells [10].

We will now describe our observations regarding the absence of autologous mixed lymphocyte reaction (MLR) in patients with active SLE. When non-T lymphocytes from normal individuals are mixed with autologous T cells, a proliferative response of the T cells is observed [6, 8, 11]. This autologous MLR has recently been reported to demonstrate both immunological specificity and memory [15] and it has been proposed that 'autologous MLR reflects a mechanism by which T lymphocytes regulate lymphocyte function' [6]. As noted above, we observed that this reaction was absent in patients with active SLE and was diminished in patients with inactive SLE. In contrast, patients with SLE were found to have an adequate allogeneic MLR [11].

The defect in autologous MLR could not be explained by a lack of stimulating cells since the percentage of B cells, L cells and monocytes in normals and patients with SLE were in the same range [11]. Patients with SLE often have a decrease in the number of circulating T cells; however, the same absolute number of responder T cells were used in the in vitro assay of autologous MLR in normals and patients with SLE. Thus, the defect in the autologous MLR observed was not due to an absence of sufficient number of T cells in the assay.

To further examine the role of responder SLE T cells in the abnormal autologous MLR, T cells were fractionated into T cells bearing Fc(IgG) receptors (Fc$^+$ T cells) and those not bearing Fc(IgG) receptors (Fc$^-$ T cells) by using preferential ability of Fc$^+$ T cells to form rosettes with IgG-coated ox erythrocytes [7]. Responding ability of these fractionated T cells was then studied in the autologous MLR.

In normal individuals, Fc$^+$ T cells as well as Fc$^-$ T cells responded well in both autologous and allogeneic MLR. Patients with inactive SLE, whose unfractionated T cells responded in autologous MLR to a normal or almost normal degree were then tested for the responding capacity of their fractionated T cells. The Fc$^-$ T cell fractions obtained from these patients responded perfectly well in both autologous and allogeneic MLR. In contrast, only minimal responses were obtained with Fc$^+$ T cell fractions from the inactive patients either in autologous MLR or allogeneic MLR. When active SLE patients were studied, the Fc$^+$ T cell fractions also responded abnormally in autologous MLR and in the allogeneic MLR. Finally, the Fc$^-$ T cells from the active patients were not stimulated in the autologous MLR.

In summary, responding lymphocytes from SLE patients were defective, and this defect appeared to be most prominent in the Fc$^+$ T fraction.

The relationship between Con A-induced suppressor T cell activity and autologous MLR was next examined. Con A-induced suppressor T cell activity of patients with SLE was studied by a procedure previously described in detail [9, 10]. Seven patients with active SLE were studied simultaneously for suppressor T cell activity and autologous MLR. In every case, both suppressor cell generation and autologous MLR were markedly defective. Lymphocytes from 6 normal individuals studied at the same time demonstrated normal activity for both functions [11].

Thus, in patients with active SLE, a suppressor T cell (previously noted to be of the Fc$^+$ subclass), as well as the Fc$^+$ T responder cell in the autologous MLR, both appear to be defective. Whether these are actually the same cells remains to be determined.

Obvious questions for future study are the relationships between the defective Fc$^+$ T cells and the overproduction of auto-antibodies observed in SLE as well as the role of serum factors (especially immune complexes and anti-T cell antibodies) with regard to these defective T cell functions.

References

1 Abdou, N. I.; Sagawa, A.; Pascual, E.; Hebert, J., and Sadeghee, S.: Suppressor T-cell abnormality in idiopathic systemic lupus erythematosus. Clin. Immunol. Immunopath. 6: 192–199 (1976).
2 Bardana, E. J.; Harbeck, R. J.; Hoffman, A. A.; Pirofsky, B., and Carr, R. I.: The prognostic and therapeutic implications of DNA: anti-DNA immune complexes in systemic lupus erythematosus. Am. J. Med. 59: 515–522 (1975).
3 Bresnihan B. and Jasin, H. E.: Suppressor function of peripheral blood mononuclear cells in normal individuals and in patients with systemic lupus erythematosus. J. clin. Invest. 59: 106–116 (1977).
4 Horowitz, S.; Borcherding, W.; Moorthy, A. V.; Chesney., R.; Schulte-Wissermann, H.; Hong, R., and Goldstein, A.: Induction of suppressor T cells in systemic lupus erythematosus by thymosin and cultured thymic epithelium. Science 197: 999–1001 (1977).
5 Kunkel, H. G. and Tan, E. M.: Autoantibodies and disease. Adv. Immunol. 4: 351–395 (1964).
6 Kuntz, M. M.; Innes, J. B., and Weksler, M. E.: Lymphocyte transformation induced by autologous cells. IV. Human T-lymphocyte proliferation induced by autologous or allogeneic non-T lymphocytes. J. exp. Med. 143: 1042–1054 (1976).
7 Moretta, L.; Webb, S. R.; Grossi, C. E.; Lydyard, P. M., and Cooper, M. D.: Functional analysis of

two human T-cell subpopulations: help and suppression of B-cell responses by T cells bearing receptors of IgM or IgG. J. exp. Med. 146: 184–200 (1977).
8 Opelz, G.; Kiuchi, M.; Takasuge, M., and Terasaki, P. I.: Autologous stimulation of human lymphocyte subpopulations. J. exp. Med. 142: 1327–1333 (1975).
9 Sakane, T. and Green, I.: Human suppressor T cells induced by concanavalin A: suppressor T cells belong to distinctive T cell subclasses. J. Immun. 119: 1169–1178 (1977).
10 Sakane, T.; Steinberg, A. D., and Green, I.: Studies of immune functions of patients with systemic lupus erythematosus. I. Failure of suppressor T cell activity related to impaired generation of, rather than response to, suppressor cells. Arthritis Rheum. 21: 657–664 (1978).
11 Sakane, T.; Steinberg, A. D., and Green, I.: Failure of autologous mixed lymphocytes reactions between T and non-T cells in patients with systemic lupus erythematosus, Proc. natn. Acad. Sci. USA 75: 3464–3468 (1978).
12 Shou, L.; Schwartz, S. A., and Good, R. A.: Suppressor cell activity after concanavalin A treatment of lymphocytes from normal donors. J. exp. Med. 143: 1100–1110 (1976).
13 Steinberg, A. D. and Klassen, L. W.: Role of suppressor T cells in lymphopoietic disorders. Clin. Haemat. 6: 439–478 (1977).
14 Stobo, J. D. and Loehnen, C. P.: Immunoregulation and autoimmunity. Mayo Clin. Proc. 51: 479–483 (1976).
15 Weksler, M. E. and Kozak, R.: Lymphocyte transformation induced by autologous cells. V. Generation of immunologic memory and specificity during the autologous mixed lymphocyte reaction. J. exp. Med. 146: 1833–1838 (1977).

Dr. I. Green, The Laboratory of Immunology, National Institute of Allergy and Infections Diseases, National Institutes of Health, Bethesda, MD 20014 (USA)

Immunopathology. 6th Int. Convoc. Immunol., Niagara Falls, N.Y., 1978, pp. 185–190 (Karger, Basel 1979)

Type C RNA Viral Genome Expression in Systemic Lupus Erythematosus (SLE)

The New Zealand Mouse Model and the Human Disease[1]

Robert C. Mellors and Jane W. Mellors

The Hospital for Special Surgery affiliated with the New York Hospital-Cornell University Medical College, New York, N.Y.

Introduction

SLE is a prototype of human systemic autoimmune disease. The possibility that the expression of a type C RNA viral genome might be implicated in the multifactorial pathogenesis of SLE is suggested by studies of the autoimmune New Zealand Black (NZB) mouse model [3, 7] of the human disease (table I). Immunopathological studies have shown that the spontaneous development of lupus-like immune-complex glomerulonephritis of New Zealand mice is related not only to nuclear antigen-antibody complexes [7, 11] but also to the glomerular deposition of a 70,000-dalton viral envelope glycoprotein, gp70 [24, 29]. gp70 is encoded by endogenous xenotropic type C viral genes that are discordantly expressed in these mice [12, 29]. Evidence for the expression of type C viral genomes in human SLE has been sought by several groups of workers [13–15, 17, 18, 25]. In this laboratory, postmortem immunopathological studies of a subset of patients with lupus diffuse proliferative glomerulonephritis have shown that an antigen which was recognized by monospecific goat antisera against viral core (p30) proteins of

mammalian and subhuman primate type C RNA viruses was deposited in the renal glomerular lesions along with host immunoglobulins in an immune-complex pattern [14, 15]. An attempt has been made to support and extend this finding by eluting host immunoglobulins from the immune deposits and assaying them for the presence of type C virus-reactive antibody. We have recently reported [16] that human immunoglobulins with specific anti-viral p30 activity and separated from anti-nuclear antibodies were eluted from the glomerular immune deposits in 2 patients with lupus glomerulonephritis known from previous work to have deposits of viral p30-related antigen in the same tissue lesions. A brief review of the progress of this new development is given in the present paper.

Materials and Methods

The starting materials for this study [16] were renal cortical tissues obtained at postmortem examination on 3 patients with lupus glomerulonephritis and showing diffuse glomerular deposits of human immunoglobulins (Igs) and C3 (table II). Focal glomerular deposits of viral p30-related antigen were present in 2 of the 3 cases. Human Igs were eluted from the glomeruli in two fractions according to the method of *Koffler et al.* [9] by sequential treatment with DNase to elute anti-DNA antibodies followed by acid buffer (pH 2.4) to elute any

[1] Supported by Grant CA-14928 awarded by the National Cancer Institute.

Table I. Comparison of murine and human SLE

	Murine SLE	Human SLE
Genetic factors	(polygenic)	(concordance of findings in identical twins)
Autoantibodies		
LE-cell inducing	+	+
Anti-deoxyribo-nucleoprotein	+	+
Anti-DNA (double/single-stranded)	+	+
Anti-RNA (double/single-stranded)	+	+
Anti-erythrocyte	+	+
Anti-thymocyte (T-cell)	+	+
Pathology and pathogenesis		
Immune-complex disease		
Glomerulonephritis	+	+
Systemic vasculitis	+	+
Autoimmune hemolytic anemia	+	+
Lymphoma/leukemia	+	±
Type C virus genome expression		
Virus-like particles	+	(normal and SLE placentas)
Viral antigens		
Internal (p30, etc.)	+	(+)[1]
Envelope (gp70)	+	
Infectious virus	xenotropic MuLV	
Virus antibodies	+	(+)[1]

[1] Tentative.

remaining antibodies. The eluted Igs were precipitated with ammonium sulfate, dialyzed and reconstituted to constant volume and normal pH and were assayed for Igs and for antibody activities as noted. The Ig concentrations were about equal in DNAase and acid-buffer eluates, approximately 0.1 mg/ml, and mainly of the IgG class. The DNAase eluates uniformly contained fluorescent antinuclear antibody with high specific activity compared to serum in the same case, as shown by the work of *Koffler et al.* [9]. Acid-buffer eluates in 2 of the 3 cases contained anti-p30 antibody as shown by immunofluorescence assay (IF) and enzymoimmunoassay (EIA) [16], which latter is the focus of this paper.

The familiar microplate indirect ELISA method [5, 28] was developed for detection and measurement of anti-p30 activity against viral p30 proteins. Briefly, purified p30 antigen on solid phase was incubated with antibody source (reference goat antisera or human lupus glomerular eluates) in liquid phase. Antibody uptake to antigen was quantitated by addition of alkaline phosphatase-conjugated anti-Ig and substrate. Antibody detection by EIAs is generally reported to be in the ng/ml range, comparable to radioimmunoassays.

Results

Table III records the antibody titers (endpoint dilutions) of reference goat anti-p30 sera as determined by EIA against homologous and heterologous p30 proteins of murine, feline, and primate (simian sarcoma-associated) infectious type C viruses and against p30 protein of feline endogenous virus RD-114 which is closely related to the baboon endogenous virus [20]. As expected, each antiserum had the highest titer against the homologous viral antigen and gave lower titers against heterologous viral antigens, in keeping with the extent of cross-reaction and relatedness of the viral p30 proteins [22, 26].

Table IV shows the anti-p30 antibody titers of human immunoglobulins eluted from lupus glomeruli by acid-buffer in 2 of the p30

Table II. Plan of study

Human SLE kidney   →   IF analysis of glomerular
  tissues (3 cases)   immune deposits:
       ↓   Hum Ig   (+, +, +)
Homogenate (discard)   Hum C3   (+, +, +)
       ↓   Viral p30   (+, +, −)
Sediment (containing
  glomeruli)
       ↓

Human Ig and antibody elution (in two fractions)[1]
       ↓

DNAase elution (anti-DNA antibodies)
       ↓

Acid buffer (pH 2.4) elution (other antibodies)
       ↓

Ig and antibody assays
       ↓

  IF: anti-nuclear, anti-cytoplasmic, anti-p30
            blocking activity
    ↓

  EIA[2]:   anti-p30 activity

[1] Method of *Koffler et al.* [9].
[2] Method of *Engvall and Perlman* [5].

Table III. Antibody titers (end-point dilutions) of goat anti-p30 sera determined by EIA[1]

Antigen	Anti-R-MuLV p30	Anti-RD-114 p28	Anti-SSAV p28
R-MuLV p30	*1,000,000*	10,000	30,000
FeLV p27	200,000	10,000	20,000
RD-114 p20	100,000	*64,000*	NT
SSAV p28	125,000	16,000	*1,000,000*

[1] Source of reagents: antisera from *R. Wilsnack*; R-MuLV p30 and FeLV p27 from *S. Oroszlan*; RD-114 p28 and SSAV p28 from *C. J. Sherr.*

Table IV. Anti-p30 antibody activity in human SLE glomerular eluates determined by EIA

Antigen	Acid eluates	
	dilution	$A^{400}/60$ min
RD-114 p28	160	0.83
"	*320*	*0.56*
"	640	0.32
"	1,280	0.22
R-MuLV p30	*80*	*0.53*
"	160	0.33
"	320	0.10
SSAV p28	*80*	*0.52*
AMV p27	20	<0.1
MMTV p28	20	<0.1
DNA	20	<0.1
RNA	20	<0.1
FCS	20	<0.1

tigen, and about 80 against the p30 antigens of murine and simian sarcoma associated viruses, consistent with weaker cross-reaction with more distantly related virus groups. There was no antibody activity measurable by EIA against the p30 antigens of avian myeloblastosis virus (a prototype avian type C virus) and mouse mammary tumor virus (a prototype murine type B virus), nor against single or double-stranded DNA and RNA, nor against fetal cell serum proteins (FCS). DNAase eluates from each case and acid-buffer eluate from the p30 antigen-negative case did not react with RD-114 or any other viral protein.

Koffler et al. [9] have developed a sensitive hemagglutination assay (HA) for measurement of anti-nucleic acid antibodies in human lupus glomerular eluates. Their data, recalculated and expressed in terms of minimum IgG concentration giving a positive assay, are summarized in table V along with the present findings on anti-p30 antibody. With due reservations for comparing results obtained by different methods and materials, it is noteworthy that the specific anti-p30

antigen-positive cases. The starting Ig concentrations of the eluates before dilution were in the range of 0.1 mg/ml, that is, about $\frac{1}{100}$ of the normal serum Ig concentration. Human anti-p30 antibody titers, conservatively evaluated as underlined, were in the range of about 320 against the p30 antigen of RD-114 virus, apparently a more closely related an-

Table V. Specific activity of antibodies in human SLE glomerular eluates expressed as minimum IgG concentration at end-point dilution

Antibody specificity	Assay	Min. IgG, μg/ml		Reference
		average	range	
Anti-nDNA	HA	15.9	1.3–94	[9]
Anti-ssDNA	HA	4.2	0.3–23	[9]
Anti-RNA Pr	HA	0.9	0.2–1.2	[9]
Anti-RD 114 p28	EIA	0.3	0.3	[this study]
Anti-R-MuLV p30	EIA	1.0	1.0	[this study]
Anti-SSAV p28	EIA	1.0	1.0	[this study]

activity measured by EIA in the present study was equivalent to the highest activity reported by *Koffler* and co-workers for anti-ssDNA antibodies in lupus glomerular eluates, namely, 0.3μg IgG/ml.

Discussion

The specificity of the reaction observed between human anti-p30 antibody and RD-114 antigen on solid phase was confirmed by inhibiting the antibody activity by absorption with minute concentrations (order of 100 ng/ml) of the same p30 antigen in liquid phase. It can also be remarked that the measured human anti-p30 activity was probably only a rough estimate of the true value, because, first, some of the potential anti-p30 activity in the acid eluates was probably absorbed at neutral pH by recombination with any remaining homologous antigen; and, secondly, anti-p30 activity in the eluates was assayed against RD-114, presumably a cross-reacting antigen rather than the putative homologous human viral antigen.

Several comprehensive papers in the literature have reported conflicting findings suggesting the presence and the absence of mammalian and subhuman primate-related type C viral nucleic acids [2, 6, 19], protein antigens [21, 23, 25, 27], and antibodies [1, 4, 8, 10, 23] in human tissues and sera in states of health and disease, including cancer and SLE. Critical evidence still lacking in human SLE tissue studies include: the detection of proviral sequences in normal cellular DNA if endogenous type C viral genes are present; evidence of structural homology between a putative viral antigen and an authentic viral protein if subinfectious antigenic expression is involved; isolation and characterization of a human type C virus if a fully infectious virus is implicated. Nonetheless, the possibility remains that the findings reported here on SLE might lead to biologically or clinically useful information.

In conclusion, human immunoglobulins showing anti-p30 antibody activity particularly against p30 antigen of feline endogenous virus RD-114 and to a lesser extent against the p30 antigens of murine and simian sarcoma-associated type C viruses were eluted from the glomerular immune deposits in 2 patients with lupus proliferative glomerulonephritis who had deposits of p30-related antigen in the same tissue lesions.

References

1 Aoki, T.; Walling, M. J.; Bushar, G. S.; Lui, M., and Hsu, K. C.: Natural antibodies in sera from healthy humans to antigens on surface of type C RNA viruses and cells from primates. Proc. natn. Acad. Sci. USA 73: 2491–2495 (1976).

2 Benveniste, R. A. and Todaro, G. J.: Evolution of type C viral genes. I. Nucleic acid from baboon type C virus as a measure of divergence among primate species. Proc. natn. Acad. Sci. USA 71: 4513–4518 (1974).

3 Bielschowsky, M.; Helyer, B. J., and Howie, J. B.: Spontaneous haemolytic anemia in mice of the NZB/BL strain. Proc. Univ. Otago med. School 37: 9–11 (1959).

4 Charman, H. P.; Kim, N.; White, M., and Gilden, R. V.: Failure to detect in human sera antibodies cross-reactive with group-specific antigens of murine leukemia virus. J. natn. Cancer Inst. 52: 1409–1413 (1974).

5 Engvall, E. and Perlmann, P.: Enzyme-linked immunosorbent assay, ELISA. III. Quantitation of specific antibodies by enzyme-labelled anti-immunoglobulin in antigen-coated tubes. J. Immun. 109: 129–135 (1972).

6 Hehlmann, R.; Kufe, D., and Spiegelman, S.: RNA in human leukemic cells related to the RNA of a mouse leukemia virus. Proc. natn. Acad. Sci. USA 69: 435–439 (1972).

7 Helyer, B. J. and Howie, J. B.: Renal disease associated with positive lupus erythematosus tests in a cross-bred strain of mice. Nature, Lond. 197: 197 (1963).

8 Hirsch, M. S.; Kelly, A. P.; Chapin, D. S.; Fuller, T. C., and Black, P. H.: Immunity to antigens associated with primate C type oncoviruses in pregnant women. Science 199: 1337–1340 (1978).

9 Koffler, D.; Agnello, V., and Kunkel, H. G.: Polynucleotide immune complexes in serum and glomeruli of patients with systemic lupus erythematosus. Am. J. Path. 74: 109–124 (1974).

10 Kurth, R.; Teich, N. M.; Weiss, R., and Oliver, R. T. D.: Natural human antibodies reactive with primate type-C viral antigens. Proc. natn. Acad. Sci. USA 74: 1237–1241 (1977).

11 Lambert, P. H. and Dixon, F. J.: Pathogenesis of the glomerulonephritis of NZB/W mice. J. exp. Med. 127: 502–522 (1968).

12 Levy, J. A.: Xenotropic viruses: murine leukemia viruses associated with NIH Swiss, NZB and other mouse strains. Science 182: 1151–1153 (1973).

13 Lewis, R. M.; Tannenberg, W.; Smith, C., and Schwartz, R. S.: C-type viruses in systemic lupus erythematosus. Nature, Lond. 252: 78–79 (1974).

14 Mellors R. C. and Mellors, J. W.: Antigen related to mammalian type-C RNA viral p30 proteins is located in renal glomeruli in human systemic lupus erythematosus. Proc. natn. Acad. Sci. USA 73: 233–237 (1976).

15 Mellors, R. C. and Mellors, J. W.: Type C RNA virus expression in systemic lupus erythematosus: New Zealand mouse model and human disease. Arthritis Rheum. 21: suppl. pp. S68–S75 (1978).

16 Mellors, R. C. and Mellors, J. W.: Type C RNA virus specific antibody in human systemic lupus erythematosus demonstrated by enzymoimmunoassay. Proc. natn. Acad. Sci. USA 75: 2463–2467 (1978).

17 Panem, S.; Ordonez, N. G.; Kirsten, W. H.; Katz, A. I., and Spargo, B. H.: C-type virus expression in systemic lupus erythematosus. New Engl. J. Med. 295: 470–475 (1976).

18 Phillips, P. E.; Hargrove, R.; Stewart, E., and Sarkar, N. H.: Type C oncornavirus isolation studies in SLE. I. Attempted detection by isopycnic sedimentation of ³H-uridine-labelled virions. Ann. rheum. Dis. 35: 422–428 (1976).

19 Reitz, M. S.; Miller, N. R.; Wong-Staal, F.; Gallagher, R. E.; Gallo, R. C., and Gillespie, D. H.: Primate type-C virus nucleic acid sequences (woolly monkey and baboon types) in tissues from a patient with acute myelogenous leukemia and in viruses isolated from cultured cells of the same patient. Proc. natn. Acad. Sci. USA 73: 2113–2117 (1976).

20 Sherr, C. J. and Todaro, G. J.: Radioimmunoassay of the major group specific protein of endogenous baboon type C viruses: relation to RD-114/CCC group and detection of antigen in normal baboon tissues. Virology 61: 168–181 (1974).

21 Sherr, C. J. and Todaro, G. J.: Type C viral antigens in man. I. Antigens related to endogenous primate virus in human tumors. Proc. natn. Acad. Sci. USA 71: 4703–4704 (1974).

22 Sherr, C. J.; Fedele, L. A.; Benveniste, R. E., and Todaro, G. J.: Interspecies antigenic determinants of the reverse transcriptase and p30 proteins of mammalian type C viruses. J. Virol. 15: 1440–1448 (1975).

23 Stephenson, J. R. and Aaronson, S. A.: Search for antigens and antibodies cross-reactive with type C viruses of the woolly monkey and gibbon ape in animal models and in humans. Proc. natn. Acad. Sci. USA 73: 1725–1729 (1976).

24 Strand, M. and August, J. T.: Structural proteins of oncogenic RNA viruses: interspec II, a new interspecies antigen. J. biol. Chem. 248: 5627–5633 (1973).

25 Strand, M. and August, J. T.: Type-C RNA virus
   gene expression in human tissue. J. Virol. *14:* 1584–
   1596 (1974).
26 Strand, M. and August, J. T.: Structural proteins of
   mammalian RNA tumor viruses: relatedness of the
   interspecies antigenic determinants of the major internal protein. J. Virol. *15:* 1332–1341 (1975).
27 Todaro, G. J. and Gallo, R. C.: Immunological
   relationship of DNA polymerase from human acute
   leukemia cells and primate and mouse leukemia virus
   reverse transcriptase. Nature, Lond. *244:* 206–209
   (1973).
28 Voller, A.; Bidwell, D., and Bartlett, A.: Microplate
   enzyme immunoassays for the immunodiagnosis of

virus infections; in Rose and Friedman Manual
of clinical immunology, pp. 506–512 (Am. Society
for Microbiology, Washington 1976).
29 Yoshiki, T.; Mellors, R. C.; Strand, M., and August,
   J. T.: The viral envelope glycoprotein of murine
   leukemia virus and the pathogenesis of immune complex glomerulonephritis of New Zealand mice. J.
   exp. Med. *140:* 1011–1027 (1974).

Dr. R. C. Mellors, The Hospital for Special
Surgery affiliated with the New York Hospital-
Cornell University Medical College, New York,
NY 10021 (USA)

Immunopathology. 6th Int. Convoc. Immunol., Niagara Falls, N.Y., 1978, pp. 191–196 (Karger, Basel 1979)

Relevance of Polyclonal Antibody Formation to the Development of Autoimmunity in Particular Relation to Murine Lupus[1]

P. H. Lambert, J. A. Louis, S. Izui and T. Kobayakawa

WHO Immunology Research and Training Centre, Geneva/Lausanne

A possible role of bacterial products in the development of autoantibodies is suggested by the observation that bacterial infection can trigger manifestations of systemic lupus erythematosus or induce an increase in the titer of anti-DNA antibodies in patients suffering from this disease [12]. Evidently, several mechanisms can be involved, including a release of endogenous tissue constituents and non-specific effects on the immune system.

It has been shown that the injection of bacterial lipopolysaccharides (LPS) in mice leads to a rapid release of DNA to circulating blood and within a few days induces the formation of anti-DNA antibodies [3, 6]. In addition, it is well known that LPS trigger the proliferation and differentiation of B lymphocytes, resulting in a polyclonal formation of antibodies [1, 2]. Therefore, LPS and similar substances may induce the formation of anti-DNA antibodies either by exerting an adjuvant effect on a specific immune response to released DNA or by a non-specific triggering of B lymphocytes including cells reactive to the antigenic determinants of DNA.

[1] This work has been supported by the Swiss National Research Foundation (Grant No. 3847.0.77), the World Health Organization and the Dinu Lipatti-Dubois Ferrière Foundation.

In the present work, first the mechanisms involved in the production of anti-DNA antibodies after the injection of LPS or of other polyclonal activators were investigated. Secondly, the possible role of a polyclonal activation in the development of autoantibodies was studied during the course of African trypanosomiasis. Thirdly, the pathological manifestations associated with the autoimmune response to LPS were analyzed.

Induction of Anti-DNA Antibodies by Polyclonal B Cell Activators

The injection of bacterial LPS (10–100 µg) into mice of various strains led to the formation of anti-DNA antibodies which were already detected after 3 days [3, 6]. The maximal response was observed on day 8. Such injections also induced the appearance of DNA in circulating blood 4–24 h later. Such results could suggest that the development of anti-DNA antibodies in this system reflects an enhancement by LPS of an immune response to the released DNA. However, recent experiments indicate that the induction of anti-DNA antibodies by LPS is a direct consequence of its ability to trigger a polyclonal B lymphocyte activation. First, advantage was taken of the existence of the C3H/HeJ strain of mice which are resistant to most of the biological effects of LPS, including adjuvanticity and mitogenicity. It was observed that the injection of 50 μg of LPS into C3H/HeJ mice failed to induce either the release of DNA into circulation or the formation of anti-DNA antibodies [7]. In contrast, both phenomena were seen in similarly treated congenic LPS responder C3HeB/FeJ mice. Since the cellular defect which accounts for the lack of mitogenicity of LPS on C3H/HeJ lymphocytes is confined to the B cell compartment, the release of DNA and the formation of anti-DNA antibodies was investigated after the injection of LPS into C3H/HeJ mice after transfer of 50.10⁶ C3HeB/FeJ spleen cells. In these mice, there was no detectable release of DNA into blood, but high titers of anti-DNA antibodies were measured. The reconstitution of the responsiveness to LPS of C3H/HeJ mice was not affected by the removal of T lymphocytes from the spleen cell inoculum. These results indicate that the formation of anti-DNA antibodies after LPS injection does not require a release of DNA into circulation.

Secondly, the ability of various substances to induce a polyclonal antibody synthesis was compared to their capacity to trigger the formation of anti-DNA antibodies and to provoke the release of DNA into circulation. It was observed that the injection of more than 0.1 μg of LPS, 200 μg of dextran sulfate (DS) or 10 μg of poly I-poly C led to the appearance of DNA in circulating blood, while doses as high as 2 mg of purified protein derivative of tubercule bacteria RT 32 (PPD) were inefficient in that respect. Anti-DNA antibodies were found in the serum of mice injected with more than 10 μg LPS or 1 mg DS and also in mice receiving 2 mg PPD. However, there were no detectable anti-DNA antibodies in mice injected with poly I-poly

C. The ability of various doses of LPS, DS, PPD and poly I-poly C to induce in vivo polyclonal antibody synthesis was studied by measuring the number of splenic antibody-producing cells (PFC) against sheep red blood cells (SRBC) or trinitrophenylated SRBC (TNP-SRBC), and by titrating serum antibodies to dinitrophenylated bovine serum albumin (DNP-BSA). Values obtained in these three test systems increased significantly after the injection of at least 10 μg LPS, 1 mg DS or 2 mg PPD, but not in mice injected with poly I-poly C (fig. 1). A further point which merits emphasis is that the kinetics of anti-DNP antibodies in serum after injection of 50 μg LPS were similar to those of anti-DNA antibodies. Anti-DNA and anti-DNP antibodies were shown by Sephadex G-200 gel filtration analysis to belong mainly to the IgM class. These results indicate that the doses of LPS, DS or PPD which induce a polyclonal antibody synthesis in mice also trigger a parallel formation of anti-DNA antibodies. In contrast, there was no correlation between the ability of the tested substances to provoke the release of DNA into circulating blood and the ability to induce anti-DNA antibodies. Therefore, the formation of anti-DNA antibodies in mice injected with LPS seems to be the direct result of the stimulation of polyclonal antibody synthesis. Recently, anti-lymphocyte antibodies were also detected in the serum of mice injected with LPS [8]. It is possible that polyclonal B cell activation induced by a variety of naturally occurring triggering events leads to the development of various autoantibodies. The intensity and the specificity of the autoimmune response are likely to depend on the number of B cells which are specific for the corresponding autoantigens. This hypothesis is in agreement with the demonstration of the genetic control of the formation of anti-DNA antibodies after stimulation with LPS in various strains of mice [3].

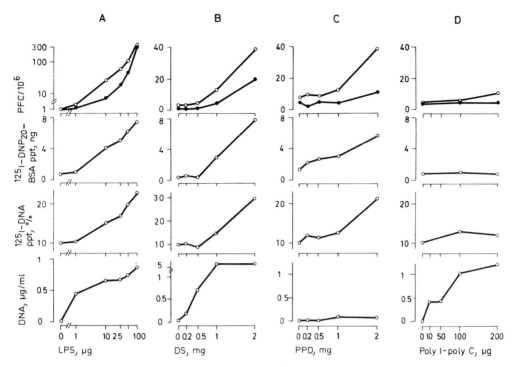

Fig. 1. *In vivo* polyclonal antibody formation after injection of PBA and comparison with the capacity of PBA to induce anti-DNA antibodies and to cause the release of DNA in circulating blood. Various doses of different PBA–LPS (A), DS (B), PPD (C) and poly I-poly C (D)–were injected i.p. in C57BL/6 mice on day 0. PFC against SRBC (●) and TNP-SRBC (○) per 10^6 spleen cells were measured 4 days after injection of LPS or 2 days after injection of other PBA. Each point represents the mean values in five to seven mice.

Polyclonal Antibody Synthesis and Formation of Autoantibodies in African Trypanosomiasis

The possible association of polyclonal antibody synthesis with autoimmune responses has been investigated in mice and in human subjects infected with African trypanosomiasis. Indeed, this disease represents a model of infection in which there is an increased level of serum immunoglobulins and a concomitant occurrence of autoantibodies.

The activation of polyclonal antibody synthesis was tested after infection of mice with *T. brucei* by measuring the number of splenic PFC against SRBC, TNP-SRBC, or fluoresceinated SRBC (FITC-SRBC) [9]. The values obtained in these three test systems began to increase 3 days after the injection of 10^5 trypanosomes. The number of PFC per spleen reached a maximum by day 17, while a peak was observed on day 6 when these values were expressed as PFC/10^6 spleen cells. It should be noted that the total number of lymphocytes in the spleen of infected animals is increased 15 times three weeks after the onset of the disease.

The necessity for T cells in this non-specific induction of proliferation and differentiation of B lymphocytes was investigated using Balb/c athymic nude mice (nu/nu). Since the number of PFC against SRBC or TNP in nu/nu mice was similar to that observed in heterozygous nu/+mice, the B lymphocyte activation associated with trypanosomiasis does not appear to be dependent on a negative or a positive influence of T cells.

In view of this evidence for an intense polyclonal B cell activation during the early stages of trypanosomiasis, the possible existence of a concomitant formation of autoantibodies has been investigated [9]. First, it was found that mice infected with 10^5 *T. brucei* developed a significant anti-DNA response. The titers of anti-SS DNA reached a peak by day 10, then decreased slowly (fig. 2). These antibodies were of the IgM class. Secondly, during such infections a sharp increase in the number of antibody-producing spleen cells directed to bromelin-treated syngeneic mouse red blood cells was observed. Since treatment of mouse red blood cells with bromelin reveals hidden autoantigens, these PFC are the expression of an autoimmune response. Thirdly, antibodies cytotoxic for syngeneic and allogeneic thymocytes were detected using a complement-mediated cytotoxicity assay [9]. Maximal thymocytotoxic activity was observed in the serum of mice infected 30 days previously; it was still detectable at a dilution of 1:64 and was due to IgM antibodies. It should be stressed that the formation of autoantibodies to DNA, to bromelin-treated murine red blood cells and to thymocytes followed the same kinetics. It was also parallel to the development of anti-SRBC, TNP and FITC antibodies indicating the polyclonal B cell activation.

These results suggest that in experimental African trypanosomiasis, the development of autoantibodies is an expression of a generalized polyclonal B cell activation.

Recently, it was found in 24 patients with various stages of human African trypanosomiasis that the infection is associated with the development of anti-DNP, anti-phosphorylcholine (PC), anti-SRBC and anti-

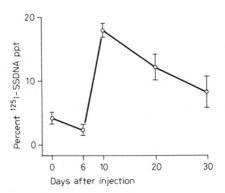

Fig. 2. Induction of anti-DNA in mice infected with *T. brucei*. Anti-DNA levels are expressed as % of ^{125}I-SSDNA precipitated.

DNA antibodies. There is a very significant correlation (p < 0.001) between the anti-DNA and the anti-PC antibody titers, suggesting that polyclonal B cell activation may be the common triggering event. Therefore, naturally occurring polyclonal B cell activation appears in man and in animals as a potential mechanism for the development of autoantibodies.

Features of Murine Lupus after Induction of Polyclonal Antibody Synthesis

There is good evidence for an indirect pathogenic role of anti-DNA antibodies when they form immune complexes with DNA released into circulating blood or into extravascular spaces. The involvement of DNA-anti-DNA complexes in the development of human and murine lupus nephritis has been demonstrated [10, 11]. The injection of bacterial lipopolysaccharides in mice was shown to induce a release of DNA into circulating blood followed by a polyclonal antibody synthesis including the formation of anti-DNA antibodies. The possibility that immune complexes could be formed between released DNA and anti-DNA antibodies and cause tissue injury after the injection of LPS has been investigated [6]. It was found that DNA released in blood 4–24 h after the injection of LPS can react with the anti-DNA antibodies appearing 3 days later. This DNA had a density similar to mammalian DNA, was 4–6 S in size and probably represented a mixture of single-stranded DNA and double-stranded DNA.

In serum, DNA-anti-DNA complexes were not detected although unidentified circulating immune complexes were demonstrated 5–8 days after the injection of LPS. In tissues, particularly in renal glomeruli, fine granular immune complex-type immunoglobulin deposits appeared along the glomerular capillary walls and in the mesangium 3 days after the injection of LPS. There is a direct correlation between the level of anti-DNA antibodies and the intensity of glomerular deposits. About 40% of immunoglobulins eluted from kidneys are anti-DNA antibodies, indicating that some of the immune complexes localized in kidneys are DNA-anti-DNA complexes [6]. In view of the long period between on one hand the release of DNA, and on the other hand the appearance of anti-DNA antibodies and their localization in glomeruli, the following hypothetical mechanism for the glomerular localization of DNA-anti-DNA complexes after injection of LPS is proposed. First, the released DNA might bind to renal glomeruli, probably through the high affinity of the collagen component of glomerular basement membrane for DNA [5]. Secondly, circulating anti-DNA antibodies which appear later might react with the glomerular-bound DNA and form immune complexes independently of circulating immune complexes.

Therefore, agents or infections which are capable of simultaneously inducing a release of autoantigens, such as DNA, and an activation of polyclonal antibody synthesis leading to the formation of the corresponding autoantibodies, should be considered as potential candidates for the triggering of autoimmune tissue injury.

Summary

There is an induction of anti-DNA antibodies in mice following the administration of bacterial lipopolysaccharides, dextran sulfate and PPD, which is closely associated with the property of these substances to trigger a polyclonal B cell activation. In the experimental model of African trypanosomiasis, there is also an intense polyclonal antibody synthesis paralleled by the formation of several autoantibodies: anti-DNA, anti-bromelin-treated mouse red blood cells, and anti-thymocyte antibodies. The pathogenic significance of the autoimmune responses induced by naturally occurring B cell activators is suggested by the observation of some features of systemic lupus in mice injected with bacterial lipopolysaccharides. Such substances may cause the release of autoantigens, such as DNA, and, later, the formation of corresponding autoantibodies. They consequently should be considered as potential candidates for the triggering of autoimmune tissue injury.

References

1 Andersson, J.; Sjöberg, O., and Möller, G.: Mitogens as probes for immunocyte activation and cellular cooperation. Transplantn. Rev. 11: 131–177 (1972).

2 Coutinho, A. and Möller, G.: Thymus-independent B cell induction and paralysis. Adv. Immunol. 21: 113–236 (1975).

3 Fournié, G. J.; Lambert, P. H., and Miescher, P. A.: Release of DNA in circulating blood and induction of anti-DNA antibodies after injection of bacterial lipopolysaccharides. J. exp. Med. 140: 1189–1206 (1974).

4 Houba, V. and Allison, A. C.: M-antiglobulins (rheumatoid factor-like globulins) and other gamma-globulins in relation to tropical parasitic infections. Lancet i: 848–852 (1966).

5 Izui, S., Lambert, P. H., and Miescher, P. A.: In vitro demonstration of a particular affinity of glomerular basement membrane and collagen for DNA. A possible basis for a local formation of DNA-anti-DNA complexes in systemic lupus erythematosus. J. exp. Med. 144: 428–433 (1976).

6 Izui, S.; Lambert, P. H.; Fournié, G. J.; Türler, H., and Miescher, P. A.: Features of systemic lupus erythematosus in mice injected with bacterial lipopolysaccharides. Identification of circulating DNA and renal localization of DNA-anti-DNA complexes. J. exp. Med. *145:* 1115–1130 (1977).

7 Izui, S.; Zaldivar, N. M.; Scher, I., and Lambert, P. H.: Mechanism for induction of anti-DNA antibodies by bacterial lipopolysaccharides in mice. I. Anti-DNA induction by LPS without significant release of DNA in circulating blood. J. Immun. *119:* 2151–2156 (1977).

8 Izui, S.; Kobayakawa, T.; Louis, J., and Lambert, P.H.: Induction of thymocytotoxin auto-antibodies after injection of bacterial lipopolysaccharides in mice. Eur. J. Immunol. *9:* 339–340 (1979).

9 Kobayakawa, T.; Louis, J.; Izui, S., and Lambert, P. H.: Autoimmune response to DNA, red blood cells and thymocyte antigens in association with polyclonal antibody synthesis during experimental African trypanosomiasis. J. Immun. *122:* 296–301 (1979).

10 Koffler, D.; Schur, P. H., and Kunkel, H. G.: Immunological studies concerning the nephritis of systemic lupus erythematosus. J. exp. Med. *126:* 607–623 (1967).

11 Lambert, P. H. and Dixon, F. J.: Pathogenesis of the glomerulonephritis of NZB/W mice. J. exp. Med. *127:* 507–521 (1968).

12 Miescher, P. A.; Paronetto, F., and Lambert, P. H.: Systemic lupus erythematosus; in Miescher and Müller-Eberhard, Textbook of immunopathology; 2nd ed., pp. 963–1001 (Grune & Stratton, New York 1976).

Dr. P. H. Lambert, WHO Immunology Research and Training Centre, Centre de Transfusion, Hôpital Cantonal, CH-1211 Genève 4 (Switzerland)

Immunopathology. 6th Int. Convoc. Immunol., Niagara Falls, N.Y., 1978, pp. 197–201 (Karger, Basel 1979)

Disordered Immunologic Regulation and Autoimmunity in NZB and NZB/NZW F₁ Mice[1]

N. Talal and J. Roubinian

Department of Medicine, University of California, and Section of Clinical Immunology, Veterans Administration Hospital, San Francisco, Calif.

Introduction

New Zealand Black (NZB) and NZB/NZW F₁ (B/W) mice have served as laboratory models for spontaneous autoimmune disease for over 20 years. Genetic [24], viral [10], and immunologic [20] factors are implicated in their disease. Our laboratory has found that sex hormones also affect the course of the murine autoimmune disorder. Although exact pathogenetic mechanisms are uncertain, it seems likely that the genetic abnormality is expressed very early in lymphocyte differentiation.

We are beginning to see the immune system as an intricate network of signals and receptors which are in constant communication. This communication is based on self-recognition of idiotype and MHC antigens present on the cell surface. Thus, self-recognition appears to be physiologic. The network may be in a state of perpetual readjustment as it responds to signals which arise from either within or without the organism. When the immune response is functioning normally, the events of antibody formation, delayed hypersensitivity, and self-nonself discrimina-tion present a harmonious and effective appearance. When the immune system is functioning abnormally, autoimmunity may result.

The potential for autoimmunity exists in normal individuals. Lymphocytes capable of binding thyroglobulin [2] or DNA [3] are present in healthy people, although patients with thyroiditis or SLE have more of these cells. Similarly, normal strains of mice have lymphocytes which bind erythrocyte autoantigens [11] or RNA [17]. Furthermore, polyclonal B cell mitogens such as lipopolysaccharide (LPS) can indiscriminately activate such cells *in vivo*, causing the production of measurable concentrations of serum autoantibodies [8, 13]. These LPS-induced autoimmune states tend to be self-limiting. There is no autoimmune disease, and the autoantibodies disappear within a few days after the last LPS injection [7]. This may represent the reestablishment of immunologic control as the system returns to its customary state of regulatory equilibrium.

The Autoimmune Disease of NZB and NZB/NZW F₁ Mice

If auto-recognition is physiologic, autoimmune disease may perhaps best be thought

[1] Supported by the Medical Research Service of the Veterans Administration, by US Public Health Service Grant AM 16140, by a grant from the Kroc Foundation, and a contract from the State of California.

of as representing a breakdown in the functioning of the immunologic network. In autoimmune disease, the immune system behaves in a deranged manner. Autoantibodies of various kinds are produced, immune complexes formed, and organs may undergo immunologic attack.

NZB and B/W mice develop LE cells, anti-nuclear factor, antibodies to nucleic acids such as DNA and RNA, autoimmune hemolytic anemia, and immune complex glomerulonephritis [21]. In addition, they exhibit a generalized infiltration of many organs by lymphocytes and plasma cells. The autoimmune (Coombs-positive) hemolytic anemia is most severe in NZB mice.

Like human SLE, the disease in New Zealand mice is characterized by the formation of antibodies to nucleic acids. The nephritis in B/W mice is related to the glomerular deposition of these antibodies as immune complexes and complement; in this, it resembles human diffuse proliferative lupus nephritis. Not all autoantibodies have the same tendency to deposit in the kidney. As in human SLE, DNA-containing immune complexes are concentrated in the renal deposits, implicating this antibody in the pathogenesis of the murine nephritis. Immune complexes resulting from the response to the murine leukemia virus also deposit in the glomeruli of these strains.

Autoantibodies in these mice make their clinical appearance at about 2–3 months. Antibodies to erythrocytes and to lymphocyte surface antigens appear in almost every NZB mouse, whereas antibodies to nucleic acids are found in B/W mice. An antibody cytotoxic to T lymphocytes occurs commonly in young NZB mice, is characteristically IgM, and does not distinguish NZB T cells from other T lymphocytes. This antibody occurs less often in B/W mice, a strain in which individual animals may develop antibodies to nucleic acids without detectable serum levels of antibodies to T cells.

B/W mice exhibit a marked sex difference, females developing severe immune complex glomerulonephritis and dying approximately 4 months before males. The accelerated pace of the disease in female B/W mice is associated with earlier appearance and greater amounts of IgG antibodies to DNA and to RNA.

Disordered Immunologic Regulation and Autoimmunity

Some experimental evidence suggests that B cell and helper T cell functions are increased in NZB and B/W mice, whereas suppressor T cell activity is decreased [21]. The simplest explanation would be a defect in suppressor T cells or factors which consequently fail to regulate helper T cells and B cells. However, the actual situation may be somewhat more complicated.

Cantor and Boyse [4] have identified three different murine T cell subpopulations based on surface membrane Ly alloantigens. T cells expressing the Ly 1^+23^- surface phenotype act to promote immune responses (helper effect). Conversely, T cells expressing the Ly 1^-23^+ surface phenotype act to depress immune responses (suppressor effect). The activities of these two cell types is in turn controlled by a third T cell (Ly 123^+) that demonstrates feedback regulation [5]. These latter cells are induced by Ly 1^+23^- to generate Ly 1^-23^+ cells: i.e. helper T cells lead to the generation of suppressor T cells. In this manner, a regulatory balance is maintained and excessive responses are avoided. Although many details of this T cell network remain to be worked out, it is already clear that a harmonious model of cellular interactions exists which is fundamental to immunoregulation. Whether the response to any given antigen will be expressed as immunity or tolerance is probably determined by the regulatory equilibrium established by this network. This equilibrium appears to be controlled by immune response genes linked to the MHC [22, 23].

In the case of NZB and B/W mice, a fundamental immunologic disequilibrium is exhibited. Within the first days or weeks of life, these mice demonstrate adult levels of immune competence [6], synthesize large amounts of immunoglobulin [12], and are relatively resistant to the establishment of immunologic tolerance [18]. These immunologic abnormalities antedate the development of autoimmunity. A fundamental disorder of immunologic regulation has long been suspected in these animals [9, 20]. A deficiency of thymic hormone has been suggested [1]. *Cantor et al.* [5] have recently found a decreased number of Ly 123$^+$ cells and a related impairment of feedback regulation in very young NZB mice prior to the onset of autoimmune disease. This finding suggests a major derangement in the T cell network which may relate to a primary genetic abnormality predisposing to spontaneous autoimmunity.

B cell abnormalities are also present early in the life of NZB and B/W mice [18]. It is difficult to know whether these abnormalities are primary or secondary to the disordered state of T cell regulation.

Sex Hormones and Autoimmunity

Autoimmunity develops earlier and with greater severity in female than in male B/W mice. Our laboratory has recently been interested in this latter point, and specifically in the possible modulation of the autoimmune disease by sex hormones.

To investigate this sex difference, we castrated males prepubertally at 2 weeks of age [14]. Significantly, castrated males died more rapidly than the sham-operated males and showed a survival rate identical to that of the sham-operated females. The castrated females showed no difference from sham-operated females: almost all were dead by the age of 9 or 10 months. This experiment suggested a possible protective effect of androgenic hormones.

In a second experiment, prepubertal castration was combined with the sustained administration of either male or female hormones [15]. There was a prolongation of survival in mice given androgen. Thus, female mice castrated and given androgen lived significantly longer than sham-operated females. By contrast, there was a significantly decreased survival of animals given estrogen. In general, these results suggested that the genetic sex of the experimental animals made little difference. The significant factor determining survival was the nature of the sex hormones given to the mice.

These changes were reflected in other parameters used to measure autoimmunity. One of the more significant parameters is the amount of IgG antibodies to DNA present in serum. The development of IgG antibodies to DNA was accelerated by estrogen and delayed by androgen. Similar results were seen with antibodies to RNA. The kidneys from these animals were examined by light, immunofluorescent, and electron microscopy. Mice given androgen showed less immune complex deposition than mice given estrogen.

It was important to study the effects of delayed androgen treatment initiated at a time when autoimmune disease was more developed. We found that delayed androgen treatment started at 3 and 6 months of age also prolonged survival in female B/W mice [16]. An interesting feature of these experiments is the fact that mice have less immune complex nephritis even though there is no significant reduction in levels of anti-DNA antibodies.

The mechanisms responsible for survival in the face of high concentration of antibodies to DNA might involve actions of the complement system or the ability of treated mice to eliminate immune complexes. An effect on antibody formation itself seems less likely. A clinical parallel to this situation might be patients with SLE who have large amounts of antibodies to DNA and yet minimal or no evidence of significant renal disease. These mice in whom androgen treatment is delayed might serve as a laboratory model for study of the complicated mechanisms involved in the pathogenesis of lupus nephritis.

We are currently studying the mechanisms by which sex hormones exert these effects. Studies of immune responses in normal mice to experimental antigens suggest that the thymus is necessary in order to demonstrate these effects of sex hormones. Similarly, we found in B/W mice that the thymus must be present if certain effects resulting from castration are to occur.

In conclusion, we have shown that sex hormones modulate the expression of murine lupus as determined by survival, concentration of antibodies to nucleic acids, and severity of immune complex nephritis. Androgens suppress and estrogens accelerate disease. These results probably explain the female predominance of human lupus and the increased incidence of autoimmunity in patients with Klinefelter's syndrome [19]. The immunoregulatory function of the thymus as well as the complement system may be involved in the action of male hormones. Our results support the thesis that lupus is a disorder of immunologic regulation and that the administration of androgens might create a more physiologic immunologic equilibrium. Androgen therapy for human autoimmune disease may be a possible outcome of this work.

Summary

The immune system is an intricate network of communicating signals and receptors which are based, in large part, on recognition of self antigens located on cell surface membranes. For example, self-recognition of idiotypic determinants of immunoglobulins and antigens specified by genes in the major histocompatibility complex are important elements in immunologic regulation. Autoimmune disease probably represents a breakdown in the homeostatic functioning of the immunologic network. Evidence supports the concept of a derangement in the function of T regulatory cells in NZB and NZB/NZW mice, strains which are genetically susceptible to the development of spontaneous autoimmune diseases. Sex hormones modulate the development of autoimmunity in NZB/NZW mice as determined by survival, concentration of antibodies to nucleic acids, and severity of immune complex nephritis. Androgens suppress and estrogens accelerate disease. Mechanisms responsible for these effects of sex hormones are currently under investigation. It appears that both thymus-dependent and thymus-independent mechanisms are probably involved.

References

1 Bach, J. F.; Dardenne, M., and Salomon, J. C.: Studies of thymus products. IV. Absence of serum thymic activity in adult NZB and (NZB × NZW) F$_1$ mice. Clin. exp. Immunol. 14: 247–256 (1973).
2 Bankhurst, A. D.; Torrigiani, G., and Allison, A. C.: Lymphocytes binding human thyroglobulin in healthy people and its relevance to tolerance for antigens. Lancet i: 226–230 (1973).
3 Bankhurst, A. D. and Williams, R. C.: Identification of DNA-binding lymphocytes in patients with systemic lupus erythematosus. J. clin. Invest. 56: 1378–1385 (1975).
4 Cantor, H. and Boyse, E. A.: Regulation of cellular and humoral immune responses by T cell subclasses. Cold Spring Harb. Symp. quant. Biol. 41: 119–127 (1976).
5 Cantor, H.; McVay-Boudreau, L.; Hugenberger, J.; Naidorf, K.; Shen, F. W., and Gershon, R. K.: Immunoregulatory circuits among T cell sets. II. Physiologic role of feedback inhibition in vivo: absence in NZB mice. J. exp. Med. 147: 1116–1125 (1978).
6 Evans, M. M.; Williamson, W. G., and Irvine, W. J.: The appearance of immunological competence at an early age in New Zealand black mice. Clin exp. Immunol. 3: 375–383 (1968).

7 Fischbach, M.; Roubinian, J. R., and Talal, N.: Lipopolysaccharide induction of IgM antibodies to polyadenylic acid in normal mice. J. Immun. *120:* 1856–1861 (1978).

8 Fournie, G. J.; Lambert, P. N., and Miescher, P. A.: Release of DNA in circulating blood and induction of anti-DNA antibodies after injection of bacterial lipopolysaccharides. J. exp. Med. *140:* 1189–1206 (1974).

9 Howie, J. B. and Helyer, B. J.: The immunology and pathology of NZB mice. Adv. Immunol. *9:* 215–266 (1968).

10 Levy, J. A.: C-type RNA viruses and autoimmune disease; in Talal Autoimmunity: genetic, immunologic, virologic and clinical aspects, pp. 404–456 (Academic Press, New York 1977).

11 Linder, E. and Edgington, T. S.: Immunobiology of the autoantibody response. II. The lipoprotein-associated soluble HB erythrocyte autoantigen of NZB mice. J. Immun. *110:* 53–62 (1973).

12 Moutsopoulos, H. M.; Boehm-Truitt, M.; Kassan, S. S., and Chused, T. M.: Demonstration of activation of B lymphocytes in New Zealand Black mice at birth by an immunoradiometric assay for murine IgM. J. Immun. *119:* 1639–1644 (1977).

13 Primi, D.; Smith, E. C.; Hammarstrom, L., and Mollar, G.: Characterization of self-reactive B cells by polyclonal B-cell activators. J. exp. Med. *145:* 21–30 (1977).

14 Roubinian, J. R.; Papoian, R., and Talal, N.: Androgenic hormones modulate autoantibody responses and improve survival in murine lupus. J. clin. Invest. *59:* 1066–1070 (1977).

15 Roubinian, J. R.; Talal, N.; Greenspan, J. S.; Goodman, J. R., and Siiteri, P. K.: Effect of castration and sex hormone treatment on survival, antinucleic acid antibodies, and glomerulonephritis in NZB/NZW F$_1$ mice. J. exp. Med. *147:* 1568–1583 (1978).

16 Roubinian, J. R.; Greenspan, J., and Talal, N.: Delayed androgen treatment prolongs survival in murine lupus. J. clin. Invest. (in press).

17 Sawada, S.; Pillarisetty, R. J.; Michalski, J. P.; Palmer, D. W., and Talal, N.: Lymphocytes binding polyriboadenylic acid and synthesizing antibodies to nucleic acids in autoimmune and normal mice. J. Immun. *119:* 355–360 (1977).

18 Staples, P. J. and Talal, N.: Relative inability to induce tolerance in adult NZB and NZB/NZW F$_1$ mice. J. exp. Med. *129:* 123–139 (1969).

19 Stern, R.; Fishman, J.; Brusman, H., and Kunkel, H. G.: Systemic lupus erythematosus associated with Klinefelter's syndrome. Arthritis Rheum. *20:* 18–22 (1977).

20 Talal, N.: Immunologic and viral factors in the pathogenesis of systemic lupus erythematosus. Arthritis Rheum. *13:* 887–893 (1970).

21 Talal, N.: Disordered immunologic regulation and autoimmunity. Transplantn. Rev. *31:* 240–263 (1976).

22 Tada, T.; Taniguchi, M., and David. C. S.: Suppressive and enhancing T-cell factors as I-region gene products: properties and the subregion assignment. Cold Spring Harb. Symp. quant. Biol. *41:* 119–127 (1976).

23 Theze, J.; Kapp, J. A., and Benacerraf, B.: Immunosuppressive factor(s) extracted from lymphoid cells of non-responder mice primed with L-glutamic acid[60]-L-alanine[30]-L-tyrosine[10] (GAT). III. Immunochemical properties of the GAT-specific suppressive factor. J. exp. Med *145:* 184–194 (1957).

24 Warner, N. L.: Genetic aspects of autoimmune disease in animals; in Talal Autoimmunity: genetic, immunologic, virologic and clinical aspects, pp. 33–62 (Academic Press, New York 1977).

Dr. Norman Talal, Immunology Arthritis, VA Hospital (151T), 4150 Clement Street, San Francisco, CA 94121 (USA)

Immunopathology. 6th Int. Convoc. Immunol., Niagara Falls, N.Y., 1978, pp. 202–206 (Karger, Basel 1979)

Systemic Heterologous Immune Complex Disease in Rabbits[1]

J. Brentjens, B. Albini, D. Mendrick, C. Neuland, D. O'Connell, E. Ossi, L. Accinni and G. A. Andres

State University of New York at Buffalo, Departments of Pathology, Microbiology, and Medicine, Buffalo, N.Y.

Introduction

The establishment in the late fifties and the early sixties of a model of chronic serum sickness (CSS) in the rabbit contributed decisively to our understanding of the pathogenesis of chronic glomerulonephritis in man [10, 12]. From the animal model, it became clear that circulating immune complexes (IC) could induce not only acute but also chronic renal lesions. The generally accepted view that the majority of human glomerulonephritides results from the deposition of circulating IC, is largely based on the findings in experimental CSS. Recently, the possible pathogenetic significance of *in situ* formation of IC in the glomeruli has also been recognized [13].

Until a few years ago, all the immunopathologic studies on CSS in the rabbit were focused on the kidney. In a classic study on the induction of CSS by *Dixon et al.* [10], the daily single intravenous dose of bovine serum albumin (BSA) was tentatively adjusted to the degree of the antibody response. In rabbits with a moderate antibody response, circulating IC were found to localize mainly in the renal glomeruli and splenic arteries [9]. Development of CSS in animals with a high antibody response was seldom observed. This was explained by assuming that in these animals large IC are formed, which are rapidly phagocytized by the reticuloendothelial system, thereby being prevented from localizing in tissue [9, 10, 12]. Raising the daily dose of BSA in these animals in an attempt to match antibody production results in high mortality from anaphylaxis. This problem of anaphylactic death may be largely circumvented by dividing a high daily dose of BSA into several injections [6]. In rabbits with a high antibody response this immunization procedure often induces a systemic disease, characterized by deposition of IC not only in renal glomeruli, but also in other tissues [1, 4–6].

This paper summarizes the findings obtained in 161 rabbits immunized daily with intravenous injections of BSA. Special attention will be given to rabbits generating a vigorous antibody response in which a systemic deposition of IC is frequently observed [4].

Materials and Methods

Albino rabbits weighing 2–3 kg were purchased from a local breeder.

The intravenous immunization with crystallized BSA was initiated in all animals with 12.5 mg of BSA

[1] Supported by Grant AI-10334 from the National Institutes of Health and by Contract 91271 of the New York State Health Research Council.

in physiologic saline per day. Subsequently, the daily doses of BSA given to different rabbits were varied in an attempt to match the antibody response [10]. Daily doses of BSA higher than 50 mg were divided into two or three equal parts slowly injected at intervals of 4–8 h. Further details of the immunization procedure and laboratory tests done on rabbit sera and urines have been described previously [6]. Direct immunofluorescence of rabbit tissues for presence of rabbit IgG and C3, and for BSA, and the preparation of tissues for light and electron microscopic studies were performed according to methods reported elsewhere [1, 6].

Results and Discussion

Of the 161 rabbits immunized daily with intravenous injections of BSA, 12% never developed precipitating antibodies against BSA, 18% were sacrificed in the acute phase of serum sickness, and 6% died from anaphylaxis in the period between the phase of acute and chronic serum sickness. In 24% of these 161 rabbits, 12.5–25 mg of BSA per day sufficed to match the antibody response ('low responders'). In 40% of the animals, daily BSA doses ranging from 50 to 150 mg were required ('high responders').

Animals which did not make precipitating antibodies showed at no time during the chronic immunization tissue localization of BSA-anti-BSA IC. When responder rabbits were examined during the acute phase of serum sickness, IC deposition was found in the renal glomeruli and serous membranes [1] only. In rabbits with either a low or a high production of precipitating antibodies, sacrificed between the acute and chronic phase of serum sickness, IC could sometimes be observed in the mesangial areas of the glomeruli, but no other structures were involved. In most of the 'low responders' with CSS, tissue localization of IC was confined to the glomeruli [4]. If present at extraglomerular renal sites or in organs or structures other than the kidney, the IC deposition was very limited in extent. In

Table I. Deposition of IC in CSS 'high responders'

Organ/structure	% positive	Positive/ total number
Glomerulus	100	55/55
Spleen, arteries	88	42/48
Ovary	86	19/22
Eye[1]	82	14/17
Lung	75	41/55
Heart	74	29/39
Uterus[1]	71	12/17
Extraglomerular deposition in the kidney	69	38/55
Serous membranes	69	27/39
Submandibular gland[1]	65	15/23
Lacrimal gland[1]	63	10/16
Testis	60	3/5
Choroid plexus	59	15/27
Bone marrow, vessels[1]	52	15/29
Liver, periportal areas	51	26/51
Intestine	49	22/45
Synovia	48	13/27
Adrenal, thyroid, pancreas	47	17/36
Spleen, sinusoidal walls	42	20/48
Liver, sinusoidal walls	20	10/50
Skin, dermo-epidermal junction	0	0/48

[1] Unpublished observations.

contrast, 'high responder' rabbits with CSS showed a systemic deposition of IC although the extent and amount of deposition varied considerably from one organ or structure to another (table 1; fig. 1, 2). Studies with radiolabeled BSA in 'high responder' rabbits with CSS showed that the deposition of BSA in the lung was similar to that in the kidney and thus appear to confirm the immunofluorescent findings [15].

In all but one of the organs and structures studied, the immune deposits were composed of BSA and rabbit IgG and C3. In the lung, however, C3 was never demonstrated by immunofluorescence technique [4, 6]. This suggests either that complement is removed from the IC during or after deposition in

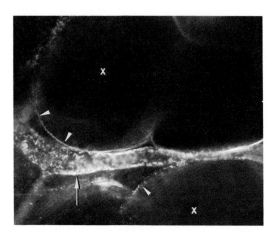

Fig. 1. A micrograph of the peritoneum of a rabbit with systemic IC disease, stained by the direct immunofluorescence method for BSA [1]. Granular deposits are present in the wall of small lymph channels (arrow heads) running around fat islands (X), and in the wall of an arteriole (arrow). × 165.

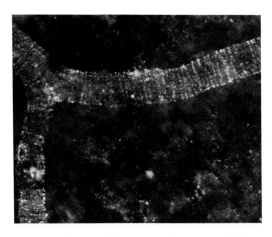

Fig. 2. A micrograph of the same peritoneum as shown in figure 1 stained for IgG. Granular deposits are visible in the wall of a medium-sized artery. Peritoneal macrophages also contain IgG (and BSA) as these cells phagocytize immune complexes. × 165.

lung tissue, or that circulating IC which become deposited in the lung have a composition different from IC localizing in other tissues. Consistent with the latter interpretation is the observation that the percentage of 'high responder' rabbits with CSS showing IC deposition in the lung, increased with the duration of the CSS phase (table II). During CSS, the antibody response invariably decreased [2]. This event might be accompanied by the formation of circulating IC more likely to localize in organs other than the kidney. However, it is also conceivable that extrarenal IC deposition may require the presence of very large amounts of IC, circulating for prolonged periods of time.

The histologic appearance of organs and structures showing IC deposition varied widely [1, 4–6]. There were severe lesions in the kidney, in the lung, and in the serous membranes. Extensive changes were also noted in the spleen, but at least part of these alterations appear to be the consequence of chronic immunization. On the other hand, in many other organs as the intestines, the endocrine glands, the eye, and the choroid plexus, the histologic lesions were usually minimal or absent. However, absence of inflammatory changes does not preclude functional abnormalities. Unfortunately, in 'high responders' with CSS, the functional studies of organs other than the kidney are hindered by uremia.

What then is the significance of this experimental model of systemic IC disease for human pathology? A remarkable similarity has been established between the immunopathologic findings observed in 'high responder' rabbits with CSS and in patients with systemic lupus erythematosus (SLE) [3, 7, 8, 14, 16–18]. This suggests that the extraglomerular immune deposits in SLE are also the result of deposition of IC. Therefore, this experimental model of systemic IC disease may be useful for the study

Table II. The relationship between positive IF findings (%) and duration of proteinuria in CSS, 'high responders'

	< 1 week				1–2 weeks				> 2 weeks			
	+++	++	+	T%	+++	++	+	T%	+++	++	+	T%
Glomerular BM	100	0	0	100	100	0	0	100	100	0	0	100
Tubular BM	43	14	0	57	20	25	35	80	25	29	18	72
Alveolar BM	14	0	0	14	35	25	15	75	39	39	11	89

Number of rabbits with proteinuria less than 1 week, 7; between 1 and 2 weeks, 20; and more than 2 weeks, 28. The extent of IC deposition was graded as follows: + = slight; ++ = moderate; +++ = marked. BM = Basement membrane; T = total.

of the pathogenesis of human systemic diseases associated with circulating IC. The recent observation that circulating IC may preferentially localize and induce injury in organs other than the kidney, as in the lungs of some patients with idiopathic interstitial pneumonia [11], stresses the importance to develop and study the pathogenesis of experimentally induced systemic IC diseases.

References

1 Albini, B.; Ossi, E., and Andres, G. A.: The pathogenesis of pericardial, pleural, and peritoneal effusions in rabbits with serum sickness. Lab. Invest. *37:* 64–78 (1977).

2 Albini, B., Drentjens J.; Olson, K.; Ossi, E., and Andres, G. A.: Studies on the immune response in rabbits and chickens with chronic serum sickness (this volume, pp. 207–211).

3 Atkins, C. J.; Kondon, J. J.; Quismorio, F. P., and Frion, G. J.: The choroid plexus in systemic lupus erythematosus. Ann. intern. Med. *76:* 65–72 (1972).

4 Brentjens, J. R.; O'Connell, D. W.; Albini, B., and Andres, G. A.: Experimental chronic serum sickness in rabbits that received daily multiple and high doses of antigen: a systemic disease. Ann. N.Y. Acad. Sci. *254:* 603–613 (1975).

5 Brentjens, J. R.; O'Connell, D. W.; Pawlowski, I. B., and Andres, G. A.: Extraglomerular lesions associated with deposition of circulating antigen-antibody complexes in kidneys of rabbits with chronic serum sickness. Clin. Immunol. Immunopath. *3:* 112–126 (1974).

6 Brentjens, J. R.; O'Connell, D. W.; Pawlowski, I. B.; Hsu, K. C., and Andres, G. A.: Experimental immune complex disease of the lung. The pathogenesis of a laboratory model resembling certain human interstitial lung diseases. J. exp. Med. *140:* 105–125 (1974).

7 Brentjens, J. R.; Sepulveda, M.; Baliah, T.; Bentzel, C.; Erlanger, B. F.; Elwood, C.; Montes, M.; Hsu, K. C., and Andres, G. A.: Interstitial immune complex nephritis in patients with systemic lupus erythematosus. Kidney int. *7:* 342–350 (1975).

8 Brentjens, J.; Ossi, E.; Albini, B.; Sepulveda, M.; Kano, K.; Sheffer, J.; Vasilion, P.; Marine, E.; Baliah, T.; Jockin, H., and Andres, G. A.: Disseminated immune deposits in lupus erythematosus. Arthritis Rheum. *20:* 962–968 (1977).

9 Dixon, F. J.: The role of antigen-antibody complexes in disease. Harvey Lect. *58:* 21–52 (1963).

10 Dixon, F. J.; Feldman, J. D., and Vazquez, J. J.: Experimental glomerulonephritis: the pathogenesis of a laboratory model resembling the spectrum of human glomerulonephritis. J. exp. Med. *113:* 899–919 (1961).

11 Dreisin, R. B.; Schwarz, M. I.; Theofilopoulos, A. N., and Stanford, R. E.: Circulating immune complexes in idiopathic interstitial pneumonias. New Engl. J. Med. *298:* 353–357 (1978).

12 Germuth, F. G., jr. and Rodriquez, E.: Immunopathology of the renal glomerulus (Little, Brown, Boston 1973).

13 Izui, S.; Lambert, P.-H., and Miescher, P. A.: *In vitro* demonstration of a particular affinity of glomerular basement membrane and collagen for DNA. A possible basis for a local formation of DNA-antibody complexes in systemic lupus erythematosus. J. exp. Med. *144:* 428–443 (1976).

14 Koffler, D.; Agnello, V.; Thoburn, R., and Kunkel,

H. G.: Systemic lupus erythematosus: prototype of immune complex nephritis in man. J. exp. Med. *134:* 169s–179s (1971).

15 Neuland, C.; Albini, B.; Andres, G.; Brentjens, J.; Ossi, E.; Steinbach, J., and Blau, M.: The kinetics of immune complex deposition in rabbits with chronic serum sickness. Abstr. 10th Annu. Meet. American Society of Nephrology, Washington.

16 Ordóñez, N. G.; Panem, S.; Aronson, A.; Dalton, H.; Katz, A. I.; Spargo, B. H., and Kirsten, W. H.: Viral immune complexes in systemic lupus erythematosus. C-type viral complex deposition at extrarenal sites. Virchows Arch. Abt. B Zellpath. *25:* 355–366 (1977).

17 Rodriguez-Iturbe, B.; Garcia, R.; Rubio, L., and Serrano, H.: Immunohistologic findings in the lung in systemic lupus erythematosus. Archs Path. Lab. Med. *101:* 342–344 (1977).

18 Schocket, A. L.; Lain, D.; Kohler, P. F., and Steigerwald, J.: Immune complex vasculitis as a cause of ascites and pleural effusions in systemic lupus erythematosus. J. Rheum. *5:* 33–38 (1978).

Dr. J. Brentjens, Department of Pathology, State University of New York at Buffalo, Buffalo, NY 14214 (USA)

Immunopathology. 6th Int. Convoc. Immunol., Niagara Falls, N.Y., 1978, pp. 207–211 (Karger, Basel 1979)

Studies on the Immune Response of Rabbits and Chickens with Chronic Serum Sickness[1]

B. Albini, J. Brentjens, K. Olson, E. Ossi and G. A. Andres[2]

Departments of Microbiology, Pathology, and Medicine, State University of New York at Buffalo, Buffalo, N.Y.

The research into immune complex-mediated diseases has been primarily directed towards investigating factors which influence the localization of immune complexes in tissues and understanding the mechanisms involved in immune complex (IC)-mediated tissue injury [6]. In contrast, little is known about the immune response in patients and experimental animals with IC diseases. This is especially true for IC-mediated diseases induced by heteroimmunization of immunologically normal subjects, i.e. in serum sickness; the research on the immune response has been almost exclusively concerned with systemic lupus erythematosus (SLE) and the disease of NZB/W mice, both pathological conditions, in which autoimmune reactivity plays an essential role. In such conditions, however, it is very difficult to dissect the derangement of the immune system pertaining to the mechanisms of autoimmunity from that possibly facilitating IC formation or caused by IC in circulation.

In the following, studies on the immune response of rabbits with systemic chronic serum sickness (SCSS) [3] and of chickens with chronic serum sickness (CSS) induced by immunization with bovine serum albumin (BSA) will be summarized.

Parameters of the Immune Response in Rabbits with Systemic Chronic Serum Sickness (SCSS)

SCSS was induced in rabbits by multiple daily injections of BSA as described elsewhere in this volume [4]. 68 rabbits with SCSS and 14 untreated rabbits were included in these studies. The stages of the disease have been defined on the basis of absence or presence of overt proteinuria and of BSA and antibodies to BSA in circulation (table I).

Precipitating and Hemagglutinating Antibodies to BSA [2]. Precipitating antibodies to BSA were first detected during the acute phase proteinuria (AcSS), 9–15 days after the first injection of BSA. Antibodies were titrated in a tube immunoprecipitation test using serial dilutions of BSA. The strongest precipitation was seen in the early stages of disease in the tubes with high concentrations of BSA. Later, strong precipitation was observed with the rabbit sera and low BSA concentrations also. During the chronic phase proteinuria, precipitation was again primarily seen with high concentrations of BSA (table I). These experiments which

[1] These studies were supported by the United States Public Health Service Grant AI-10334 and a grant from the Buswell Foundation.

[2] The technical assistance of Mrs. *Irene Pawlowski*, Miss *Ingrid Glurich*, and Mrs. *Joy Luchyshyn* is gratefully acknowledged.

Table I. The immune response in rabbits with SCSS

	Stages of disease							
	acute phase proteinuria			'in-between phase' (between acute and chronic phases)	chronic phase proteinuria			recovery phase
	early	middle	late		early	middle	late	
Proteinuria	+	+	+	0	+	+	+	0
Precipitating antibody	0	±	+	+ +	+	±	0	0
BSA in circulation	+	±	0	0	0	±	+	+
Precipitating antibodies:								
Titers	1^1	2	4	6	4	1	1	1
Reaction with high BSA concentrations	0	+	+ +	+ +	+ +	+	0	0
Reaction with low BSA concentrations	0	0	+	+ +	+	±	0	0
Hemagglutinating antibodies:								
Titers	2^1	8	11	13	14	10	1	1
IgM/IgG ratio	H^2	HL	L	L	L	HL	0	H
Cells with IgG membrane receptors for BSA	±	±	+	+ +	+ +	+	±	0
Cells with IgM membrane receptors for BSA	+	+	+	±	±	+ +	+ +	0
Plasmacells: IgM/IgG ratio	H	HL	HL	L	L	L	HL	H

[1] Titers are expressed as log 2 of highest dilutions giving a positive reaction.
[2] H = High; L = low; HL = medium.

suggest that the avidity of precipitating antibodies in circulation may first increase and then again decrease in the progress of the disease are in agreement with previous studies [6].

In selected animals, the serum precipitin titer was determined using the concentration of BSA which had given the strongest reaction with undiluted serum. The results are summarized in table I.

Interestingly, rabbits surviving CSS did not have any demonstrable precipitins in circulation. In these animals, the production of precipitating antibodies to BSA could not be induced despite continuous injections of BSA for over 2 years. Neither immunization with low or high doses of BSA without or with complete or incomplete Freunds adjuvant, nor discontinuation of BSA injections for 14–31 days prior to reinjection resulted in antibody production. This phase of unresponsiveness of the humoral immune response to BSA was specific, as the rabbits were able to respond to unrelated antigens, e.g. chicken γ-globulin, and even developed acute serum sickness. Rabbits in which the

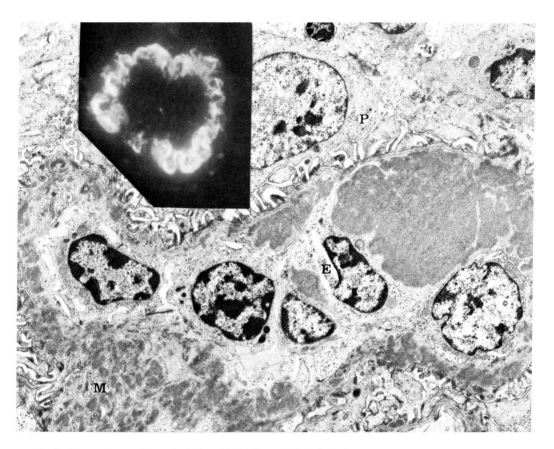

Fig. 1. Glomerular capillary of chicken 55 (CSS). Electron-dense deposits are seen in subendothelial localization and in the mesangial region. ×6,600. E = Endothelial cell; M = mesangial region; P = podocyte. The insert shows immunofluorescent staining for BSA of a glomerulus. ×230.

injections of BSA were discontinued during early phases of chronic serum sickness remained responsive to BSA reimmunization.

Eight animals were first immunized with BSA in complete Freund's adjuvant three times in 14-day intervals; BSA was then given in increasing doses subcutaneously to avoid anaphylactic reactions, and after 7–10 days, BSA was given daily i.v. Such animals usually had high titers of precipitating antibodies and, although they did not develop an acute proteinuric phase, their immune re-sponse in the course of disease was comparable to that of animals injected only intravenously.

Hemagglutinating antibodies showed a pattern comparable to that of the precipitins (table I). In the unresponsive phase, however, hemagglutination was positive in titers up to 1:2. The antibodies to BSA first were predominantly of the IgM class; very soon, in AcSS, the bulk of antibodies was IgG. IgM antibody increased only late in the disease. The hemagglutinating antibodies occasionally seen in very low titers during the unresponsive phase were always of the IgM class (table I).

Cells with Surface Immunoglobulin and Plasma Cells in the Spleen. Sequential spleen biopsies (up to four in a single animal) were performed. Spleen cell suspensions and tissue sections were studied as described elsewhere [*Albini et al.*, in preparation]. A summary of the results is given in table I. These results indicate that in the CSS, cells bearing IgM receptors for BSA and cells producing IgM antibodies to BSA relatively increase in number, whereas cells bearing IgG receptors and cells producing IgG antibodies to BSA become less frequent. In animals surviving CSS, no cells with BSA immunoglobulin receptors can be detected in the spleen. Nevertheless, very few plasma cells with intracytoplasmatic IgM antibody to BSA (2–3 cells per 10 visual fields at a magnification of × 250) persist throughout the 'unresponsive phase' (see above). This switch back to IgM production seen in rabbits with SCSS may reflect a mechanism similar to that described for other simpler systems of immunization by *Weigle* [5].

In the phase just preceding CSS, in some of the animals studied, the plasma cells of the spleen include: (a) many cells producing IgG-class antibodies to antigens other than BSA and (b) some plasma cells producing antibodies to BSA of immunoglobulin classes other than IgG or IgM. It is interesting to note that, at the same time, the rabbits are most prone to develop anaphylaxis [*Brentjens et al.*, unpublished observation], and that in animals without overt clinical anaphylaxis, intravascular precipitates of BSA and antibody form in vessels of the serosae, the placenta, in the glomerular capillaries and in lung and spleen vasculature [*Albini et al.*, unpublished observation].

The obvious change in the pattern of antibodies to BSA produced may account for some of the differences seen in the capacity of phagocytic cells to remove immune complexes localized in basement membranes. In the disease stage just preceding CSS, immune complexes seem to localize, albeit to a limited extent, in the basement membrane of glomerular capillary loops, but are apparently removed, presumably by mesangial cells very fast and are not seen 24 h after injection of the antigen. In contrast, in CSS, the disappearance of immune complexes from the basement membranes is much slower [*Neuland et al.*, unpublished observations].

The Effect of Thymectomy on Chronic Serum Sickness in Chickens

The model of serum sickness in chickens and the effects of thymectomy and bursectomy on its course will be described in detail elsewhere [*Albini and Andres*, in preparation]. The glomerular immune complex deposits in CSS in chickens are found mainly in subendothelial localization and resemble wire loop lesions seen in some forms of human SLE (fig. 1). Subepithelial deposits of BSA-anti-BSA antibody complexes are seen much less frequently [1].

The findings obtained with thymectomized chickens are summarized in table II. Whereas thymectomy does not have any detectable effect on the frequency of disease if high doses of BSA are injected i.v., it seems that in animals receiving low doses of BSA, thymectomy significantly enhances the predisposition to develop CSS.

Table II. The effect of thymectomy on the frequency of CSS in chickens

Daily BSA dose, mg	Normal animals, %	n	Thymectomized animals, %	n
20	60	10	56	9
5	21	38	68	40

Conclusions

From the findings reported here, it appears that: (1) normal rabbits in which immune complex formation is elicited by high doses of a foreign antigen react to prolonged circulation of immune complexes by a 'shut-off' of antibody production; (2) this 'shut-off' of antibody production is preceded by the reappearance in the spleen of cells producing IgM antibodies to BSA; and (3) thymectomy in chickens increases the predisposition to develop CSS.

References

1 Albini, B. and Andres, G.: Serum sickness in the chicken. Abstr. 9th Annu. Meet. of the American Society of Nephrology, 1976, p. 61.

2 Albini, B.; Brentjens, J.; O'Connell, D., and Andres, G. A.: Antibody production in rabbits with chronic serum sickness (CSS) (abstr.). Proc. Fed. Am. Socs exp. Biol. 35: 2587 (1976).

3 Brentjens, J. R.; O'Connell, D.; Albini, B., and Andres, G. A.: Experimental chronic serum sickness in rabbits that received daily multiple and high doses of antigen; a systemic disease. Ann. N.Y. Acad. Sci. 254: 603–613 (1975).

4 Brentjens, J.; Albini, B.; Mendrick, D.; Neuland, C.; O'Connell, D.; Ossi, E.; Accini, L., and Andres, G. A.: Systemic heterologous immune complex disease in rabbits (this volume, pp. 202–206).

5 Weigle, W. O.: Cyclical production of antibody as a regulatory mechanisms in the immune response. Adv. Immunol. 21: 87–111 (1975).

6 Wilson, C. B. and Dixon, F. J.: The renal response to immunological injury; in Brenner and Rector The kidney, pp. 838–940. (Saunders, Philadelphia 1976).

Dr. Boris Albini, 240 B Cary Hall, Department of Microbiology, State University of New York at Buffalo, Buffalo, NY 14214 (USA)

Immunopathology. 6th Int. Convoc. Immunol., Niagara Falls, N.Y., 1978, pp. 212–216 (Karger, Basel 1979)

The Mononuclear Phagocyte System in Immune Complex Diseases[1]

Mart Mannik and Richard A. H. Jimenez

Division of Rheumatology, Department of Medicine, University of Washington, Seattle, Wash.

Circulating immune complexes have been demonstrated in human immune complex diseases with many sensitive methods. The concentration of circulating immune complexes at any given time depends on the rate of immune complex formation in the circulation and the rate of immune complex removal from the circulation. No information is available on these parameters in human diseases. Even in animal models of spontaneous immune complex diseases, these rates have not been determined. The administration of preformed immune complexes to animals, however, has provided quantitative information on the processes responsible for the removal of circulating immune complexes. Uptake by the mononuclear phagocyte system (MPS), tissue deposition, and yet unidentified catabolic processes account for removal of circulating immune complexes. The uptake of immune complexes by the MPS is influenced by variables including the lattice structure of the complexes, the status of the MPS, and the nature of antigens and antibodies in the complexes.

Influence of the Lattice of Immune Complexes on the Fate of Circulating Immune Complexes

The lattice of immune complexes, defined as the number of antigen and antibody molecules in a given complex, influences the biological properties of soluble complexes containing IgG class of antibodies [9]. Large-latticed immune complexes, defined as complexes containing more than two antibody molecules, are relatively rapidly removed from the circulation. On the other hand, small-latticed immune complexes, defined as complexes containing two or one antibody molecules, persist longer in circulation but are catabolized faster than antibodies alone. These conclusions were reached by injecting small doses of antigen-antibody complexes with known degrees of lattice formation [2] into rabbits, monkeys [12], and mice [7]. In these studies, the composition of the injected complexes and of the complexes remaining in circulation was examined by sucrose density gradient ultracentrifugation. In this manner, the half-lives of circulating complexes with varying degrees of lattice formation were determined. Studies in mice established that the dose of large-latticed immune complexes influenced their half-life [7]. With increasing doses of complexes, the

[1] The work reported herein was supported in part by Research Grant AM 11476 and Research Training Grant AMO 7108, both from the National Institute of Arthritis, Metabolism and Digestive Diseases.

rate of their removal decreased. When the clearance velocity was determined, saturation of the removal mechanism was demonstrated. As will be discussed below, the quantity of large-latticed complexes removed from the circulation approximated the quantity of complexes taken up by the hepatic MPS (Kupffer cells) [1, 7]. The tissues responsible for the catabolism of small-latticed immune complexes, and for that matter for IgG, have not been determined.

The problem of re-equilibration of lattice during *in vivo* experiments must be considered during experiments with immune complexes. In the above cited studies, this was not a major factor since the amount of complexes removed from the circulation was recovered in the liver and no increase in small-latticed complexes or antibodies was noted. Nevertheless, investigators have turned to preparing covalently cross-linked immune complexes to permit isolation of immune complexes with discrete degrees of lattice formations [16; *Mannik*, unpublished observations]. Experiments with such preparations have further corroborated the role of lattice in removal of immune complexes from the circulation.

The Mononuclear Phagocyte System in Removal of Circulating Immune Complexes

The hepatic MPS was the major organ in rabbits, mice, and monkeys for removal of soluble, large-latticed immune complexes, containing IgG class of antibodies [1, 7, 12]. The MPS in the liver consists of Kupffer cells that were at least partly replenished by marrow-derived monocytes [11]. The Kupffer cells were not covered by endothelial cells [20] and thus are in contact with and suited for removal of circulating materials. Fc receptors were demonstrated on isolated

Kupffer cells by rosetting techniques with sensitized erythrocytes [13]. The uptake of soluble immune complexes by the spleen was only a small fraction of complexes taken up by the liver in rabbits and monkeys after the injection of small doses of complexes [1, 12]. Therefore, it is likely that the Fc receptors on Kupffer cells play a major role in removal of circulating immune complexes. In contrast, the spleen played the major role in removal of IgG-sensitized red cells from the circulation, unless the cells were heavily sensitized [5].

In mice with increasing doses of injected immune complexes, saturation kinetics were demonstrated for the removal of circulating immune complexes parallel with a maximum specific hepatic uptake of immune complexes [7]. These observations indicated that in acute experiments the hepatic MPS became saturated, thereby prolonging the circulation of large-latticed immune complexes and enhancing tissue deposition [10]. Similarly, during the presence of circulating immune complexes in serum sickness of rabbits, the MPS function was depressed as measured by aggregated albumin [19] or by aggregated IgG [18]. All these observations indicate that a decreased hepatic uptake of immune complexes due to saturation prolongs their circulation and enhances tissue deposition. Therefore, the assessment of the capacity of MPS to remove circulating immune complexes during the course of human immune complex diseases seems relevant for better understanding of pathogenic events and design of novel therapeutic interventions. Besides saturation of the Fc receptors or a total decrease in Kupffer cells, the hepatic MPS function could be altered by changes in the regional blood flow in the liver by reducing contact between circulating immune complexes and Kupffer cells.

The saturability of hepatic MPS uptake was first shown with carbon particles, and more recently competitive inhibition of several different substances (carbon particles, aggregated albumin, lipid emulsion, formalinized foreign red cells and latex particles) for uptake by MPS was shown in rats [14], suggesting lack of specificity among various substances. Observations in other species indicated particle specificity for inhibition of uptake by MPS [17]. The competitive uptake of immune complexes and various previously used substances for MPS uptake has not been determined.

An entirely satisfactory probe for the ability of the MPS in humans to remove circulating immune complexes has not yet been proposed. The MPS activity was evaluated with lipid emulsion in patients with rheumatoid arthritis or systemic lupus erythematosus [15] and with radiolabeled, aggregated human serum albumin in patients with active glomerulonephritis [3]. With active disease, these test substances were more quickly removed in patients than in control groups. It is not certain if these test substances adequately test the MPS ability to take up immune complexes. Recently, *Frank et al.* [6] showed that the removal of autologous red blood cells, sensitized with Rh(D) antibodies, was decreased in patients with active SLE while high levels of circulating immune complexes were present. With improvement these parameters returned towards normal. Of particular interest was the observation that the removal of aggregated albumin was not altered, indicating that the MPS function for uptake of immune complexes should be measured with Fc receptor specific probes.

What should be the ideal probe for testing the ability of human MPS to remove circulating immune complexes? The removal of sensitized red cells is a function of antibody density on the red cells, these cells are primarily removed by the spleen [5] and the presence of antibodies to test cells may alter

the results. Large-latticed, soluble, immune complexes are not satisfactory for this purpose since previous immunity to a given antigen will influence the results. The use of a neoantigen in immune complexes will limit the use of such an agent to a single test due to subsequent immunity. Therefore, in our opinion, the most likely candidate for clinical investigation is the development of stable, reproducible, and limited aggregates of human IgG as a surrogate for soluble immune complexes. Since commercial preparations of IgG with aggregates have been administered to humans for passive immunizations for several decades, the use of small quantities of this material should be safe. The utility of such a probe for MPS Fc receptor function can easily be tested in acute or chronic experimental models of immune complex diseases with known degrees of MPS saturation or with presence of known quantities of circulating immune complexes.

The Influence of Antigens and Antibodies on the Uptake of Immune Complexes by the MPS

Variations in antigenic molecules, particularly the valence of antigens, influence the degree of lattice formation and thereby the uptake by the MPS and deposition in tissues [9]. In addition, other properties of antigens can alter the fate of circulating immune complexes independent of the degree of lattice formation.

As an example, the degree of conjugation of 4-fluoro-3-nitrophenyl azide (abbreviated NAP) to human serum albumin (HSA) increased the rapidity of removal of these molecules as a function of epitope density. Small-latticed, covalently cross-linked immune complexes were prepared with antibodies to NAP and HSA with different densities of NAP. Small-latticed complexes

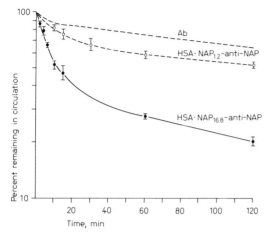

Fig. 1. Disappearance of covalently cross-linked, small-latticed (Ag_2Ab_2 or smaller) immune complexes, prepared with antigens with varying epitope (NAP = 4-fluoro-3-nitrophenyl azide) density. The HSA·$NAP_{16.8}$-anti-NAP and the HSA·$NAP_{1.2}$-anti-NAP complexes were prepared with purified antibodies to NAP, covalently cross-linked by photoactivation and the small-latticed complexes were obtained by gel filtration. The injected complexes contained 17.3 μg of $NAP_{16.8}$ and 35 μg of $NAP_{1.2}$ antigen, respectively. The small-latticed complexes prepared with the high epitope density antigen were more quickly removed from circulation than complexes with comparable lattice but containing the antigen with low epitope density.

containing the antigen with high epitope density were removed from circulation due to the fast removal of the antigen alone (fig. 1). Of particular interest to the study of systemic lupus erythematosus is the observation that single-stranded DNA injected into mice was removed and degraded by the liver many times faster than large-latticed immune complexes [4]. One might expect that small-laticed immune complexes with this antigen are also quickly removed from circulation because of the nature of the antigen. These observations point out the need for studying the influence of antigens on the fate of immune complexes in human diseases.

The class and subclass of antibody molecules influence the efficacy of their interaction with monocyte receptors *in vitro* [9]. These studies suggest that large-latticed immune complexes, composed of antibodies that bind ineffectively with monocyte receptors, would circulate longer than complexes containing antibodies that bind effectively with these receptors. This question has not been examined with varying classes or subclasses of antibodies. IgG molecules with reduced and alkylated interchain disulfide bonds, however, have served as a model since immune complexes made with such antibodies formed lattices comparable to those obtained with intact molecules [8]. Such large-latticed complexes interacted ineffectively with monocyte receptors *in vitro* [9], persisted in circulation due to decreased uptake by MPS [1, 7, 8, 12] and caused extensive deposits in renal glomeruli [10]. Similar findings can be anticipated in human diseases with large-latticed complexes that are ineffective in reacting with receptors on Kupffer cells.

References

1 Arend, W. P. and Mannik, M.: Studies on antigen-antibody complexes. II. Quantification of tissue uptake of soluble complexes in normal and complement-depleted rabbits. J. Immun. *107*: 63–75 (1971).

2 Arend, W. P.; Teller, D. C., and Mannik, M.: Molecular composition and sedimentation characteristics of soluble antigen-antibody complexes. Biochemistry, N.Y. *11*: 4063–4071 (1972).

3 Drivas, G.; Kerr, D. N. S., and Wardle, C. N.: Reticulo-endothelial phagocytosis in patients with nephritis. Br. med. J. *i:* 321 (1976).

4 Emlen, W. and Mannik, M.: Kinetics and mechanisms for removal of circulating single-stranded DNA in mice. J. exp. Med. *147:* 684–699 (1978).

5 Frank, M. M.: Pathophysiology of immune hemolytic anemia. Ann. intern. Med. *87:* 210–222 (1977).

6 Frank, M. M.; Jaffe, C. J.; Kimberly, R. P.; Lawley, T. J., and Plotz, P. H.: An immunospecific clearance defect in patients with systemic lupus erythematosus (SLE) related to the levels of circulating immune complexes (IC) (abstr.). Clin. Res. *25:* 357A (1977).

7 Haakenstad, A. O. and Mannik, M.: Saturation of the reticuloendothelial system with soluble immune complexes. J. Immun. *112:* 1939–1948 (1974).

8 Haakenstad, A. O. and Mannik, M.: The disappearance kinetics of soluble immune complexes prepared with reduced and alkylated antibodies and with intact antibodies in mice. Lab. Invest. *35:* 283–292 (1976).

9 Haakenstad, A. O. and Mannik, M.: The biology of immune complexes; in Talal Autoimmunity, pp. 277–360 (Academic Press, New York 1977).

10 Haakenstad, A. O.; Striker, G. E., and Mannik, M.: The glomerular deposition of soluble immune complexes prepared with reduced and alkylated antibodies and with intact antibodies in mice. Lab. Invest. *35:* 293–301 (1976).

11 Howard, J. G.: The origin and immunological significance of Kupffer cells; in van Furth Mononuclear phagocytes, pp. 178–199 (Davis, Philadelphia 1970).

12 Mannik, M. and Arend, W. P.: Fate of preformed immune complexes in rabbits and rhesus monkeys, J. exp. Med. *134:* 19s–31s (1971).

13 Munthe-Kaas, A. C.; Berg, T.; Seglon, P. O., and Seljelid, R.: Mass isolation and culture of rat Kupffer cells. J. exp. Med. *141:* 1–10 (1975).

14 Norman, S. J.: Kinetics of phagocytosis. II. Analysis of *in vivo* clearance with demonstration of competitive inhibition between similar and dissimilar foreign particles. Lab. Invest. *31:* 161–169 (1974).

15 Salky, N. K.; Mills, D., and Di Luzio, N. R.: Activity of the reticuloendothelial system in diseases of altered immunity. J. Lab. clin. Med. *66:* 952–960 (1965).

16 Segal, D. M., and Hurwitz, E.: Dimers and trimers of immunoglobulin G covalently cross-linked with a bivalent affinity label. Biochemistry, N.Y. *15:* 5253–5258 (1976).

17 Wagner, H. N., jr. and Iio, M.: Studies of the reticuloendothelial system (RES). III. Blockade of the RES in man. J. clin. Invest. *43:* 1525–1532 (1964).

18 Wardle, E. N.: Reticuloendothelial clearance studies in the course of horse serum induced nephritis. Br. J. exp. Path. *55:* 149–152 (1974).

19 Wilson, C. B. and Dixon, F. J.: Quantitation of acute and chronic serum sickness in the rabbit. J. exp. Med. *134:* 7s–18s (1971).

20 Wisse, E. and Daems, W. T.: Fine structural study on the sinusoidal lining cells of rat liver; in van Furth Mononuclear phagocytes, pp. 200–210 (Davis, Philadelphia 1970).

Dr. Mart Mannik, Department of Medicine
RG-20, University of Washington, Seattle,
WA 98195 (USA)

Immunopathology. 6th Int. Convoc. Immunol., Niagara Falls, N.Y., 1978, pp. 217–223 (Karger, Basel 1979)

Pathology and Pathogenesis of Rheumatoid Arthritis[1]

Nathan J. Zvaifler

Department of Medicine, School of Medicine, University of California San Diego, San Diego, Calif.

The pathology and pathogenesis of rheumatoid arthritis can be considered in three distinct stages: (1) The initiation of synovitis by the primary etiological factor; (2) subsequent immunological events that perpetuate the initial inflammatory reaction, and (3) transition of the inflammatory allergic reaction in the synovium to a proliferative, destructive granulation tissue (pannus).

The earliest events in rheumatoid arthritis are difficult to document, but the available studies suggest that microvascular injury and mild synovial cell proliferation are the first lesions [22, 30]. *Schumacher* [30] described the synovial membrane and joint fluid changes in 8 patients seen during the first 6 weeks of an arthritis that could subsequently be classified as definite or classical rheumatoid arthritis. All showed mild lining cell proliferation and perivascular lymphocytes by light microscopy. Polymorphonuclear leukocytes, when present, were in the superficial synovium; plasma cells were rarely noted. Vascular lesions were prominent. Small blood vessels were obliterated by inflammatory cells and organized thrombi. Electron microscopic examination disclosed gaps between vascular endothelial cells and

endothelial cell injury. Virus-like particles were seen in association with the endothelial lesions in 4 patients. Phagocytosis was prominent in proliferating synoviocytes and in large mononuclear cells.

In contrast to established rheumatoid arthritis, the synovial fluids from these early cases usually showed more mononuclear cells than polymorphonuclear leukocytes. Inclusions were not demonstrated in the neutrophils. This conforms with the experience of others [11].

These observations have obvious implications for the initiation of rheumatoid arthritis. Microvascular changes are probably non-specific since they are seen in other acute inflammatory joint diseases. The morphological changes suggesting viral particles are interesting, but they are difficult to distinguish from altered cell components and, at least to date, there is no compelling evidence supporting a viral etiology for rheumatoid arthritis [23]. However, these early findings do suggest that the responsible etiological factor(s) is carried to the joint by the circulation.

The histopathologic features of established rheumatoid arthritis and the immunological events that perpetuate the primary synovial inflammatory reaction are well described [10, 12, 38]. Grossly, the synovium appears

[1] Supported in part by grants from the United States Public Health Service (AM 14916 and AM 07062) and the Kroc Foundation

edematous and protrudes into the joint cavity as slender villous projections. Light miscroscopic examination of the established rheumatoid synovitis discloses a characteristic but not pathognomonic constellation of histological changes. There is hyperplasia and hypertrophy of the synovial lining cells which may reach to a depth of 6–10 cells; normally, there are only 1–3 cell layers. Focal or segmental vascular changes are a regular feature of rheumatoid synovitis. Venous distention results from swollen endothelial cells. Capillary obstruction is common. Arterial walls are infiltrated with neutrophils and areas of thrombosis and perivascular hemorrhage are seen. The connective tissue stroma of the normal synovial villous has few cells. In rheumatoid arthritis, it is packed with mononuclear cells, some collected into aggregates or follicles, particularly around small blood vessels. True germinal centers are rare. Lymphocytes predominate in these follicles with a mantle of plasma cells about their periphery. Polymorphonuclear leukocytes, common in the early lesions, are only occasionally seen. Multinucleated giant cells, when present, are usually located in areas of synovial lining cell hyperplasia. Fibrin-like material is deposited on the synovial cell surface and in the intracellular matrix.

The fine structure of the rheumatoid synovium has been examined by electron microscopy [3, 27]. Hyperplasia of synoviocytes results from an increase in both A (reticulo-endothelial-like) and B type cells. The former show large accumulations of residual bodies and altered lysosomes. Superficially, the synoviocytes appear to form an uninterrupted layer, but in reality no true basement membrane separates them from the underlying connective tissue. Rather, it is the interdigitation of their cytoplasmic processes that provides the continuity of the lining cell layer. For this reason, the joint cavity communicates directly with the subsynovial space. The intracellular matrix beneath the lining layer contains amorphous granular deposits and fine fibrillar material. Some of this is fibrin and as noted below, immunoglobulins are common in this region.

The most conspicuous finding in the subsynovial space is round cell accumulation. *Ziff* and his co-workers have studied these cells in detail [18]. In some places, particularly around small blood vessels, lymphocytes predominate; in others, plasma cells are the dominant type. Transitional areas have also been identified and show an intermingling of macrophages, lymphocytes and plasma cells. Blast cells are uncommon in the first two regions, constituting less than 5% of the cells in either the lymphocyte rich or plasma cell rich zones. But in the transitional areas, two thirds of the cells are blast cells, suggesting that antibodies and the products of activated lymphocytes and macrophages are generated there.

Immunological methods have been used to further define the lymphocytes in the rheumatoid synovium. The majority of cells stain with anti-human T cell serum [2] and in cyto-adherence studies bind sheep erythrocytes (E) but not red cells coated with antibody and the third component of complement (EAC) [35]. Similar results were obtained with lymphocytes isolated from rheumatoid synovium by dispersion with collagenase and deoxyribonuclease. Most of the cells lack surface immunoglobulin and EAC receptors, but form E rosettes [1, 24]. It is possible that the enhanced recovery of T lymphocytes is artifactual due to the greater difficulty of extracting cells committed to antibody production or because plasmablasts lose their cell surface markers. Alternatively, their receptors may be blocked by immune complexes. Whatever the reasons for the failure to demonstrate B cells or plasma cells, their presence in the synovium can be inferred from the findings of local antibody production.

The rheumatoid synovium contains large amounts of immunoglobulin when examined by immunofluorescent techniques [9]. IgG and IgM single or in combination is demonstrable in synovial lining cells, blood vessels, and in the interstitial connective tissues. The IgG, generally found in abundance, is in areas that also stain for C3 and C4, whereas IgM is in lesser amounts and not identified with complement [38]. Immunofluorescent analysis of the plasma cells in the subsynovium shows IgG to be the predominant immunoglobulin, but few have anti-Ig activity when tested with fluorescien-labeled, aggregated IgG [25]. After pepsin treatment, the number staining for rheumatoid factor increases significantly. This suggests that many of the plasma cells in the rheumatoid synovium make an IgG rheumatoid factor which combines in the cytoplasm with similar IgG molecules ('self-associating IgG'). Results were similar in pepsin-digested tissues from both seronegative or seropositive patients, namely 20–60% of the IgG plasma cells showed anti-Ig activity [26].

Additional observations indicating that the B cells in the synovium of patients with rheumatoid arthritis make immunoglobulins include the demonstration of in vivo IgG synthesis [31] and de novo immunoglobulin synthesis by rheumatoid synovial explants or continuous cultures of lymphocytes from synovium [32].

Based on these observations, two pathogenetic mechanisms have been advanced to explain rheumatoid synovitis. The first—the 'extra-vascular immune complex hypothesis' —proposes an interaction of antigens and antibodies in synovial tissues and fluid [39]. The antibodies are, in general, locally produced, especially the self-associating dimers and higher multiples of the IgG-anti IgG complex. Other potentially important com-

plexes are those in which the antigens are constituents of articular· tissues or byproducts of the inflammatory process, such as collagen, cartilage, fibrinogen or fibrin, partially digested IgG (pepsin agglutinator), DNA and soluble nucleoproteins [38]. The reaction of antigen with antibody in the joint tissues initiates the complement sequence, generating a number of biologically active products. Some, by virtue of their ability to increase vascular permeability, allow an influx of serum proteins and cellular blood elements into the site where the complexes reside. Polymorphonuclear leukocytes are attracted by complement derived chemotactic factors and the complexes are attached to their cell surfaces by receptors for IgG and C3. Engulfment follows with a subsequent release of large quantities of hydrolytic enzymes. It is these lysosomal enzymes that are directly responsible for the inflammation and tissue damage [36].

There is an alternative hypothesis, namely that rheumatic joint disease results from cellular hypersensitivity [29]. The accumulation of lymphocytes in the rheumatoid synovium is reminiscent of a delayed type of hypersensitivity reaction. The identification of a large number of these lymphocytes as T cells, and the finding of soluble factors derived from T cells (lymphokines) support this view. For instance, rheumatoid synovial fluids inhibit the migration of guinea pig macrophages. A similar MIF-like material was found in supernatents from cultures of rheumatoid synovial explants [33]. Rheumatoid joint fluids contain substances which stimulate spleen cells to incorporate tritiated thymidine [34]. It is worth noting, however, that none of these factors has been isolated and compared to known lymphokines and that synovial fluids contain neutral proteases which can inhibit macrophage migration and stimulate mitogenesis. Despite these reservations, it is hard to deny that cellular

immune reactions play some role in rheumatoid synovitis.

Chronic rheumatoid arthritis is characterized by destruction of articular cartilage,
ligaments, tendons and bone. The damage
results from a dual attack—from without by
enzymes in the synovial fluid and from above
and below by granulation tissue. An appreci-
ation of the characteristics of the tissues
involved is helpful in understanding this
process.

Cartilage and other articular connective
tissues are comprised primarily of a ground
substance (proteoglycans) and collagen. The
former consists of repeating disaccharide
subunits linked covalently to a protein core.
The earliest evidence of cartilage injury is a
loss of metachromatic staining due to a
leaching out of the proteoglycans [13]. Cartilage that has lost ground substance has a
diminished capacity to resist deformation
and is at risk for permanent damage through
mechanical disruption. Proteoglycan loss is
reversible, and complete recovery is possible,
but once collagen, which forms the structural
skeleton, is lost, cartilage disintegration
becomes irreversible [17].

A number of potentially damaging enzymes released from phagocytic synoviocytes
and polymorphonuclear leukocytes are in
the fluid that continually bathes the cartilage
surfaces [39]. These include acid and neutral
proteases that can split proteoglycan from
its protein matrix and collagenases [4, 14,
28]. Collagen, when in its triple helical configuration, resists degradation by non-specific
proteases. However, specific collagenases
derived from polymorphonuclear leukocytes
and rheumatoid synovial cells can cleave the
collagen polypeptide chains into two fragments, exposing them to further degradation
by proteolytic enzymes [16]. The observation
of proteoglycan depletion and collagen degradation in normal appearing cartilage at
sites distant from the advancing margin of

the proliferating synovial membrane is additional confirmation of the importance of
enzymes in articular damage [13, 19].

An important feature of the pathology
of rheumatoid arthritis is the formation of
pannus, a vascular granulation tissue composed of proliferating fibroblasts, numerous
small blood vessels, and various numbers of
inflammatory cells [10, 12]. Three types have
been described [20]. The first, a cellular
pannus, has the appearance of synovium and
infiltrates the cartilage with proliferating
blood vessels and perivascular mononuclear
cells. Collagen and proteoglycans seem to
be dissolved in the region immediately surrounding the nests of cells. A second type
resembles a granulation tissue composed of
monocytic cells and fibroblasts. Multiple
filopodia extend from these cells into the
cartilage matrix and degradation proceeds
around them. Another variety of pannus is
composed of a dense avascular, acellular,
fibrous tissue tightly adherent to cartilage.

The first type of pannus, which has the
appearance of an 'activated' synovial membrane, appears to produce cartilage destruction by enzymatic digestion [15, 20]. The
second 'cellular' form of pannus may operate
the same way, but its similarity to granulation tissue seen at other sites of injury suggests
the alternate possibility that this cellular and
fibrous infiltrate is the result of cartilage
injury, rather than the cause. The third type
of pannus probably acts as a mantle inter-
fering with cartilage nutrition. Although the
three types of pannus can be found simultaneously in the same joint, it is not clear that
they represent a sequential phenomenon or
that each develops independently.

A better understanding of the chronic
synovitis of rheumatoid arthritis is developing from studies of the effects of lymphocytes,
macrophages and their products upon target
cells in the synovium, cartilage and bone.
Cultured explants of rheumatoid synovial

fragments produce large quantities of collagenase and prostaglandins [8, 21]. The responsible cells are large, measuring 30 nm in diameter or greater, with abundant cytoplasm, a large nucleus and dendritic processes which given them a stellate appearance [6]. They do not produce lysosyme and lack the conventional surface markers of macrophages. When placed in continuous culture, they initially make both collagenase and prostaglandin (PGE_2), but the collagenase decreases after trypsinization and serial passage of the cells. This enzyme activity is renewed by the addition of an incubation medium from peripheral blood leukocytes to the cultures [7]. Plant lectins further increase the amount of stimulating factor. Fractionation studies reveal that a monocyte and/or macrophage is the cell responsible for the basal production of the stimulating factor. But this is not increased by lectins, suggesting the participation of other cell types. This is supported by the observation that T cells which ordinarily produce little stimulating factor markedly increase the collagenase production of synoviocytes when cultured with 5% mononuclear cells and lectin [5]. There is limited information as yet about the substance released from the peripheral blood mononuclear cells.

On the other hand, there is considerable new information about the collagenase produced by cultured synovial cells. The collagenase is released from isolated synovial cells in an inactive or latent form. Treatment with trypsin or plasmin can activate the latent enzyme [37]. Plasmin is potentially important *in vivo* because plasminogen activator is demonstrable in cultured rheumatoid synovial cells. Further, it appears that the latent collagenase binds to collagen fibrils and it is this species which is activated by plasmin. Finally, α_2-macroglobulin is an important inhibitor of active collagenase [37].

Based on these findings, the following scheme has been proposed. The lymphocytes and macrophages in the rheumatoid synovium, individually or in consort, release soluble products that cause tissue inflammation, permeability of synovial blood vessels, and the production of latent collagenases by synovial cells. The same population of synovial cells produces plasminogen activator which can convert serum plasminogen that has entered the inflamed joint tissues to plasmin. Plasmin saturates α_2-macroglobulins and other circulating inhibitors of collagenase and activates the latent enzyme bound to collagen fibrils. This leads to a rapid destruction of collagen-containing tissues. Alternatively, the latent collagenase could be released, but escape activation and remain bound to fibrils. At some later time, plasminogen activators produced by the endothelial cells of small blood vessels in the pannus could initiate the collagenolytic process. It is quite likely that these mechanisms are not unique to rheumatoid arthritis, and in fact may represent a generalized biological response to chronic inflammation. It does, however, provide a system which is amenable to regulation and control, and could lead to the development of important new therapies for rheumatoid arthritis.

References

1 Abrahamsen, T. B.; Froland, S. S.; Natvig, J. B., and Pahle, J.: Elution and characterization of lymphocytes from rheumatoid inflammatory tissue. Scand. J. Immunol. *4:* 823–830 (1975).
2 Bankhurst, A. D.; Husby, G., and Williams, R. C., jr.: Predominance of T cells in lymphocytic infiltrates of synovial tissues in rheumatoid arthritis. Arthritis Rheum. *19:* 555–562 (1976).
3 Barland, P.; Novikoff, A. B., and Hamerman, D.: Fine structure of the rheumatoid synovial membrane with special reference to lysosomes. Am. J. Path. *44:* 853–866 (1964).
4 Barrett, A. J.: The enzymic degradation of cartilage matrix; in Burleigh and Poole Dynamics of connec-

tive tissue macromolecules, pp. 189–226 (North Holland, Amsterdam 1975).

5 Dayer, J. M. and Krane, S. M.: The interaction of immune competent cells and chronic inflammation as exemplified by rheumatoid arthritis. Clin. Rheum. Dis. *4:* 517–537 (1978).

6 Dayer, J. M.; Krane, S. M.; Russell, R. G. G., and Robinson, D. R.: Production of collagenase and prostaglandins by isolated adherent rheumatoid synovial cells. Proc. natn. Acad. Sci. USA *73:* 945–949 (1976).

7 Dayer, J. D.; Robinson, D. R., and Krane, S. M.: Prostaglandin production by rheumatoid synovial cells. Stimulation by a factor from human mononuclear cells. J. exp. Med. *145:* 1393–1404 (1977).

8 Evanson, J. M.; Jeffrey, J. J., and Krane, S. M.: Studies on collagenase from rheumatoid synovium in tissue culture. J. clin. Invest. *47:* 2639–2651 (1968).

9 Fish, A. J.; Michael, A. F.; Gewurz, H., and Good, R. A.: Immunopathologic changes in rheumatoid arthritis synovium. Arthritis Rheum. *9:* 267–280 (1966).

10 Gardner, D. L.: The pathology of rheumatoid arthritis (Arnold, London 1972).

11 Gatter, R. A. and Richmond, J. D.: The predominance of synovial lymphocytes in early rheumatoid arthritis. J. Rheum. *2:* 340–345 (1975).

12 Hamerman, D.; Barland, P., and Janis, R.: The structure and chemistry of the synovial membrane in health and disease; in Bittar and Bittar The biological basis of medicine, vol. 3, pp. 269–310 (Saunders, Philadelphia 1969).

13 Hamerman, D.; Janis, R., and Smith, C.: Cartilage matrix depletion by rheumatoid synovial cells in tissue culture. J. exp. Med. *126:* 1005–1012 (1967).

14 Harris, E. D., jr.; Dibona, D. R., and Krane, S. M.: Collagenases in human synovial fluid. J. clin. Invest. *48:* 2104–2113 (1969).

15 Harris, E. D.; Glauert, A. M., and Merrley, A. H.: Intracellular collagen fibers at the pannus cartilage junction in rheumatoid arthritis. Arthritis Rheum. *20:* 657–665 (1977).

16 Harris, E. D., jr. and Krane, S. M.: Collagenases. New Engl. J. Med. *291:* 557–563, 605–609, 652–661 (1974).

17 Harris. E. D., jr.; Parker, H. D.; Radin, E. L., and Krane, S. M.: Effects of proteolytic enzymes on structural and mechanical properties of cartilage. Arthritis Rheum. *15:* 497–503 (1972).

18 Ishikawa, H. and Ziff, M.: Electron microscopic observations of immuno-reactive cells in the rheumatoid synovial membrane. Arthritis Rheum. *19:* 1–14 (1976).

19 Kimura, H.; Tateishi, H., and Ziff, M.: Surface ultrastructure of rheumatoid articular cartilage. Arthritis Rheum. *20:* 1085–1097 (1977).

20 Kobayashi, I. and Ziff, M.: Electron microscopic studies of the cartilage-pannus junction in rheumatoid arthritis. Arthritis Rheum. *18:* 475–483 (1975).

21 Krane, S. M.: Collagenase production by human synovial tissues. Ann. N.Y. Acad. Sci. *265:* 289–303 (1975).

22 Kulka, J.P.; Bocking, D.; Ropes, M. W., and Bauer, W.: Early joint lesions of rheumatoid arthritis. Archs Path. *59:* 129–150 (1955).

23 Marmion, B. P.: Infectious agents and the immunopathology of rheumatoid arthritis. Clin. Rheum. Dis. *4:* 565–586 (1978).

24 Meijer, C. J.; Putte, L. B. Van De; Eulderink, F.; Dleinjan, R.; Lafeber, G., and Bots, G. Th.: Characteristics of mononuclear cell populations in chronically inflamed synovial membranes. J. Path. *121:* 1–11 (1976).

25 Munthe, F. and Natvig, J. B.: Immunoglobulin classes, subclasses and complexes of IgG rheumatoid factor in rheumatoid plasma cells. Clin. exp. Immunol. *12:* 55–70 (1972).

26 Natvig, J. B. and Munthe, E.: Self-associating IgG rheumatoid factor represents a major response of plasma cells in rheumatoid inflammatory tissue. Ann. N.Y. Acad. Sci. *256:* 88–95 (1975).

27 Norton, W. L. and Ziff, M.: Electron microscopic observations on the rheumatoid synovial membrane. Arthritis Rheum. *9:* 589–610 (1966).

28 Oronsky, A. L.; Ignarro, L., and Perper, R. J.: Release of cartilage mucopolysaccharide degrading neutral protease from human leukocytes. J. exp. Med. *138:* 461–472 (1973).

29 Pearson, C. M.; Paulus, H. E., and Machleder, H. I.: The role of the lymphocyte and its products in the propagation of joint disease. Ann. N.Y. Acad. Sci. *256:* 150–168 (1975).

30 Schumacher, H. R.: Synovial membrane and fluid morphologic alterations in early rheumatoid arthritis: microvascular injury and virus-like particles. Ann. N.Y. Acad. Sci. *256:* 39–64 (1975).

31 Sliwinski, A. J. and Zvaifler, N. J.: *In vivo* synthesis of IgG by the rheumatoid synovium. J. Lab. clin. Med. *76:* 304–310 (1970).

32 Smiley, J. D.; Sachs, C., and Ziff, M.: *In vitro* synthesis of immunoglobulin by rheumatoid synovial membrane. J. clin. Invest. *47:* 624–632 (1968).

33 Stastny, P.; Rosenthal, M.; Andreis, M., and Ziff, M.: Lymphokines in the rheumatoid joint. Arthritis Rheum. *18:* 237–243 (1975).

34 Stastny, P.; Rosenthal, M.; Andreis, M.; Cooke, D., and Ziff, M.: Lymphokines in rheumatoid synovitis. Ann. N.Y. Acad. Sci. 256: 117–131 (1975).
35 Boxel, J. A. Van and Paget, S. A.: Predominantly T-cell infiltrate in rheumatoid synovial membrane. New Engl. J. Med. 293: 517–520 (1975).
36 Weissman, G.: Lysosomal mechanisms of tissue injury in arthritis. New Engl. J. Med. 286: 141–147 (1972).
37 Werb, Z.; Mainardi, C. L.; Vater, C. A., and Harris, E. D., jr.: Endogenous activation of latent collagenase by rheumaoid synovial cells. Evidence for a role of plasminogen activator. New Engl. J. Med. 296: 1017–1023 (1977).

38 Zvaifler, N. J.: Immunopathology of joint inflammation in rheumatoid arthritis. Adv. Immunol. 16: 265–336 (1973).
39 Zvaifler, N. J.: Rheumatoid synovitis: an extravascular immune complex disease. Arthritis Rheum. 17: 297–305 (1974).

Dr. N. J. Zvaifler, Department of Medicine School of Medicine, University of California San Diego, San Diego, CA 92103 (USA)

Immunopathology. 6th Int. Convoc. Immunol., Niagara Falls, N.Y., 1978, pp. 224–229 (Karger, Basel 1979)

Anti-IgG in Rheumatoid Arthritis
Pathogenetic Potential and Stimulation by Epstein-Barr Virus

John H. Vaughan, Dennis A. Carson, Roy A. Kaplan and Laura S. Slaughter

Scripps Clinic and Research Foundation, La Jolla, Calif.

Rheumatoid arthritis (RA) is an immune complex disease characterized by a high incidence among patients of the histocompatibility antigen HLA-DW4 [15] and by the presence of autoantibodies, of which polyclonal antibodies to IgG, so-called rheumatoid factors, are predominant. This presentation will address itself to three questions: (1) Are the anti-IgG likely to be exerting a pathogenetic effect in RA? (2) Is there evidence for other antibodies contributing to the pathogenesis of the disease? (3) What sorts of mechanisms control the production of anti-IgG? For the last of these, we will consider experiments carried out with Epstein-Barr virus (EBV).

A variety of findings has suggested that anti-IgG plays a role in the pathogenesis of RA. The immune complexes deposited in the affected tissues of patients contain anti-IgG [8, 19]; anti-IgG are themselves capable of fixing and activating complement [16, 17, 21]; and IgG-anti-IgG complexes have been demonstrated both in the joint fluids [20] and in the circulation [7] of patients with RA. Preparations of anti-IgG complexes have, when injected into experimental animals, produced mesenteric [3] and pulmonary vasculitis [6].

¹ Supported by NIH grants AM 07144, AM 21175, AM 00369, RR 00833 and RR 05514.

The most frequently cited evidence against anti-IgG having a pathogenetic role is the frequency with which anti-IgG can be found in the blood of patients with diseases other than RA, sometimes even in apparently normal individuals [9]; experiments which show that anti-IgG can reduce the complement-fixing ability in some immune systems [14], which has been interpreted as giving anti-IgG a protective role; and the ability of anti-IgG to accelerate the clearance of virus-antibody complexes from the circulation [12], again interpreted as a protective role.

Materials and Methods

Anti-IgG. Antibodies (of the IgM and IgG class) to IgG were quantified in a solid phase radioimmunoassay [4]. For antibodies of the IgM class, whole sera were added to tubes to which IgG had been preadsorbed, and the attached IgM anti-IgG was detected with a radiolabelled burro anti-Fcμ. For antibodies of the IgG class, the fraction of RA sera that passed through a DE52 column at $0.005 \, M \, PO_4$ pH 8.0 was added to tubes to which Fcγ had been pre-adsorbed, and the attached IgG anti-IgG was detected with a radiolabelled rabbit anti Fabγ.

To measure the ability of anti-IgG to activate complement, a hemolytic assay was used [16]. The system involved sheep cells sensitized with rabbit amboceptor which had been reduced and alkylated, so that the sheep cells were not lysed by complement except when anti-IgG was added to the system.

Complement Turnover Studies. The rates of consumption of C4 or factor B in our patients was determined by injecting them with highly purified C4 or Factor B labeled with ^{125}I or ^{131}I by the iodomonochloride method [10] and following the disappearance of the label from the serum and its appearance in the urine over a 10-day period. The consumption, measured as fractional catabolic rate (FCR), was calculated by Nosslin's intergrated rate equations [11].

Lymphocyte Cultures. 50 ml of heparinized blood was obtained from each of 11 patients with seropositive RA and from 10 control persons. The mononuclear cells were isolated by centrifugation in a Ficoll-Hypaque gradient, the interface cells washed to remove excess surface immunoglobulin, exposed for 1 h to EBV from the B95-8 marmoset line at 37 °C, washed once again, and cultured in RPMI-1640 with 10% fetal bovine serum. Supernatant fluids from the cultured cells were removed at intervals thereafter and examined for total IgM and IgM anti-IgG by radioimmunoassay.

Statistics. The data were expressed as means ± SEM. Correlation coefficients were calculated by Spearman's non-parametric rank correlation [5].

Results and Discussion

Complement Activation by Anti-IgG. A dose-response relationship between degree of hemolysis and dilution of serum was clearly seen when increasing dilutions of RA sera containing anti-IgG were examined in the presence of complement (fig. 1a). Comparable results were obtained with isolated 19S fractions but not with 7S fractions of the sera. The hemolysis depends on the activation of the classical complement pathway and

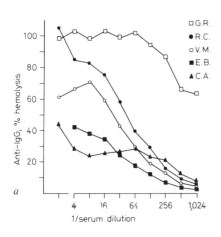

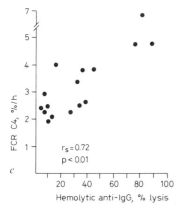

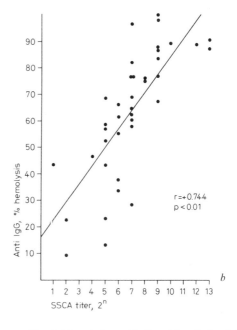

Fig. 1. Hemolytic anti-IgG. *a* Hemolysis of sheep cells sensitized with reduced and alkylated rabbit IgG by increasing dilutions of five RA sera containing anti-IgG. From [13]. *b* Correlation between hemolytic and agglutinating activities of anti-IgG in various RA sera. *c* Correlation between fractional catabolic rate of C4 (FCR-C4) in RA patients with titer of hemolytic anti-IgG activity.

involves the consumption of C4 [16]. Pro-zones were occasionally seen when serum was used at dilutions less than 1/16. Our standard assay was carried out at the single dilution of 1/20 and the degree of hemolysis seen at this dilution was taken to estimate the quantity of hemolytic anti-IgG present.

Although a generally positive correlation exists between the titer of hemolytic anti-IgG and anti-IgG measured by agglutinating titer, a considerable variation in degree of hemolysis was seen for different sera at given agglutinating titers. This variation is due to qualitative differences of the IgM anti-IgG in the different sera [13] (fig. 1b).

Metabolism of Complement in Patients. The mean FCR-C4 for patients with RA was $3.41 \pm 1.19\%/h$; that for normal subjects was $2.07 \pm 0.21\%/h$. Clinically, the increased FCR-C4 in the RA patients correlated most closely with extensiveness of disease, as measured by number of manifestations of disease in tissues beyond the joints themselves, e.g. by subcutaneous nodules, various cutaneous manifestations of vasculitis, splenomegaly, neuropathy, pleuritis, or pericarditis.

When we investigated the relation between the FCR-C4 and the serum IgM or IgG anti-IgG measured in a solid phase radioimmunoassay, or with anti-IgG measured in our hemolytic assay, we found that the fractional catabolic rate correlated somewhat ($r_s = 0.45$) with IgM anti-IgG, better ($r_s = 0.57$) with IgG anti-IgG, but best ($r_s = 0.71$) with hemolytic anti-IgG (fig. 1c).

We have also examined the fractional catabolic rate of factor B (the alternative pathway) in a number of patients to get some estimate of the degree to which this pathway of complement activation may be involved in the disease. These studies have shown that, while the mean FCR factor B is elevated in RA, FCR-C4 is significantly more elevated than FCR-FB. We believe that these observations tell us that the classical pathway of complement activation is the pathway predominantly involved in RA and that hemolytic anti-IgG probably makes a significant contribution through this pathway. Involvement of the alternative pathway, as represented by the elevated FCR-FB, may occur entirely by recruitment from the classical pathway by the C3b positive feedback loop,

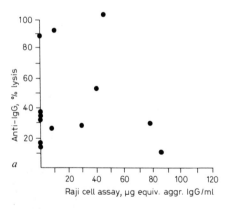

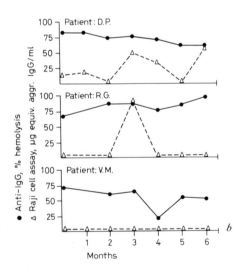

Fig. 2. Immune complexes by Raji cell assay. Lack of correlation of Raji cell assay to quantities of hemolytic anti-IgG. *a* In various RA sera. *b* In serial studies on three individual sera.

or may depend upon other as yet unknown mechanisms.

Other Immune Complexes. No correlation was found between anti-IgG and immune complexes detected with the Raji cell assay in individual RA sera (fig. 2a). We have followed 22 patients at monthly intervals for 6 months, examining simultaneously the presence of immune complexes in the Raji cell assay and the hemolytic anti-IgG titers. Three examples are given in figure 2b. The bottom panel presents the results with the serum of a patient who had a persistently negative Raji cell assay throughout the 6-month period while continuously exhibiting elevated hemolytic anti-IgG titers. The middle panel shows the results with the serum of a patient who had a positive Raji cell assay at only a single visit, the hemolytic anti-IgG being continuously and steadily elevated throughout the period. The top panel summarizes the results with the serum of a patient who had a positive Raji cell assay with fluctuating titer throughout the period of observation, but again without change in quantities of hemolytic anti-IgG. In our entire series, 4/22 patients were persistently negative in the Raji cell assay like the patient represented in the bottom panel, 12/22 were intermittently positive like that in the middle panel, and 6/22 consistently positive like that in the top panel. The peaks and valleys in the sequences of Raji cell titers were not reflected by any consistent changes in the patients' clinical status.

The variations in the results obtained with the Raji cell assay are undoubtedly important and probably signal some unknown, intermittent antigenic events in the disease with consequent immune complex formation. The exact nature of these events, however, is not yet known. Although immune complexes may ultimately be critical in keeping the disease active, it is the anti-IgG that is continuously present and apparently more predominant in activating complement in the patients. Mechanisms influencing the production of the anti-IgG seem therefore to be important.

Production of Anti-IgG by Cultured Cells. We have carried out *in vitro* studies on anti-IgG production using EBV, which is known to be a potent polyclonal activator of human B lymphocytes. EBV is of interest in RA also because of the recent demonstration by *Alspaugh and Tan* [2] that 70% of RA patients have antibodies to an EBV-associated antigen present in B cell lines, and the further demonstration by *Alspaugh et al.* [1] that EBV induces the development of the same nuclear antigen in normal lymphocytes.

Figure 3a shows the amounts of IgM anti-IgG released into the supernatant fluids of the infected and uninfected cells. It may be seen that: (1) EBV provoked the production of anti-IgG not only by the lymphocytes of patients with RA but also by lymphocytes of normal individuals, although the RA lymphocytes made significantly more anti-IgG than did normal lymphocytes; (2) the peak anti-IgG production occurred at 18 and 24 days after the initiation of culture in both groups; (3) in the absence of EBV, the lymphocytes of normal donors produced little or no anti-IgG, while the lymphocytes from RA patients produced small but significant quantities in an early (6–12 days) period.

The lymphocytes from patients with RA made more IgM anti-IgG relative to the amount of IgM produced than did cells from normal individuals. This is shown graphically in figure 3b. By our assays, about 30% of the IgM produced in the RA cell cultures was IgM anti-IgG. On the other hand, only about 2% of the IgM of the early supernatants of the normal cells was anti-IgG. This rose to around 7.5% at 30 days.

During these studies, we noted another fact which interested us. The RA lymphocytes

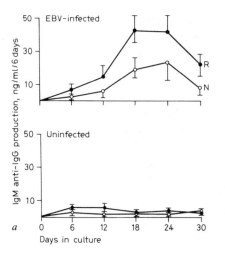

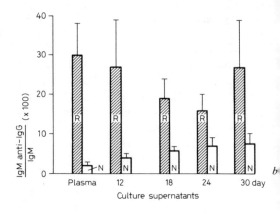

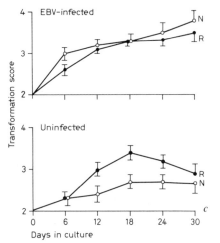

Fig. 3. In vitro culture of RA (R) and normal (N) peripheral blood mononuclear cells with and without Epstein-Barr Virus (EBV). *a* Production of IgM anti-IgG, as measured by quantities in supernatants at successive 6-day intervals. *b* Proportion of total IgM accountable as IgM anti-IgG. *c* Degree of transformation of the cells by Thorley-Lawson score [18]. Reproduced from [14a].

had an unusual tendency to transform spontaneously in culture in the absence of superimposed EBV infection (fig. 3c, bottom panel). Six of 11 RA cell cultures developed into established lines. This compares to a normal incidence that generally is of roughly 10%. Two of our 10 controls developed into lines.

We interpret our data as indicating that in RA there are many B cells in the circulation capable of producing anti-IgG, that RA lymphocytes are continuously activated and differentiating, and that they are already producing at their maximum at the times they are put into culture. In normals, however,

there are few or no B cells in the circulation actively engaged in anti-IgG production, and those that can produce anti-IgG upon stimulation are not fully expressed but respond to a maturation event, or derepression, when they are put into culture with EBV.

What factors are responsible for the high rate of transformation of the RA lymphocytes *in vitro*, is not known. The demonstrations by *Alspaugh and Tan* [2] and *Alspaugh et al.* [1] suggest, however, that EBV may play a special role in RA. This role could be simply that of a polyclonal B cell activator, the peculiar selection of autoantibodies in the disease being due to a corresponding peculiarity in their T cell suppressors, which in turn are probably under the control of Ir genes in the HLA-D region. Our system for studying anti-IgG production *in vitro* should allow critical experiments to test this latter possibility.

If EBV is important in RA as a polyclonal B cell stimulator, it is probably not alone in this property. Other microbial polyclonal stimulators, such as ASO, PPD, lipopolysaccharides, and dextrans, may deserve similar considerations, both in RA and in other autoimmune disorders.

References

1 Alspaugh, M. A.; Jensen, F. C.; Rabin, H., and Tan, E. M.: Lymphocytes transformed by Epstein-Barr virus. Induction of nuclear antigen reactive with antibody in rheumatoid arthritis. J. exp. Med. *147:* 1018–1027 (1978).

2 Alspaugh, M. A. and Tan, E. M.: Serum antibody in rheumatoid arthritis reactive with a cell-associated antigen. Arthritis Rheum. *19:* 711–719 (1976).

3 Baum, J.; Stastny, P., and Ziff, M.: Effects of the rheumatoid factor and antigen-antibody complexes on the vessels of the rat mesentery. J. Immun. *93:* 985–992 (1964).

4 Carson, D. A.; Lawrance, S.; Catalano, M. A.; Vaughan, J. H., and Abraham, G.: Radioimmunoassay of IgG and IgM rheumatoid factors reacting with human IgG. J. Immun. *119:* 295–300 (1977).

5 Colton T.; Statistics in medicine; 1st ed., p. 223 (Little, Brown, Boston 1974).

6 DeHoratius, R. J. and Williams, R. C.: Rheumatoid factor accentuation of pulmonary lesions associated with experimental diffuse proliferative lung disease. Arthritis Rheum. *15:* 293–301 (1972).

7 Franklin, E. C.; Holman, H. R.; Müller-Eberhard, H. J., and Kunkel, H. G.: An unusual protein component of high molecular weight in the serum of certain patients with rheumatoid arthritis. J. exp. Med. *105:* 425–438 (1957).

8 Kaplan, M. G. and Vaughan, J. H.: Reaction of rheumatoid sera with synovial tissue as revealed by fluorescent antibody studies. Arthritis Rheum. *2:* 356–358 (1959).

9 Lawrence, J. S.: Epidemiology of rheumatoid arthritis. Arthritis Rheum. *6:* 166–171 (1963).

10 McFarlane, A. S.: Efficient trace labeling of proteins with iodine. Nature, Lond. *182:* 53 (1958).

11 Nosslin, B.: Analysis of disappearance time-curves after single injection of labeled proteins; in Protein turnover. Ciba Found. Symp., pp. 113–130 (Associated Scientific Publishers, New York 1973).

12 Notkins, A. L.: Infectious virus-antibody complexes: interaction with anti-immunoglobulins, complement, and rheumatoid factor. J. exp. Med. *134:* 41s–51s (1971).

13 Robbins, D. L.; Moore, T. L.; Small, D., and Vaughan, J. H.: Complement fixation by rheumatoid factor (manuscript in preparation).

14 Romeyn, J. A. and Bowman, D. M.: Inhibition of complementary lysis by rheumatoid sera. Nature, Lond. *216:* 180–181 (1967).

14a Slaughter, L.; Carson, D. A.; Jensen, F. C.; Holbrook, T. L.; and Vaughan, J. H.: *In vitro* effects of Epstein-Barr virus on peripheral blood monocells from patients with rheumatoid arthritis and normal subjects. J. exp. Med. *148:* 1429–1434 (1978).

15 Stastny, P.: HLA-D typing in rheumatoid arthritis. Arthritis Rheum. *20:* S45–S49 (1977).

16 Tanimoto, K.; Cooper, N. R.; Johnson, J. S., and Vaughan, J. H.: Complement fixation by rheumatoid factor. J. clin. Invest. *55:* 347–445 (1975).

17 Tesar, J. T. and Schmid, F. R.: Conversion of soluble immune complexes into complement fixing aggregates by IgM-rheumatoid factor. J. Immun. *105:* 1206–1214 (1970).

18 Thorley-Lawson, D. A.; Chess, L., and Strominger, J. L.: Suppression of *in vitro* Epstein-Barr virus infection. J. exp. Med. *146:* 495–508 (1977).

19 Vaughan, J. H.; Jacox, R. F., and Noell, P.: Relation of intracytoplasmic inclusions in joint fluid leukocytes to anti-γG globulins. Arthritis Rheum. *11:* 135–144 (1968).

20 Winchester, R. J.; Agnello, V., and Kunkel, H. G.: Gammaglobulin complexes in synovial fluids of patients with rheumatoid arthritis. Partial characterization and relationship to lowered complement levels. Clin. exp. Immunol. *6:* 689–706 (1970).

21 Zvaifler, N. J. and Schur, P. H.: Reactions of aggregated mercaptoethanol treated gamma globulin in rheumatoid factor-precipitin and complement-fixation studies. Arthritis Rheum. *11:* 523–536 (1968).

Dr. J. H. Vaughan, Scripps Clinic and Research Foundation, 10666 North Torrey Pines Road, La Jolla, CA 92037 (USA)

Immunopathology. 6th Int. Convoc. Immunol., Niagara Falls, N.Y., 1978, pp. 230–235 (Karger, Basel 1979)

T Cell-Mediated Immunity to Intracellular Parasites
Role of the Major Histocompatibility Gene Complex and of the Thymus[1]

R. M. Zinkernagel

Scripps Clinic and Research Foundation, La Jolla, Calif.

Introduction

Cell immunity plays a major role in protecting higher vertebrates against viruses and intracellular bacteria, whereas humoral immunity—antibodies, complement and related mechanisms—deal predominantly with extracellular antigens, toxins, and extracellular bacteria [8, 12]. The evolutionary need for a system that discriminated self from nonself probably arose quite early in phylogeny. It may well be that cell-mediated immunity in the higher vertebrates developed out of such a primitive self-nonself recognition system which prevented phagocytes from engulfing themselves or their progeny, but allowed them to phagocytize foreign antigenic material [for excellent reviews of these issues, see 2, 3, 8, 11]. Whether this speculation is correct or not, modern T cells seem to have conserved two basic qualities in their receptor(s). One is to recognize self and another is to recognize foreign antigens or X. Such recognition could occur via one receptor, which specializes in recognizing 'modification' or 'alterations' of self, or via two re-

[1] This is Publication Number 1557 from the Immunology Departments, Scripps Clinic and Research Foundation, La Jolla, CA 92037. This work was supported by United States Public Service Grants AI-07007, AI-13779, AI-00248.

ceptors, one for self and one for X [10, 19]. Neither theory is provable at the moment.

All T cell functions studied so far in mice are specific not only for antigen but also differentially for cell surface structures coded by the major histocompatibility gene complex (MHC, H-2 in mice, HLA in humans) [5, 10, 19]. Furthermore, the activities of T cells from inbred mice, rats and chickens are clearly MHC-restricted, and some proof of this restriction exists for outbred individuals including humans.

Speculations on the Function of Major Transplantation Antigens

The self-specificity of T cells varies according to their function: Cytolytic T cells, which *in vitro* lyse target cells expressing foreign antigenic determinants (virus, major or minor transplantation antigens), are restricted to the *K* or *D* region products in mice (or *A*, *B* in humans) [5, 10, 19]. These products seem to be identical with the serologically defined major transplantation antigens that are associated with rejection of histoincompatible transplants. In contrast, nonlytic T cells—such as helper T cells or T cells involved in delayed type hypersensitivity—are restricted generally to products of the *I*-region of *H-2*

[6, 10] a region which also codes the immune response (*Ir*) genes that control antibody production [1]. Interestingly, T cells involved in activating macrophages during the specific T cell-dependent immune response against an intracellular bacterium, *Listeria mono-cytogenes*, are restricted to the same *I* region [15]. Overall, these patterns of restriction specificities expressed by various functional subclasses of T cells fit the following teleological argument [20]:

The many kinds of viruses infect differentially and with strong preference vertebrate cells of particular tissues, and also both phagocytic and nonphagocytic cells. Moreover, viruses undergo an eclipse phase during their infectious cycle, i.e. after absorption and penetration a virus is not an infectious entity until its progeny reassemble. Therefore, during the eclipse phase, cell lysis is synonymous with the elimination of virus. Because of the fact that viruses can actively infect all cells, theoretically, the receptor through which T cells transmit the lytic signal must be expressed ubiquitously on phagocytic and nonphagocytic cells. It is no coincidence then that the *K*, *D* structures, which are defined serologically as major transplantation antigens and serve as lytic targets are also expressed on all somatic cells tested so far, although in different quantities.

In contrast, facultative intracellular bacteria infect only phagocytic cells and do not undergo an eclipse phase. In this case, lysis of infected cells is not protective for the host, since lysis results in release, not destruction, of the bacteria. *Mackaness* [9] showed that intracellular bacteria are eliminated by T cells which are specifically sensitized to activate or release lymphokines. In turn, the lymphokines stimulate macrophages to nonspecifically increased digestive and bactericidal activity resulting in *intra*cellular destruction of bacteria in phagolysosomes. Similarly, antibodies can be viewed as opsonins that facilitate phagocytosis of extracellular bacteria or as neutralizing factors that inactivate bacterial toxins. Thus, T cells deal with these latter types of antigens only in association with phagocytes (monocytes, macrophages) or with precursors to antibody-producing B cells. The *I* region markers, which are differentially expressed by B, T and phagocytic cells, may thus serve as receptors for T cell-directed differentiation signals that are operated or triggered in an antigen-dependent and, therefore, specific manner. On macrophages, certain *I* structures may serve as receptors to increase enzyme production, or to induce more efficient types of digestive enzymes. On B cells, *I* structures may signal the start of immunoglobulin (Ig) production or switch the type of production from IgM to IgG, etc.

The dual specificity of T cells in recognizing a receptor for cell-specific differentiation signals on target B cells, target macrophages, target T cells or any other somatic target cells, then, has developed to trigger certain cell functions differentially and in an *antigen-specific* fashion.

Characteristics of Virus-Specific Cytotoxic T Cells

Immune cytotoxic T cells generated *in vivo*: (1) kill target cells by direct contact; (2) are virus-specific; (3) are clonally specific for *K* or *D* region coded surface structures; (4) act anti-virally by lysing virus infected cells during the viral eclipse phase, and (5) are probably identical with antiviral effector T cells *in vivo* [19].

The specificity of cytotoxic T cells for virus is probably comparable to that of antibodies [10]. However, the nature of the virally induced cell surface antigen, which serves as the target for cytotoxic T cells, is not well known. It is reasonable to assume that hemagglutinin and the matrix protein of influenza virus each serves as a distinct target antigen [4]. Similarly, the hemagglutinin of Sendai virus seems to be recognized by T cells, and the glycoprotein of vesicular stomatitis virus is probably its major if not its exclusive target antigen [7, 16]. Whether H-2 coded cell surface molecules undergo alterations during viral infection, for example, by glycosylation, is conjectural. To date, no studies exist on antigen binding by virus-specific cytotoxic T cells. The questions whether T cells recognize viral determinants as such, and if so which ones and how, are still open.

The specificity of cytotoxic T cells for self $H-2K$ or D is exquisite. In fact, structural differences caused by just a few amino acid changes in K or D products of $H-2$ mutants distinguishes their restricting self-markers from that of the wild type [19]. Also, cross-reactivity between $H-2^k$, $H-2^b$ and $H-2^d$ restricted, virus-specific T cells is usually less than 1%.

Influence of the Thymus on MHC-Restricted, Virus-Specific Cytotoxic T Cells

Recent experiments indicate that the specificity for self-$H-2$ is selected in the thymus, independently of antigen, during T cell generation [17]. This notion derives from the following experimental observations: irradiated mice A became bone marrow chimeras after type $A \times B$ bone marrow cells were used to reconstitute A mice. These chimeric mice were then infected with virus, and their spleen cells were tested for cytotoxic activity on infected A or infected B targets. Only infected A target cells were lysed. Therefore, tolerance alone is insufficient to allow sensitization against virus plus tolerated B, and the host A must exert a determining role on the restriction specificity of T cells as they mature and differentiate from stem cells. The chimeric host influences selection of the restriction specificity via the thymus as follows: mice of $(A \times B)F_1$ type, which lacked a thymus or mature T cells, were grafted with a thymus from parent A. Thereafter, the effector T cell specificity generated in the thymuses of these chimeras was only for A plus antigen. The B parental graft produced reactivity only for B plus antigen.

Chimeras produced another important result. After $A \to (A \times B)F_1$ chimeras were infected experimentally, they generated virus-specific cytotoxic activity for A infected targets only. However, after adoptive sensitization of these $[A \to (A \times B)]$ chimeric lymphocytes against infected $(A \times B)F_1$ macrophages, activity was against both A and B infected target cells. Thus, lethal irradiation apparently wiped out the $(A \times B)F_1$ chimeric hosts' supply of antigen-presenting cells, and these were replaced by cells derived from lymphohemopoietic stem cells A [18].

This finding is dramatized in completely allogeneic chimeras $A \to B$ that are functionally immunoincompetent, i.e. they cannot mount an immune response against virus [18]. In such chimeras, T cells are selected to recognize B as self. Since all the reconstituting B cells and macrophages are of A type, multiple lymphocyte interactions are not possible and immunoincompetence ensues. For immunocompetence to evolve, transferred stem cells and recipient must share at least the I-region if antibody is to be produced, or they must share K or D plus the I region if cytotoxic T cells are to be generated.

These experiments demonstrate: (1) that only cells belonging to the lymphoreticular system, probably macrophages and monocytes, are immunogenic and that other somatic cells such as infected skin or liver cells are *not*, (2) that the $H-2$ type of lymphoreticular cells selects the specificity of effector T cells, out of the restriction imposed in the thymus, and (3) that *I*-restricted T cells must be present to induce virus-specific cytotoxic T cells readily. These findings are more compatible with a dual receptor than with a single receptor model of immune recognition, however, do not formally exclude the latter. The nature of T cell recognition remains unknown.

H-2 Polymorphism, Ir Gene Expression and the Thymic Selection of Restriction Specificity

Ir genes that regulate T cell responsiveness map to the same *H-2* regions as the restricting *H-2* structures that are recognized by T cells. Thus, *I* restricted T helper cells are regulated by *Ir* genes in *H-2 I*; *K* or *D* restricted virus-specific cytotoxic T cells are regulated by *Ir* genes in *H-2K, D*. Whether these restricting elements and *Ir* gene products are identical is suggested by the data but remains unknown. Several groups of researchers recently found that the intimate relationship between these phenomena was dictated by the *H-2* type of the thymus [13, 14]. Chimeras were formed by reconstituting irradiated responder or nonresponder parental mice with bone marrow stem cells from (responder × nonresponder) F_1 mice. The responder phenotype of the chimeric T cells was that of the irradiated host. Therefore, it seems as if selection of the restriction specificity of T cells for a particular *H-2* coded self-structure also determines responsiveness. This may indicate that recognition of a foreign determinant X depends on (1) the receptor repertoire that is left or arises after the receptor for self-recognition has been selected, and (2) the degree to which foreign antigen X mimicks self-antigens (tolerance) [for further discussion, see 1, 6, 8, 13, 14].

Whatever the mechanism, it becomes clear that if only one *K* or *D* self-marker existed, viruses could quickly adapt and escape immunosurveillance. Polymorphism of MHC products is therefore crucial to guarantee survival of the species. Since polymorphism causes heterozygosity at MHC, the individual's chance of resisting infection by cell-mediated immunity is enhanced, particularly if gene duplication further expands responsiveness by diminishing the chances of low or nonresponsiveness to one particular virus; very interestingly similar polymorphism has evolved in the Ig system and also guarantees maximal responsiveness, e.g. to bacterial toxins such as lipopolysaccharides. T cell restriction and immune responsiveness are thus interdependent, and the polymorphism of *H-2* may have evolved to offer species and individuals optimal and maximal immune responsiveness against intracellular parasites.

Practical Implications

(1) Further analysis of the link between MHC-restriction and immune responsiveness may, together with the definition of T cell receptors, clarify the association between certain HLA haplotypes and susceptibility to disease. A clear knowledge of how the MHC relates to lack of responsiveness, to insufficient immune protection, or to immunologic hyperresponsiveness that induces immunopathology offers tremendous potential benefits with respect to medical diagnosis, prognosis and, most important, preventive measures.

(2) The results of studying irradiation bone marrow chimeras and thymus chimeras are so compelling that they should be considered in approaches to reconstitute immunodeficient patients. Our experiments suggest that the three immunologically distinguishable

cellular groups of higher vertebrates, i.e. thymus cells, lymphohemopoietic stem cells and the remaining somatic cells, must share at least one haplotype of the I (HLA-D) region and at least one of either K or D (HLA-A or B) region to form a functional T cell immune system. That is, if only thymus and stem cells are compatible, then viruses can infect other somatic cells without control. This observation may be crucial for planning therapy in which fetal liver or thymus is used to reconstitute immunodeficient patients. These fetal cells and organs have been transplanted without HLA matching but induced no graft-versus-host reaction (GVHR), because of their immunologic immunoincompetence. Nevertheless, few patients were reconstituted adequately to defeat infectious disease. Consideration of the proposed mechanisms and rules above may well improve the rate of success [17, 18].

Conclusion

Many aspects of immunology are poorly understood, e.g. tolerance is a mystery as are T cell receptors. Yet, studies of T cell-mediated immunity to intracellular parasites have proven fruitful over the years and have improved our understanding not only of basic immunologic mechanisms and T cell physiology, but also of disease, of its immunopathologic basis and of factors influencing resistance to disease.

References

1 Benacerraf, B. and Germain, R. N.: The immune response genes of the major histocompatibility complex. Immunol. Rev. 38: 71–119 (1978).

2 Bodmer, W. F.: Evolutionary significance of the HL-A system. Nature, Lond. 237: 139–145 (1972).

3 Burnet, F. M.: 'Self-recognition' in colonial marine forms and flowering plants in relation to the evolution of immunity. Nature, Lond. 232: 230–235 (1971).

4 Effros, R. B.; Doherty, P. C.; Gerhard, W., and Bennink, J.: Generation of both cross-reactive and virus-specific T-cell populations after immunization with serologically distinct influenza a viruses. J. exp. Med. 145: 557–568 (1977).

5 Goulmy, E.; Termijtelen, A.; Bradley, B. A., and Rood, J. J. van: Y-antigen killing by T cells of women is restricted by HLA. Nature, Lond. 266: 544–545 (1976).

6 Katz, D. H. and Benacerraf, B.: The function and interrelationship of T cell receptors, Ir genes and other histocompatibility gene products. Transplantn Rev. 22: 175–195 (1975).

7 Koszinowski, U.; Gething, M. J., and Waterfield, M.: T-cell cytotoxicity in the absence of viral protein synthesis in target cells. Nature, Lond. 267: 160–163 (1977).

8 Langman, R. E.: Cell-mediated immunity and the major histocompatibility complex. Rev. Psy. Bioch. Pharm. 81: 1–37 (1978).

9 Mackaness, G. B.: The influence of immunologically committed lymphoid cells on macrophage activity in vivo. J. exp. Med. 129: 973–992 (1968).

10 Paul, W. E. and Benacerraf, B.: Functional specificity of thymus-dependent lymphocytes. Science 195: 1293–1300 (1977).

11 Theodor, J. L.: Distinction between 'self' and 'nonself' in lower invertebrates. Nature, Lond. 227: 690–692 (1970).

12 The immune response to infectious diseases. Transplantn Rev. 19 (1974).

13 Boehmer, H. von; Haas, W., and Jerne, N.: Major histocompatibility complex-linked immune responsiveness is acquired by lymphocytes of low responder mice differentiating in thymus of high responder mice. Proc. natl. Acad. Sci. USA 75: 2439–2442 (1978).

14 Zinkernagel, R. M.; Althage, A.; Cooper, S.; Callahan, G., and Klein, J.: In irradiation chimeras, K or D regions of the chimeric host, not of the donor lymphocytes determine immune responsiveness of antiviral cytotoxic T cells. J. exp. Med. 148: 805–810 (1978).

15 Zinkernagel, R. M.; Althage, A.; Adler, B.; Blanden, R. V.; Davidson, W. F.; Kees, U.; Dunlop, M. B. C., and Shreffler, D. C.: H-2 restriction of cell-mediated immunity to an intracellular bacterium. Effector T cells are specific for Listeria antigen in association with H-2I region coded self-markers. J. exp. Med. 145: 1353–1367 (1977).

16 Zinkernagel, R. M.; Althage, A., and Holland, J. J.: Target antigens for H-2 restricted vesicular stomatitis virus-specific cytotoxic T cells. J. Immun. 121: 744–748 (1978).

17 Zinkernagel, R. M.; Callahan, G. N.; Althage, A.;
   Cooper, S.; Klein, P. A., and Klein, J.: On the
   thymus in the differentiation of 'H-2 self-recognition'
   by T cells: evidence for dual recognition? J. exp.
   Med. *147:* 882–896 (1978).

18 Zinkernagel, R. M.; Callahan, G. N.; Althage, A.;
   Cooper, S.; Streilein, J. W., and Klein, J.: The
   lymphoreticular system in triggering virus-plus-self-
   specific cytotoxic T cells: evidence for T help. J. exp.
   Med. *147:* 897–911 (1978).

19 Zinkernagel, R. M. and Doherty, P. C.: Major
   transplantation antigens virus and specificity of surveillance T cells. The 'altered self' hypothesis. Con-
   temp. Topics Immunobiol. *7:* 179–220 (1977).

20 Zinkernagel, R. M.: Role of the H-2 gene complex
   in cell-mediated immunity to infectious disease.
   Transplantn Proc. *9:* 1835–1838 (1977).

Dr. R. M. Zinkernagel, Scripps Clinic and
Research Foundation, La Jolla,
CA 92037 (USA)

Immunopathology. 6th Int. Convoc. Immunol., Niagara Falls, N.Y., 1978, pp. 236–241 (Karger, Basel 1979)

Immunopathology of Hepatitis B Virus Infection[1]

P. L. Ogra, K. R. Beutner, M. L. Tiku and G. M. Makhdoomi

Division of Infectious Disease and Virology, Children's Hospital of Buffalo, and Department of Pediatrics and Microbiology, State University of New York at Buffalo, Buffalo, N.Y.

Introduction

Recent evidence [9, 10] suggests that infection with hepatitis B virus (HBV) and subsequent synthesis of hepatitis B surface antigen (HB$_s$Ag), hepatitis B core antigen (HB$_c$Ag) and other structural components of the HBV are generally not associated with any discernable cytopathic effects in hepatocytes. It is believed that hepatocyte injury is mediated via antibody or cellular immune mechanisms. The primary targets of immunologic reactivity appear to be components of HBV which are expressed on the surface of infected hepatocyte membrane [4]. However, a number of recent observations have raised the possibility that the pathogenesis of liver damage may also be related to the induction of immune response to host liver tissue proteins [5, 7, 9]. The viral induced host immune response may mediate hepatocyte injury via a number of effector mechanisms. These may include antibody, T cell or macrophage-mediated cytotoxicity, development of antigen-antibody complexes, and antibody-mediated complement-dependent cytotoxic immune phenomena. The observations of importance relative to these effector mechanisms which have emanated during the past few years are briefly summarized in this report.

Role of Antibody Response in Hepatocyte Injury

Acute infection with HBV is characterized in most individuals by the induction of specific antibody response to HB$_s$Ag, hepatitis e antigen (HB$_e$Ag), HB$_c$Ag and other components of HBV expressed on the hepatocyte membrane. The highest levels of antibody to HB$_s$Ag (anti-HB$_s$) are seen in patients with acute HBV infection after the disappearance of HB$_s$Ag from the serum. The anti-HB$_s$ response is generally not detectable in subjects with chronic HB$_s$ antigenemia [9]. However, employing techniques which permit dissociation of antigen-antibody complexes, the presence of anti-HB$_s$ has been demonstrated in serum specimens containing HB$_s$Ag during the incubation phase or at the onset of hepatocellular damage after HBV infection. Examination of cryoprecipitates prepared from subjects with chronic HB$_s$Ag carrier state with biochemical evidence of hepatocellular damage has demonstrated the presence of circulating immune complexes, containing HB$_s$Ag in

[1] Supported by a contract (AI32511) and a grant (HD10088) from the National Institutes of Health.

71% and specific anti-HB$_s$ in 10–20% of such patients. Specific immune complexes with anti-HB$_s$ activity were not detectable in the cryoprecipitates prepared from normal and HBV seronegative controls. Many immune complex-containing cryoprecipitates were able to activate the alternate pathway of complement system [10].

A number of studies [9, 10] have indicated that patients with chronic active hepatitis may completely eliminate HB$_s$Ag and yet continue to have active liver disease. During the course of acute HBV infection, several hepatocellular antigens are detectable in the serum. Of these, the high molecular weight lipoportein antigen and liver-specific antigen have been well characterized and are localized to the hepatocyte surface [7]. Immunoglobulin binding to the hepatocytes has been observed in some patients with hepatitis and indirect evidence for the presence of circulating antibody to hepatocyte surface in patients with chronic liver disease has also been suggested. However, little or no information is available about the presence or characteristics of specific antibody response to liver-specific antigens in HBV infection. A recent study has suggested the appearance of a blocking antibody which inhibits *in vitro* development of lymphocyte-mediated cytotoxicity of autochthonous hepatocytes [8].

Although these data suggest the induction of immune complexes, specific anti-HB$_s$ and appearance of normal or HBV-induced hepatocellular antigens in patients with hepatitis, their role in the pathogenesis of hepatocyte injury in HBV infection remains to be fully elucidated.

Development of Immunoconglutinins in HBV Infection

Elevated levels of immunoconglutinins (autoantibodies to altered or fixed C$_3$ or C$_4$

complement components) have been found during the course of infections and inflammatory processes of diverse etiologic spectrum. Many of these disease states are accompanied by alterations in the levels of complement components and tissue deposition of antigen-antibody complexes [2]. Although a few recent studies have demonstrated major alterations in the complement activity in patients with HBV infection, relatively little is known about the development of immunoconglutinins in such subjects.

Groups of patients with chronic HB$_s$Ag carrier state with or without biochemical evidence of liver disease were recently studied for the levels and immunoglobulin class specificity of immunoconglutinin activity in the serum. Other subjects with juvenile rheumatoid arthritis, acute HBV infection and HBV seronegative normal children were included as controls. As shown in table I, all HB$_s$Ag-positive carriers with elevated

Table I. Distribution of immunoconglutinin activity (IK) in the serum of patients with chronic HB$_s$Ag state, juvenile rheumatoid arthritis, and HBV seronegative subjects

Patient group	Number tested	% subjects with IK titer >4	Geometric mean ± SD IK titer
Chronic HB$_s$Ag carriers			
with elevated SGPT	60	100	24 ± 4.5
with normal SGPT	34	48	9.6 ± 3.0
Juvenile rheumatoid arthritis	24	100	18.8 ± 2.3
Acute resolving HBV	10	100	30.0 ± 5.4
Naturally immune Anti-HB$_s$+ HB$_s$Ag−	29	50	3.5 ± 1.0
HBV seronegative	49	74	4.0 ± 1.5

Elevated SGPT >40 IU; normal SGPT <25 IU.

SGPT levels, patients with juvenile rheumatoid arthritis, and subjects with acute HBV infection had appreciable immunoconglutinin activity in the serum. The mean titers of immunoconglutinin in these patients were significantly higher (p < 0.01) than in naturally immune and HBV seronegative controls. Examination of several fractionated specimens of serum revealed that the immunoconglutinin activity in chronic HBsAg carriers and subjects with juvenile rheumatoid arthritis was limited to IgM immunoglobulin although such activity was associated with IgM as well as IgG immunoglobulin in patients with acute resolving hepatitis. Sequential testing of patients with acute HBV infection indicated a transient immunoconglutinin response for 2–6 weeks after the onset of infection. On the other hand, the response in subjects with chronic HBsAg carrier state persisted in high titers for as long as 13–14 weeks of observation after initial testing. These observations suggest increased and persistent immunoconglutinin response in subjects with chronic HBsAg carrier state.

Role of Cellular Immune Responses in Hepatocyte Injury

The development of specific cellular reactivity to components of HBV has been demonstrated by the induction of delayed cutaneous hypersensitivity to HBsAg in guinea pigs in *in vivo* settings and by the appearance of *in vitro* correlates of cell-mediated immunity (lymphoproliferation and leukocyte migration) to HBsAg and HBcAg [9, 10]. In addition, evidence for cell-mediated immune responses specific for hepatocellular antigens has frequently been observed in association with liver injury. The *in vitro* correlates of cellular immunity to HBsAg and liver-specific antigens (LSA) was studied

in our laboratories in groups of subjects with acute resolving and chronic HBV infection and in a population of HBV-seronegative controls, employing the technique of lymphoproliferative (LTF) response in peripheral blood T lymphocytes. LTF response to LSA or HBsAg was not observed in HBV seronegative control population. The development of LSA and HBsAg-specific cellular immunity in patients followed sequentially after the onset of acute HBV infection was characterized by the appearance of significant LTF activity during the early phase of the disease and no activity to LSA or HBsAg was detected after the disappearance of HBsAg, appearance of anti-HBs and decline of SGPT values to normal levels (patient 01, 03, and 04, table II). On the other hand, persistent LTF activity against LSA and HBsAg was observed in other patients (05, table II), who continued to have chronic HBsAg carrier state, lack of anti-HBs response and elevated SGPT levels. The association of high LTF activity with evidence of hepatocyte damage was further supported by the comparative studies in different forms of HBV infection presented in table III. 70% of subjects with chronic HBsAg carrier state and elevated SGPT levels and 79% subjects tested during the icteric phase of acute HBV infection manifested positive proliferative response to HBsAg. Of these, 29 and 57%, respectively, manifested a response to both HBsAg and LSA and many other subjects developed a response to LSA alone (table III). On the other hand, chronic HBsAg carriers with normal SGPT levels and subjects tested during convalescent (posticteric) phase of acute HBV infection had LTF activity to HBsAg in 18 and 7%, respectively, and the height of proliferative response was significantly lower than observed in icteric phase patients or chronic antigen carriers (table III).

Although the number of circulating lymphocytes in different forms of HBV infection

Table II. Representative examples of the types of lymphoproliferative and serologic responses to hepatitis B surface antigen (HB$_s$Ag), liver-specific antigen (LSA), and phytohemagglutinin (PHA), observed in patients with acute type B viral hepatitis (group 3)

Patient	Weeks after onset of jaundice	Titer HB$_s$Ag	anti-HB$_s$	SGPT, IU[1]	Stimulation index in response to LSA	HB$_s$Ag	PHA
01	0	1,024	<2	386	1.1	0.6	24
	4	32	<2	17	5.9	12.7	557
	12	<2	16	13	1.0	0.8	122
	16	<2	16	6	1.4	1.1	121
03	2	65,536	<2	1,515	4.7	9.7	27
	6	64	<2	14	4.2	20.0	646
	8	<2	<2	9	6.0	4.1	835
	16	<2	8	10	2.5	2.0	750
04	1	>65,536	<2	1,428	1.0	1.3	284
	3	>65,536	<2	1,470	2.6	1.4	752
	4	>65,536	<2	225	2.4	0.8	470
	6	8,192	<2	37	1.8	1.1	501
	32	<2	4	22	0.2	2.0	133
05	0	>65,536	<2	75	0.9	2.0	32
	2	>65,536	<2	404	4.3	3.3	400
	3	>65,536	<2	364	3.1	4.8	58
	4	>65,536	<2	422	1.2	1.2	409
	5	>65,536	<2	79	1.9	1.4	634
	8	>65,536	<2	389	4.4	4.1	140
	38	>65,536	<2	100	6.6	2.7	1,818

[1] International units.

Table III. Lymphocyte transformation (LTF) responses to hepatitis B surface (HB$_s$Ag) and liver-specific antigen (LSA) after hepatitis B virus infection

Groups	Total number studied	LTF response to HB$_s$Ag alone % subjects	mean stimulation index	LSA alone % subjects	mean stimulation index	HB$_s$Ag and LSA % subj.
1. Chronic HB$_s$Ag carriers						
(a) With elevated SGPT	17	70	4.6[1]	35	2.8[1]	29
(b) With normal SGPT	11	18	1.6	18	1.9	9
2. HB$_s$Ag negative (anti-HB$_s$-positive)	14	36	2.6[1]	21	1.9	7
3. Acute type B viral hepatitis						
(a) Acute phase	14	79	6.6[1]	64	3.8[1]	57
(b) Convalescent phase	15	7	2.0	34	2.6	7
4. HBV seronegative (control)	19	0	1.2	0	1.5	0

[1] Statistically significant response (p < 0.05). All p values calculated by two-tailed t-test against the mean stimulation index of control and study groups.

have been found to remain normal, the absolute number of E rosette-forming T cells appears to be somewhat reduced during icteric phase of HBV infection. Recent studies have indicated that a population of T cells characterized by the absence of surface immunoglobulins and E rosette markers are significantly increased during active HBV infection and such cells may account for over 25% of total blood lymphocytes during the icteric phase [3]. These cells appear to be generated either intrinsically, or as a result of a humoral factor, the rosette inhibitory factor (RIF) produced during the period of maximum transaminase activity. The abnormalities of T lymphocyte function and persistence of RIF have been associated with the development of chronic HB_sAg carrier state.

Conclusions

The observations summarized in this review provide evidence for the occurrence of immune complexes containing HB_sAg and anti-HB_s, development of immunoconglutinins and alteration in the components of the complement system, induction of specific cell-mediated immune response to HBV and hepatocellular antigens, and abnormal T lymphocyte function in association with hepatocellular injury in acute type B viral hepatitis and chronic HB_sAg carrier state.

The development of immune complexes and immunoconglutinins during acute infection and in chronic carriers may represent a meager attempt of the host immune system to terminate antigenemia. Based on the information obtained in experimental models of tumor immunity [11] and in other chronic viral infections [1], it is possible that immune complexes in HBV infection may be involved

in the regulation of cell-mediated immune response to the HBV and hepatocellular antigens. As observed in other experimental models, immune complexes in chronic HB_sAg carriers may suppress the expression of T lymphocyte function and thus limit the manifestation of hepatocellular injury in asymptomatic antigen carriers.

Cellular immunity appears to be a major effector mechanism in elimination of viruses associated with cytopathology and the development of hepatocellular injury, and liver injury in HBV infection may thus represent a consequence of T cell-mediated immunity to terminate HBV in infected hepatocytes. Such immunologically mediated cellular damage may be independent of specific antibody response to HBV components. This is supported by the observation of hepatocellular injury in agammaglobulinemic subjects with HBV infection and development of mild liver disease in chronic asymptomatic HB_sAg carriers after the administration of soluble mediators of T cell function such as transfer factor. In view of the information presented here, it is suggested that the development of viral and hepatocyte-specific immune responses may determine the course and pathogenesis of HBV infection in man.

Summary

Available information suggests that the acquisition of hepatitis B virus (HBV) infection is followed by the development of specific immune response to HBV and hepatocellular antigens. The antibody and cell-mediated immune responses and the development of immune complexes and immunoconglutinins after HBV infection have been well characterized. It is proposed that the pathogenesis and course of acute or chronic active hepatitis, or asymptomatic chronic HBV carrier state may be determined by the host immune response against HBV-induced viral or host protein antigens.

References

1 Ahmed, A.; Strong, D. M.; Sell, K. W.; Thurman, G. B.; Knudsen, R. C.; Wistar, R., and Grace, W. R.: Demonstration of a blocking factor in the plasma and spinal fluid of patients with subacute sclerosing panencephalitis. J. exp. Med. *139:* 902–924 (1974).
2 Bienenstock, J. and Block, K. J.: Some characteristics of immunoconglutinin. J. Immun. *96:* 637–641 (1966).
3 Chisari, F. V.; Routenberg, J. A.; Fiala, M., and Edgington, T. S.: Extrinsic modulation of human T lymphocyte E-rosette function associated with prolonged hepatocellular injury after viral hepatitis. J. clin. Invest. *59:* 134–142 (1977).
4 Edgington, T. S. and Ritt, D. J.: Intrahepatic expression of serum hepatitis virus-associated antigens. J. exp. Med. *134:* 871–885 (1971).
5 Hopf, U.; Meyer zum Büschenfelde, K. H., and Freudenberg, J.: Liver-specific antigens of different species. II. Localization of a membrane antigen at cell surface of isolated hepatocytes. Clin. exp. Immunol. *16:* 117–124 (1974).
6 Kohler, P. F.; Trembath, J., and Merrill, D. A.: Immunotherapy with antibody, lymphocytes and transfer factor in chronic hepatitis B. Clin. Immunol. Immunopath. *2:* 462–471 (1974).
7 Meyer zum Büschenfelde, K. H. and Miescher, P. A.: Liver specific antigens—purification and characterization. Clin. exp. Immunol. *10:* 89–102 (1972).
8 Paronetto, F.; Gerber, M., and Vernance, S. J.: Immunologic studies in patients with chronic active hepatitis and primary biliary cirrhosis. 1. Cytotoxic activity and binding of sera to human liver cells grown in tissue culture. Proc. Soc. exp. Biol. Med. *143:* 756–760 (1973).
9 Proc. Symp. on Viral Hepatitis, National Academy of Sciences (Slack, Thorofare 1975).
10 Proc. Int. Symp. on Viral Hepatitis, San Francisco (in press, 1978).
11 Tamerius, J.; Nepom, J.; Hellstrom, I., and Hellstrom, K. E.: Tumor-associated blocking factors: isolation from sera of tumor-bearing mice. J. Immun. *116:* 724–730 (1976).

Dr. P. L. Ogra, Department of Pediatrics, State University of New York at Buffalo, Buffalo, NY 14222 (USA)

Immunopathology. 6th Int. Convoc. Immunol., Niagara Falls, N.Y., 1978, pp. 242–246 (Karger, Basel 1979)

Infectious Mononucleosis: Heterophile Antibody Response[1]

Kyoichi Kano

Department of Microbiology, State University of New York at Buffalo, School of Medicine, Buffalo, N.Y.

Introduction

Infectious mononucleosis (IM) is a disease characterized by clinical, hematologic and serologic findings. In 1920, *Sprunt and Evans* [28] were the first to describe the clinical picture of IM including hematologic changes and to coin the term 'infectious mononucleosis'. *Downey and McKinley* [5] in 1923 described in detail the hematologic changes, especially the morphology of atypical lymphocytes. The discovery of the heterophile antibody was made by *Paul and Bunnell* [25] in 1932. The diagnostic value of the heterophile, Paul-Bunnell (P-B) antibody, however, was not appreciated fully until *Davidsohn* [3] established a differential test to distinguish the P-B antibody from other heterophile antibodies.

Based on their serological findings in an IM patient, *Henle et al.* [9] in 1968 claimed that the Epstein-Barr virus (EBV) was the causative agent of the disease. This was followed by extensive seroepidemiological studies to support the contention and recent attempts to isolate EBV from the patients' materials [6].

IM has attracted interest of many immunologists since IM patients exhibit rather

unique humoral and cellular immune responses [2, 6, 7, 14]. In general, cell-mediated immunity of IM patients is largely depressed, especially during the acute stage of the disease, while a variety of humoral antibodies are formed by IM patients in addition to P-B antibodies [2, 6, 7, 14]. They are heterophile antibodies different from P-B antibodies, antibodies apparently directed against unaltered cell surface antigens of human cells and antibodies to viruses. Extensive lymphoproliferative activity is always observed in IM patients as evidenced by the striking mitotic activity of atypical lymphocytes and proliferative changes in the thymus-dependent paracortical area of lymph nodes [2]. Although the lymphoproliferative changes are extensive during the acute stage of IM, most, if not all, IM patients recover from the disease without serious complications. This is why the disease is often called 'self-limiting leukemia' [2, 7, 14]. Therefore, our studies on IM have been intended to find answers to the same old question: 'What stops IM from developing into true leukemia'?

Paul-Bunnell Antigen and Antibody in Infectious Mononucleosis

Serodiagnosis of IM has been dependent solely upon the detection of P-B antibodies in the patients' sera, since they appear almost always in the patients' sera and rarely in

[1] Supported by Research Grants AM-17317 from the National Institute of Arthritis, Metabolism and Digestive Diseases, IM-24B from the American Cancer Society and RG-892B2 from the National Multiple Sclerosis Society.

other diseases [7, 14]. It has been known also for some time that the P-B antigen on bovine erythrocytes (BRBC) is by no means a single antigenic determinant [7, 14, 21].

Our studies on P-B antigen by means of double diffusion in agar gel tests with stroma particles of BRBC and sheep erythrocytes (SRBC) or crude stroma extracts clearly showed a complex nature of the antigen [20, 21]. As seen in figure 1, separation of the bovine extract lines into two, one closer to the antigen well and the other closer to the IM serum well, was often observed. Furthermore, the reaction line formed with sheep or horse stroma extracts either merged into a reaction of complete identity or a reaction of partial identity with the bovine line closer to the IM serum well. In a very few instances, a reaction of nonidentity was noted between the 'sheep line' and one of the 'bovine lines'.

The distribution of P-B antigen in cells and tissues of various mammalian species has been extensively studied in our laboratory. We have attempted to demonstrate the antigen on the surface of dissociated nucleated cells by means of cytolysis tests in agar gel and on cultured cells by mixed agglutination tests. It was found that oxen possess the antigen not only on erythrocytes but also on all other cells thus far examined [14]. It should be mentioned that bovine plasma contains very little, if any, P-B antigen as evidenced by its failure to inhibit hemagglutination of SRBC and to disperse agglutinates of SRBC formed by P-B antibodies.

Of particular interest was the distribution of the antigen on murine lymphoid cells. It was shown that murine thymocytes and Thy-1-positive lymphoma cells were lysed by P-B antibodies, and that absorption of IM sera with murine thymocytes resulted in the disappearance of P-B antibodies [17]. Significantly, the P-B antigen could not be demonstrated on spleen cells of nude mice. It was,

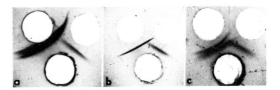

Fig. 1. Upper wells in a, b and c: Bovine stroma extract (left); sheep stroma extract (right). Lower wells: IM sera Cw (a), La (b) and Fr (c). From Milgrom et al. [21].

therefore, concluded that the P-B antigen is a marker for murine T lymphocytes.

Concerning the expression of P-B antigen in cells and tissues of man, we have found that thymocytes obtained from a Caucasian girl who had heart surgery were shown to contain P-B antigen while lymphocytes from the remaining 24 children which were included as a control in our mixed agglutination studies on spleen cells of lymphoma or leukemia patients gave negative results [12]. It is also of interest to note that Orientals never develop true P-B antibodies, even those patients who suffer from lymphoproliferative diseases similar to IM [16, 29]. Our preliminary studies on thymocytes from Japanese children by the mixed agglutination test as well as studies on sections of thymuses by autoradiography with ^{125}I-labeled P-B antibodies strongly indicated that they contain P-B antigen. It is tempting, therefore, to speculate that P-B antigen may be expressed in the early developmental stages of Orientals, and that they are, therefore, unable to form P-B antibodies.

We have investigated the possibility that P-B antigen may be expressed on lymphoid cells of IM patients. Our failure, using peripheral blood lymphocytes of IM patients, appeared to be due to the fact that at the time when specimens from such patients became available, P-B antibodies had reached their peak and combined with the antigen-carrying cells *in vivo*, so that many of such cells might have been already eliminated from the circulation. More recently, we have had an opportunity to investigate tissues of a patient with IM [1] who died of heart failure 12 days after the onset of IM when the P-B antibody titer had not yet reached its peak. P-B antibodies were eluted from spleen, liver and kidney tissues of this patient. After the elution, these tissues were shown to be able to absorb P-B antibodies from IM sera. Histologic examination of kidney tissue revealed intense infiltration with mononuclear cells, including atypical lymphocytes, in interstitial tissues. IgM deposits in the mesangium of the kidney were demonstrated by indirect immunofluorescence staining with anti-IgM conjugate. The IgM deposits could be removed from the tissue sections by elution procedures or by incubation with an excess of solubilized P-B antigen. Furthermore, after the elution of the IgM deposits, we were able to reconstitute them by incubation of sections with other IM sera or with the eluate. On the basis of these studies, one may conclude that P-B antigen is present in tissues of IM patients in the early stages of the disease, and that it forms complexes *in vivo* with the corresponding antibodies.

Several investigators have pointed out that the P-B antigen is most likely a glycoprotein [14]. Our own investigation [18] has revealed that glycoproteins extracted from BRBC stromata carry P-B antigen. The exact nature of the determinant of the molecules is currently under investigation.

The IgM nature of P-B antibodies of the vast majority of IM patients is well established [2, 7, 14]. By means of immunoelectrophoresis, using solubilized P-B antigen preparations, we [21] have demonstrated that a precipitation arc was formed with IgM of IM sera. In our studies, we have also found that serum of 1 patient did contain IgG P-B antibodies in addition to ordinary IgM antibodies. Therefore, it may be stated that P-B

antibody response in IM shows little or no IgM to IgG conversion, even during convalescence from the disease.

Recently, short-term cultures of peripheral blood lymphocytes obtained from 20 IM patients 2–4 weeks after the onset of the disease were studied for *in vitro* formation of heterophile antibodies [22]. In studying pooled supernatant fluids of lymphocyte cultures, lytic IgM antibodies of P-B specificity were demonstrated. Subsequently, plaque-forming cell (PFC) assays were performed with lymphocyte cultures. Significant numbers (60–750 per culture) of PFC-secreting antibodies against BRBC were demonstrated in lymphocyte cultures of 12 patients. The number of PFC apparently reached its peak after 5–10 days of culturing. No or only very few PFC were observed among the lymphocytes that were not cultured or in lymphocytes cultured for 3 weeks or longer. Lymphocyte cultures prepared in a similar fashion from normal individuals or patients suffering from sore throat and submandibular lymphadenopathy of other than IM origin did not produce PFC. Production of lytic zones by antibodies to BRBC secreted by PFC was inhibited by preincubation of the cultured lymphocytes with solubilized P-B antigen. Therefore, it may be concluded that antibodies involved in the PFC formation are of P-B specificity.

Other Heterophile Antibodies in Infectious Mononucleosis

Following the discovery of a new heterophile antibody engendered by injections of foreign species sera in the mid 1920s [4, 8], *Schiff* [27] coined the term 'serum-sickness' antigen to denote its corresponding antigen, and the antibodies under discussion were customarily called 'serum-sickness' antibodies. However, both *Hanganutziu* [8] and

Deicher [4], as well as *Pirofsky et al.* [26], pointed out that the appearance of these heterophile antibodies has no direct relationship to any of the clinical symptoms of serum sickness or to the volume of foreign species serum injected. Furthermore, our recent studies [15, 23] have demonstrated that many patients with various diseases, who had never received injections of foreign species serum, formed the same type of heterophile antibodies. Therefore, we [15] proposed that this type of heterophile antibodies should be called Hanganutziu-Deicher (H-D) antibodies.

Higashi et al. [10] and *Merrick et al.* [19] identified independently the determinant of the H-D antigen isolated from BRBC stromata as *N*-glycolylneuraminic acid of acidic glycosphingolipids. If such purified H-D antigen along with P-B antigen prepared from BRBC stromata were employed in double diffusion in agar gel, the distinct specificities of these two heterophile antibodies could clearly be demonstrated (fig. 2).

Sera of IM patients often contain agglutinins to erythrocytes of Rhesus monkeys which are distinct from P-B antibodies [11, 24]. Our recent studies clearly showed that the Rhesus hemagglutinins in IM sera were H-D antibodies, since absorption of the IM sera with both BRBC and guinea pig kidneys abolished their activities.

Our recent studies [30] showed that 40% of IM sera lysed murine IgM myeloma cells, MOPC-104, as well as some subpopulation of normal murine B cells. The antibodies responsible for lysis of these cells were different from P-B antibodies. Antibodies of the majority of these sera could be absorbed with BRBC or guinea pig kidneys and, therefore, were similar to or even identical with H-D antibodies. In this regard, it should be mentioned that spleen cells of some lymphoma or leukemia patients possess not only P-B antigen but also H-D antigen [12, 13].

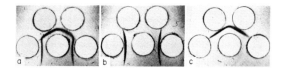

Fig. 2. Central wells: (a) crude extract; (b) P-B antigen, and (c) H-D antigen of bovine stromata; lower left and right, IM sera; upper wells, sera with H-D antibodies. From *Kasukawa et al.* [15].

Comments

During our investigation on IM for the last 15 years, we have always been tempted to speculate on the role of heterophile antibodies, especially P-B antibody, in surveillance of the disease.

In IM, cells infected with a virus, presumably EBV, acquire P-B antigen and perhaps H-D antigen as a result of transformation which immediately stimulate patients' B cells for formation of P-B and/or H-D antibodies. Simultaneously, the infected cells acquire new lymphocyte-activating determinants which stimulate patients' own T cells for blast transformation. This *in vivo* MLR-like reaction may result in elaboration of allogeneic enhancing factor which enhances production of the heterophile antibodies by the patients.

The P-B antibodies thus produced would combine with the cells carrying the antigen and accelerate their elimination. In spite of the fact that P-B antigen is expressed on spleen cells of lymphoma or leukemia patients, P-B antibody formation has never been demonstrated in these patients. The mechanism(s) preventing immune response to the neoantigen may be responsible for malignant nature of these lymphoproliferative diseases in contrast to the benign nature of IM.

References

1 Andres, G. A.; Kano, K.; Elwood, C.; Prezyna, A.; Sepulveda, M., and Milgrom, F.: Immune deposit nephritis in infectious mononucleosis. Int. Archs. Allergy appl. Immun. *52:* 136–144 (1976).

2 Carter, R. L.: Infectious mononucleosis: model for self-limiting lymphoproliferation. Lancet *i:* 846–849 (1975).

3 Davidsohn, I.: Test for infectious mononucleosis. Am. J. clin. Path. *8:* 56–60 (1938).

4 Deicher, H.: Über die Erzeugung heterospecifischer Hämagglutinine durch Injektion artfremden Serums. Z. Hyg. InfektKrankh. *106:* 561–579 (1926).

5 Downey, H. and McKinley, C. A.: Acute lymphadenosis compared with acute lymphatic leukemia. Archs intern. Med. *32:* 82–112 (1923).

6 Evans, A. S.: The history of infectious mononucleosis. Am. J. med. Sci. *267:* 189–195 (1974).

7 Glade, P. R. (ed.): Infectious mononucleosis (Lippincott, Philadelphia 1973).

8 Hanganutziu, M.: Hémagglutinines hétérogénétiques après injection de sérum de cheval. C. r. Séanc. Soc. Biol. *91:* 1457–1459 (1924).

9 Henle, G.; Henle, W., and Diehl, V.: Relation of Burkitt's tumor-associated herpes-type virus to infectious mononucleosis. Proc. natn. Acad. Sci. USA *59:* 94–101 (1968).

10 Higashi, H.; Naiki, M.; Matuo, S., and Okouchi, K.: Antigen of 'serum sickness' type of heterophile antibodies in human sera: identification as gangliosides with N-glycolylneuraminic acid. Biochem. biophys. Res. Commun. *79:* 388–395 (1977).

11 Hoyt, R. E. and Morrison, L. M.: Reaction of viral hepatitis serum with M. rhesus erythrocytes. Proc. Soc. exp. Biol. Med. *93:* 547–549 (1956).

12 Kano, K.; Fjelde, A., and Milgrom, F.: Paul-Bunnell antigen in lymphoma and leukemia spleens. J. Immun. *119:* 945–949 (1977).

13 Kano, K.; Kasukawa, R.; Fjelde, A., and Milgrom, F.: Heterophile antigens on human lymphoid cells (abstr.). Fed. Proc. Fed. Am. Socs exp. Biol. *35:* 548 (1976).

14 Kano, K. and Milgrom, F.: Heterophile antigens and antibodies in medicine. Curr. Top. Microbiol. Immunol., pp. 43–69 (Springer, Berlin 1977).

15 Kasukawa, R.; Kano, K.; Bloom, M., and Milgrom, F.: Heterophile antibodies in pathologic human sera resembling antibodies stimulated by foreign species sera. Clin. exp. Immunol. *25:* 122–132 (1976).

16 Kumagai, R. N. and Kawakita, Y.: Serological studies on infectious mononucleosis in Japan. Proc. 9th Congr. Int. Soc. Hemat., vol. I, pp. 535–547 (1962).

17 Malavé, I.; Kano, K., and Milgrom, F.: Reactions of murine lymphoma cells with infectious mononucleosis. J. Immun. *110:* 439–443 (1973).

18 Merrick, J. M.; Schifferle, R.; Zadarlik, K.; Kano, K., and Milgrom, F.: Isolation and partial characterization of the heterophile antigen of infectious mononucleosis from bovine erythrocytes. J. supramolec. Struct. *6:* 275–290 (1977).

19 Merrick, J. M.; Zadarlik, K., and Milgrom, F.: Characterization of the Hanganutziu-Deicher (serum-sickness) antigen as gangliosides containing N-glycolylneuraminic acid. Int. Archs Allergy appl. Immun. *57:* 477–480 (1978).

20 Milgrom, F. and Loza, U.: Agglutination of particulate antigens in agar gel. J. Immun. *98:* 102–109 (1967).

21 Milgrom, F.; Loza, U., and Kano, K.: Double diffusion in gel tests with Paul-Bunnell antibodies of infectious mononucleosis. Int. Archs Allergy appl. Immun. *48:* 82–93 (1975).

22 Mori, T.; Kano, K., and Milgrom, F.: Formation of Paul-Bunnell antibodies by cultures of lymphocytes from infectious mononucleosis. Cell. Immunol. *34:* 289–298 (1977).

23 Nishimaki, T.; Kano, K., and Milgrom, F.: Studies on heterophile antibodies in rheumatoid arthritis. Arthritis Rheum. *21:* 634–638 (1978).

24 O'Connell, C. J.: Rhesus erythrocyte agglutination in infectious mononucleosis. Int. Archs Allergy appl. Immun. *38:* 466–473 (1970).

25 Paul, J. R. and Bunnell, W. W.: The presence of heterophile antibodies in infectious mononucleosis. Am. J. med. Sci. *183:* 91–104 (1932).

26 Pirofsky, B.; Ramirez-Mateos, J. C., and August, A.: 'Foreign serum' heterophile antibodies in patients receiving antithymocyte antisera. Blood *42:* 385–392 (1973).

27 Schiff, F.: Heterogenetic hemagglutinins in man following therapeutic injections of immune sera produced in rabbits. J. Immun. *33:* 305–313 (1937).

28 Sprunt, T. P. and Evans, F. A.: Mononucleosis leukocytosis in reaction to acute infections (infectious mononucleosis). Johns Hopkins Hosp. Bull. *31:* 409–417 (1920).

29 Tan, D. S. K.: 'Absence' of infectious mononucleosis among Asians in Malaya. Med. J. Malaya *XXI:* 358–361 (1967).

30 Yoshida, H.; Kano, K., and Milgrom, F.: Reactions of murine myeloma cells with infectious mononucleosis. J. Immun. *114:* 1449–1453 (1975).

Dr. K. Kano, Department of Microbiology, State University of New York at Buffalo, School of Medicine, Buffalo, NY 14214 (USA)

Immunopathology. 6th Int. Convoc. Immunol., Niagara Falls, N.Y., 1978, pp. 247–252 (Karger, Basel 1979)

Streptococci and Autoimmunity

J. B. Zabriskie, H. M. Fillit and J. W. Tauber

The Rockefeller University, New York, N.Y.

Introduction

The term 'biological mimicry' was coined at least two decades ago and usually refers to that particular situation in which microbes and mammalian tissues share antigenic determinants. Among the many examples of this mimicry, the group A streptococcus stands out in this regard primarily because of the extent and diversity of its shared determinants. We will point out a few of the many examples of this mimicry and then marshall the corresponding clinical and immunological evidence to support the hypothesis that this mimicry might be responsible for certain disease states.

The main areas of shared antigenicity are schematically outlined in figure 1. On the left is a cross-section of the streptococcal cell and on the right are the different tissues which appear at least serologically to share common antigenic determinants with various cellular components of the streptococcal cell.

Hyaluronic Acid. The 'par excellence' example of this mimicry is the hyaluronic acid of joint fluid and the capsule of the streptococcus which were shown in the elegant studies of *Meyer* [9] and *McCarty* [7] to be identical in structure (repeating units of 1–3 beta linkage of glucouronic acid-N-acetyl-glucosamine). Yet, repeated attempts by *McCarty* to raise antibodies in experimental animals against the capsule have been unsuccessful [9].

Membrane Antigens. Far more is known about the cross-reactive antigens in the streptococcus which shares antigenic determinants with sarcolemmal tissues of mammalian muscle. Figure 2 (right side) is an immunofluorescent photograph of this type of binding and points out that this type of staining was primarily limited to the sarcolemmal portion of the muscle fiber. Both skeletal and cardiac muscle stained with equal intensity, and the smooth muscles of blood vessel walls also exhibited bright fluorescence. The localization of this cross-reactive antigen in the streptococcus (i.e. cell wall or cell membrane) is a matter of some dispute. At the present time, there appear to be two cross-reactive antigens. One is associated with, but not identical to, the M protein [6]. In contrast, other investigators have reported that the antigen is present in all group A streptococcal strains regardless of the presence or absence of M protein, and this antigen appears to reside in the cell membrane portion of the streptococcus [13].

More recently, *Husby et al.* [5] have shown that membrane antigens also cross-react with neuronal cells in the caudate and subthalamic fractions of the brain. This was detected when he noted that patients with chorea (a central nervous system manifestation of rheumatic

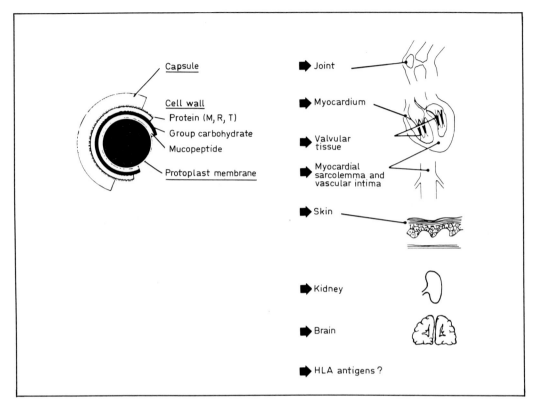

Fig. 1. A schematic drawing of the streptococcal cell and the postulated cross-reactions with mammalian antigens.

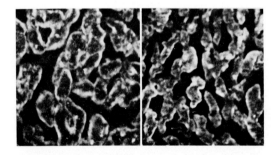

Fig. 2. A photomicrograph of immunofluorescent staining of heart tissue sections. On the left is the staining pattern observed with acute rheumatic fever serum, on the right is the staining observed with rabbit antiserum to group A streptococcal membrane.

Table I. The effect of streptococcal antigens on

Streptococcal membranes (1.3 mg/ml)		
None		
Group A		
Group D		

Lymphocyte donors: X = HLA-A1, B7; Y =

fever) had antineuronal antibodies present in their sera. This antibody was specifically absorbed out by group A streptococcal membrane structures. It was not related to the anti-nuclear antibody seen in lupus erythematosus since the latter antibody was not absorbed by the same streptococcal membrane.

Another target organ for the cross-reaction with streptococcal membrane antigens is the glomerular basement membrane. The evidence for this cross-reaction may be summarized as follows: (1) Antisera prepared against streptococcal antigens will bind preferentially to rat and human glomerular basement membrane antigens. (2) Animals sensitized to streptococcal membranes exhibit accelerated rejection of implanted renal allografts. (3) Extracts prepared from these antigens can induce nephritis in dogs and monkeys. (4) Patients with certain forms of chronic glomerulonephritis exhibit heightened cellular reactivity to these streptococcal antigens [10].

A final concomitant denominator in all these reactions may be the shared antigenicity between streptococcal antigens and transplantation antigens within or outside the major histocompatibility complex. In this respect, Dr. *Tauber* [11, 12] in our laboratory reexamined the observations made by *Hirata and Terasaki* [4] that streptococcal extracts inhibited the cytotoxicity of known HLA antisera in a non-specific manner. While M protein was part of these assays, a number of other streptococcal antigens were also present in the inhibiting material. Table I demonstrates that we were able to easily confirm the original observation by *Hirata*; namely, that streptococcal antigens did indeed inhibit HLA cytotoxic antisera in a non-specific manner. However, further experiments revealed that streptococcal antigens, in particular streptococcal membranes, were markedly anticomplementary and appeared to involve the alternate pathway of complement consumption primarily at the level of factor D.

Carbohydrate Antigens. Another candidate has been the carbohydrate portion of the streptococcal cell wall. It has now been firmly established that the antigenic specificity of the group A streptococcal carbohydrate [8] is dependent on its terminal N-acetyl glucosamine residues on rhamnose side chains. Until recently, there was essentially no evidence that these carbohydrates might be cross-reactive. However, a few

lymphocyte cytotoxicity assay

HLA antiserum										
A1	A2		A2		A2		B7		B12	
X	Y	Z	Y	Z	Y	Z	Y	X	Y	Z
++++	++++	++++	++++	++++	++++	++++	++++	++++	+++	++++
−	−	−	−	−	+	−	−	−		
++++	++++	++++	+++	++++	+++	++++	+++	++	−	++++

HLA-A2, B7, B12; Z = HLA-A2, B9, B12. + = Cells dead; − = cells alive.

years ago, *Goldstein et al.* [3] isolated a glycoprotein from heart valves which appeared to be serologically related to the streptococcal antigen. In addition, *Dudding and Ayoub* [1] have noted that the sera of patients with valvular damage continue to exhibit high levels of anti-carbohydrate antibodies, suggesting possible cross-reactivity between the carbohydrate and tissue antigens secondary to valvular disease.

Disease States

Given these examples of cross-reactions between these streptococcal antigens and mammalian tissue antigens, what is the evidence that these cross-reactions may play a role in disease states? The best example is the relationship between the group A streptococcal antigens and the host response in rheumatic fever. When the serum from a patient with acute rheumatic fever is layered over a cardiac muscle section, the staining pattern bears a striking resemblance to the pattern observed with rabbit antisera to group A streptococci (fig. 2, left side). In general, the localization of the staining, the limitation to muscle tissue and the lack of species specificity were again exhibited by this antibody.

Examination of a large number of sera from patients with recent streptococcal infection and their sequelae revealed that the majority of subjects with a recent streptococcal infection had the cross-reactive heart-staining antibody present in their sera [14]. The striking difference was that the amount detected in rheumatic fever individuals was 4–5 times greater than in patients with uncomplicated streptococcal infections.

Serial examinations of sera obtained from rheumatic patients emphasized the concept that a direct relationship does exist between the presence of heart-reactive antibody and the onset of rheumatic fever [14]. Following an initial episode of rheumatic fever, the antibody titers decline in a normal fashion over a 3- to 5-year period. However, if there is evidence of intervening streptococcal infections, as indicated by a rise in anti-streptolysin 0 titers, there appears to be a crucial turning point in these patients. The heart-reactive antibody levels tend to increase again, and a third or fourth streptococcal infection may precipitate another attack of acute rheumatic fever. Thus, it is tempting to speculate that repeated streptococcal infections (perhaps with subclinical symptoms of disease) are necessary to stimulate the production of heart-reactive antibodies. Only at the point when the titers are sufficiently elevated will the full-blown disease complex appear.

Turning to another organ, several studies have suggested that cross-reactions between streptococcal antigens and renal glomerular antigens might play a role in the disease process. Until recently, the significance of

Table II. Lymphocyte blastogenic response to glomerular basement membrane (GBM) antigens: statistical evaluation (Fisher's exact test)

Antigen	Group	Non-reactors	Reactors[1]	p
Native GBM	GN	21	3	NS
	NC	16	2	NS
	NGRD	6	1	NS
Soluble GBM	GN	15	3	
	NC	12	1	NS
	NGRD	7	0	NS
Altered GBM	GN	12	12	
	NC	17	1	0.012
	NGRD	8	0	0.002

[1] Result greater than two standard deviations above mean control.
GN = Glomerulonephritis; NC = normal controls; NGRD = non-glomerular renal disease; NS = not significant.

these findings remained unclear. The recent studies of *Fillit et al.* [2] have added substantially to our thinking in this area of cross-reactivity. Using blast transformation techniques as a measure of cellular reactivity to these antigens, he had found that patients with chronic glomerulonephritis (table II) respond to glycosidase-treated glomerular basement membrane antigens while nonglomerular renal disease patients and controls do not. When categorized as to the histologic type, those with proliferative glomerulonephritis lesions exhibited the highest reactivity to these 'altered' antigens. Pertinent to the central theme of this discussion was the observation that those who respond most avidly to the glycosidase-treated glomerular basement membrane antigens were also the highest reactors to streptococcal membrane antigens.

Summary and Conclusions

The evidence is now clear that the group A streptococcus has an enormous capacity to mimic a variety of tissue antigens. In general, this mimicry is organ-specific and it may very well be that different strains of group A streptococci vary in the amount and type of cross-reactive antigens present within the streptococcal cell. In several clinical situations, the available evidence suggests (but does not absolutely prove) that these cross-reactive antigens play a role either in the initiation or perpetuation of the disease state. Still missing in these studies are experiments in which these sensitized cells and antibodies are shown to play a direct cytopathic role in the disease process. It is conceivable that we are merely observing a fortuitous reflection of these cross-reactive antigens which is unrelated to the actual disease process and the true damage is an autoimmune reaction to the given organ.

In spite of these deficiencies, one can speculate that there is a general theme in these observations; namely, that we are dealing with what we have termed cryptoantigens. These antigens are present both in the streptococcus and buried within the matrix of a given organ. Since these appear to be common to a number of organs, one could easily envision an embryonic origin for these tissue antigens. In a native state, they are not recognized as foreign and sensitization to the streptococcal antigen will *not* provoke a reaction. However, in the case of the heart or the kidney (to cite but two examples), once an immune insult has occurred (whether a direct toxic reaction or immune complex damage), these antigens are uncovered. These cryptoantigens are now recognized as foreign and more closely resemble the streptococcal structures than the native antigen. An immune reactivity against these antigens is initiated. A vicious cycle of damage and continual release of these antigens generates a chronic autoimmune process, perhaps exacerbated by intercurrent streptococcal infections. The common denominator in all these reactions would be the close association of these streptococcal antigens to buried determinants within the organ-specific antigens.

References

1 Dudding, B. A. and Ayoub, E. M.: Persistence of streptococcal Group A antibody in patients with rheumatic valvular disease. J. exp. Med. *128:* 1081–1098 (1968).
2 Fillit, H. M.; Read, S. E.; Sherman, R. L.; Zabriskie, J. B., and Rijn, I. van de: Cellular reactivity to altered glomerular basement membrane in glomerulonephritis. New Engl. J. Med. *298:* 861–868 (1978).
3 Goldstein, I.; Rebeyrotte, P.; Parlebas, J., and Halpern, B.: Isolation from heart valves of glycopeptides which share immunological properties with *Streptococcus haemolyticus* group A polysaccharides. Nature, Lond. *219:* 866–868 (1968).

4 Hirata, A. A. and Terasaki, P. I.: Cross-reactions between streptococcal M proteins and human transplantation antigens. Science, Wash. *168:* 1095–1096 (1970).

5 Husby, G.; Rijn, I. van de; Zabriskie, J. B.; Abdin, Z. H., and Williams, R. C., jr.: Antibodies reacting with cytoplasm of subthalamic and caudate nuclei neurons in chorea and acute rheumatic fever. J. exp. Med. *144:* 1094–1110 (1976).

6 Kaplan, M. H. and Frengley, J. D.: Autoimmunity to the heart in cardiac disease. Current concepts of the relation of autoimmunity to rheumatic fever, postcardiotomy and postinfarction syndromes and cardiomyopathies. Am. J. Cardiol. *24:* 459–473 (1969).

7 McCarty, M.: Personal commun.

8 McCarty, M.: Further studies on the chemical basis for serological specificity of group A streptococcal carbohydrate. J. exp. Med. *108:* 311–323 (1958).

9 Meyer, K.: The biological significance of hyaluronic acid and hyaluronidase. Physiol. Rev. *27:* 335–359 (1947).

10 Rapaport, F. T.: The biological significance of cross-reactions between histocompatibility antigens and antigens of bacterial and/or heterologous mammalian origin; in Kahan and Reisfeld, Transplantation antigens, markers of biological individuality, pp. 181–208 (Academic Press, New York 1972).

11 Tauber, J. W.; Falk, J. A.; Falk, R. E., and Zabriskie, J. B.: Nonspecific complement activation by streptococcal structures. I. Re-evaluation of HLA cytotoxicity inhibition. J. exp. Med. *143:* 1341–1351 (1976).

12 Tauber, J. W.; Polley, M. J., and Zabriskie, J. B.: Nonspecific complement activation by streptococcal structures. II. Properdin-independent initiation of the alternate pathway. J. exp. Med. *143:* 1352–1366 (1976).

13 Zabriskie, J. B. and Freimer, E. H.: An immunological relationship between the group A streptococcus and mammalian muscle. J. exp. Med. *124:* 661–678 (1966).

14 Zabriskie, J. B.; Hsu, K. C., and Seegal, B. C.: Heart-reactive antibody associated with rheumatic fever: characterization and diagnostic significance. Clin. exp. Immunol. *7:* 147–159 (1970).

15 Zabriskie, J. B.; Read, S. E.; Ellis, R. J.; Markowitz, A. S., and Rapaport, F. T.: Cellular reactivity studies in human and experimental renal transplantation. Transplantn Proc. *4:* 259–264 (1972).

Dr. J. B. Zabriskie, The Rockefeller University, 1230 York Avenue, New York, NY 10021 (USA)

Immunopathology. 6th Int. Convoc. Immunol., Niagara Falls, N.Y., 1978, pp. 253–256 (Karger, Basel 1979)

Immunopathology and Antibacterial Immunity in Tuberculosis

G. Middlebrook

Department of Pathology, University of Maryland School of Medicine, Baltimore, Md.

Introduction

Recent studies of the host-parasite relationship in tuberculosis *in vitro* [2] and *in vivo* [1] call for information regarding the relative roles of bacteriostatic and bactericidal manifestations of antibacterial immune mechanisms in this disease. Those investigators [10, 16] who have reported observing antibacterial effects of macrophages *in vitro* with immune lymphocytes (presumably sensitive T cells) or with lymphokine preparations from such lymphocytes cultured with specific antigen, i.e. either PPD or whole mycobacterial cells, have documented only a bacteriostatic or at best a partially bacteriostatic effect with no sterilizing, bactericidal activity. On the other hand, definite bactericidal effects with evidences of physical destruction of tubercle bacilli have been documented *in vivo* [12]. This has been emphasized as a hallmark of the cellular immune mechanism in tuberculosis [1].

Therefore, it seems important to decide whether or not some as yet unrevealed bactericidal mechanism of potentially great significance for cellular immunity should be sought in cell culture studies *in vitro*. And it is the purpose of this report to describe the results of some experiments which appear to clarify this question. Evidence will be presented that in some experimental models bactericidal effects are attributable to an immunopathologic host response.

Materials and Methods

Animals. Hartley strain guinea pigs weighing 400–500 g and outbred Cob-CD-1 (Charles River Laboratories) mice were used.

Aerogenic Infection. Infections were carried out in an airborne infection apparatus [13], Model A3 (Tri-R Instruments, Inc.), with a main airflow of 2 ft.^{3}/min. *Mycobacterium tuberculosis*, H37Rv strain, was used in these experiments. The suspensions of well-dispersed bacteria (>95% as single cells) were prepared as described previously [12] and stored at −75 °C before thawing and use as recommended by *Grover et al.* [8]. The H37Rv mutant strain resistant to 10 μg streptomycin/ml was isolated from the parent population by plating out a large inoculum of same on 7H10 medium containing 10μg streptomycin/ml and subcultured like the parent susceptible strain in liquid medium 7H9 containing 0.05% Tween 80. For guinea pig infection, the dilutions of stock suspensions employed in the nebulizer were such as to yield only about 10 primary pulmonary tubercles per right lower lobe. For infection of mice a larger inoculum size was used: each mouse had a total of 10–20 lesions per lung. For counting, the numbers of viable bacteria in the guinea pig lungs at indicated intervals after primary infection with the H37Rv-SM-susceptible strain and secondary infection 3 weeks later with the streptomycin-resistant strain, the right lower lobe of each animal was removed aseptically after sacrificing the animal with chloroform, the lobe was ground in a Teflon-glass grinder (Tri-R Instruments,

Inc.) and 0.1 ml of serial dilutions were prepared. These were inoculated in sextuplicate onto 7H10 agar in order to establish the number of viable units present. Streptomycin ($10\mu g/ml$) was added to the medium for selective culture of the organisms of the secondary infection.

Skin Testing of Guinea Pigs. PPD (Lederle Laboratories) was diluted in pyrogen-free Travenol sterile saline containing 0.0005% Tween 80 and 0.3% phenol and employed at a concentration of 250 tuberculin units per 0.1 ml injected intradermally. The reactions were read at 24 h and the average diameter of erythema was recorded.

Histologic Sections of Mouse Lungs. Mice were sacrificed at 4 and 6 weeks after aerogenic infection by chloroform inhalation, and the lungs were removed, washed in saline and fixed in 10% neutral formalin. The sections for HE and acid-fast staining were $5-\mu$m thick and the Epon-mounted and toluidine blue-stained sections were $1-\mu$m thick.

Results

As shown in figure 1, *M. tuberculosis* replicates logarithmically at sites of deposition in normal guinea pig lung without inhibition for a period of 2 weeks, at the end of which time a weak but definite skin reaction of hypersensitivity to tuberculoprotein becomes manifest. During the third week of infection, there is evidence of some antibacterial effect in the lesions. During the fourth week, this effect is striking: there is actually a 10-fold loss in numbers of viable cells—a bactericidal effect—and this is accompanied by a further rise in delayed type hypersensitivity and by *central necrosis* of the lesions, a phenomenon too well known to be pictured here.

When the same guinea pigs are challenged again at 3 weeks after primary infection with the same number of bacteria which differ only in that they are streptomycin-resistant, permitting their selective cultivation, how do they behave? Surprisingly enough, they multiply as freely for the first week as did the organisms of primary infection. Thereafter, after reaching a population size of 10^3 to 10^4, they plateau off bacteriostatically at 3–5

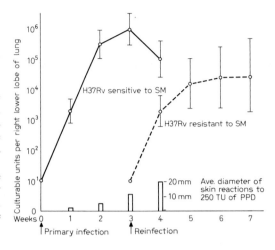

Fig. 1. Multiplication of *M. tuberculosis* in the lungs of guinea pigs after primary infection and after superinfection. 35 animals were infected aerogenically on day 0 with a number of tubercle bacilli (H37Rv strain, susceptible to streptomycin $2\mu g/ml$) calculated to deposit in their lungs about 40 viable bacilli (10 bacilli in the right lower lobe). Animals were sacrificed in groups of 5 each week and plate counts were made to determine the numbers of viable units per right lower lobe. At 3 weeks, the surviving animals were reinfected with the same number of bacilli of the streptomycin-resistant mutant strain of H37Rv. ——— = Counts of drugsusceptible organisms (on medium without streptomycin); -------- = counts of drug-resistant organisms of reinfection on medium containing $10\mu g$ streptomycin/ml. Brackets indicate 2 standard deviations from the means.

weeks at a much lower population size than did the organisms of the primary infection.

Thus, in the same lung in which a clearly bactericidal effect is being exerted in established lesions which are necrotizing in the hypersensitive host, no effect at all is observed on the multiplication of other bacteria at the cellular level at new sites. And even later at such new sites with a much lower peak load of bacteria (about 3×10^4 per lobe) than was reached by the bacteria of the first infection (about 10^6 per lobe), there is evidence only of a bacteriostatic effect of cell-mediated immunity in this species, the guinea pig [7].

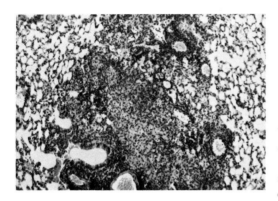

Fig. 2. Photomicrograph of HE-stained section of a pulmonary tuberculous lesion in an albino mouse 6 weeks after aerogenic infection, showing the absence of necrosis. × 65.

In contrast with the guinea pig, it is well known that tuberculous pulmonary lesions in the mouse do not show necrosis [4, 14]. This fact is illustrated in figure 2 showing an HE stained section of a mouse lung lesion 6 weeks after aerogenic infection with *M. tuberculosis*. No necrosis is seen in spite of the presence of large numbers of acid fast rods in these lesions. And those [4–6] who have followed the fate of tubercle bacilli in such lesions have noted no sudden loss of viability analogous to what I have just described in guinea pig lesions.

Discussion

The ancient controversy [17] regarding the relationship between delayed hypersensitivity and protective immunity in tuberculosis and other forms of intracellular parasitism is slowly being resolved. It is becoming clear that both immunologic phenomena are mediated by T lymphocytes but probably by different subsets of these cells and it seems likely now that distinctly different lymphokines may be involved in these two expressions of immunity [15, 18].

The observations described here can be readily fitted into this emerging picture. It is seen that delayed type hypersensitivity, when it is expressed in a species such as the guinea pig as a necrotizing response, is indeed responsible for one type of protective immune response which can involve a rapid loss of viability of parasites *in vivo*. This is probably attributable to the ischemia and anaerobiosis in such lesions with loss of viability of the strictly aerobic mycobacteria [9, 10]. It is equally clear that cellular immune mechanisms which do not involve tissue necrosis are also operable and these do not appear to entail any rapid bactericidal effect—only a bacteriostatic response. Thus, it would seem that the purely bacteriostatic effects observed in macrophages in *in vitro* studies of cell-mediated immunity [2, 3, 10, 16] are the most that can be expected from such studies, since they do not involve the immunopathology of what can appropriately be called 'lesion immunity' seen in the highly hypersensitive host.

In summary, it seems important to distinguish between the bactericidal antibacterial effects of the immunopathologic response of delayed hypersensitivity and the bacteriostatic effect of cellular immunity as manifested in living mononuclear phagocytes.

References

1 Ando, M.; Dannenberg, A. M.; Sugimoto, M., and Tepper, B.: Histochemical studies relating the activation of macrophages to the intracellular destruction of tubercle bacilli. Am. J. Path. *86:* 623–634 (1977).
2 Armstrong, J. A. and Hart, P. D'Arcy.: Phagosome-lysosome interactions in cultured macrophages infected with virulent tubercle bacilli. J. exp. Med. *142:* 1–16 (1975).
3 Berthrong, M.: The macrophage-tubercle bacillus relationship and resistance to tuberculosis. Ann. N.Y. Acad. Sci. *154:* 157–166 (1968).
4 Cohn, M. L. and Davis, C. L.: Chronic aerogenic

tuberculosis in mice. Proc. Soc. exp. Biol. Med. *131:* 805–809 (1969).

5 Collins, F. M. and Miller, T. E.: Growth of a drug-resistant strain of *Mycobacterium bovis* (BCG) in normal and immunized mice. J. infect. Dis. *120:* 517–533 (1969).

6 Costello, R. and Izumi, T.: Measurement of resistance to experimental tuberculosis in albino mice. J. exp. Med. *133:* 362–375 (1971).

7 Fok, J. S.; Ho, R. S.; Arora, P. K.; Harding, G. E., and Smith, D. W.: Host-parasite relationships in experimental airborne tuberculosis. V. Lack of hematogenous dissemination of *Mycobacterium tuberculosis* to the lungs in animals vaccinated with bacille Calmette-Guérin. J. infect. Dis. *133:* 137–144 (1976).

8 Grover, A. A.; Kim, H. K.; Wiegeshaus, E. H., and Smith, D. W.: Host-parasite relationships in experimental airborne tuberculosis. II. Reproducible infection by means of an inoculum preserved at − 70 °C. J. Bact. *94:* 832–835 (1967).

9 Guy, L. R.; Raffel, S., and Clifton, C. E.: Virulence of the tubercle bacillus. II. Effect of oxygen tension upon growth of virulent and avirulent bacilli. J. infect. Dis. *94:* 99–106 (1954).

10 Klun, C. L. and Youmans, G. P.: The effect of lymphocyte supernatant fluids on the intracellular growth of virulent tubercle bacilli. J. reticuloendoth. Soc. *13:* 263–274 (1973).

11 Loebel, R. O.; Shorr, E., and Richardson, H. B.: The influence of adverse conditions upon the respiratory metabolism and growth of human tubercle bacilli. J. Bact. *26:* 167–200 (1933).

12 Lurie, M. D.: Resistance to tuberculosis: experimental studies in native and acquired defensive mechanisms (Harvard University Press, Cambridge 1964).

13 Middlebrook, G.: Immunological aspects of airborne infection: reactions to inhaled antigens. Bact. Rev. *25:* 331–346 (1961).

14 Pagel, W.: Experimental tuberculosis. Observations on tissue reaction and natural resistance. Am. Rev. Tuberc. *42:* 58–69 (1940).

15 Patel, P. J. and Lefford, M. J.: Antigen-specific lymphocyte transformation, delayed hypersensitivity and protective immunity. Cell. Immun. *37:* 315–326 (1978).

16 Patterson, R. J. and Youmans, G. P.: Demonstration in tissue culture of lymphocyte-mediated immunity to tuberculosis. Infec. Immun. *1:* 600–603 (1970).

17 Raffel, S.: Immunity, pp. 646 (Appleton Century Crofts, New York 1961).

18 Reggiardo, Z. and Middlebrook, G.: Delayed-type hypersensitivity and immunity against aerogenic tuberculosis in guinea pigs. Infec. Immun. *9:* 815–820 (1974).

Dr. G. Middlebrook, Department of Pathology, University of Maryland School of Medicine, Baltimore, MD 21201 (USA)

Immunopathology. 6th Int. Convoc. Immunol., Niagara Falls, N.Y., 1978, pp. 257–261 (Karger, Basel 1979)

Immunopathology of Syphilis Revisited

Konrad Wicher and Victoria Wicher

Department of Microbiology, School of Medicine, State University of New York at Buffalo, and the Division of Clinical Microbiology and Immunology, Erie County Laboratory, Erie County Medical Center, Buffalo, N.Y.

In the past two decades, the immuno-pathology of some diseases has progressed from phenomenologic description of the immune response to a cellular or molecular analysis of the underlying mechanism. Syphilis, unfortunately, cannot be included in the list of such diseases. The modest progress made during the last 10 years in the field of syphilology, however, justifies a review.[1]

Morphology

The anatomy and chemistry of spirochetes has been excellently reviewed [13]. We, however, like to stress the presence of the mucoid material on the surface of virulent *Treponema pallidum*, inferred or indirectly indicated years ago by several researchers [4, 25]. More recently, *Zeigler et al.* [38] have documented the presence of an extracellular layer on *T. pallidum* from infected rabbit testes using the ruthenium-red tetroxide fixation method. The outer layer, tentatively identified as mucopolysaccharide, is not uniformly distributed; some *T. pallidum* have a thick layer, others a thin layer and still others do not have it at all. *Fitzgerald* [7] reported that injection

of the mucopolysaccharide from *T. pallidum* Nichols strain causes reactivation of skin lesions in previously infected rabbits, even in those immune to reinfection.

Attachment

The eagerness of *T. pallidum* to adhere to cells has long been known but only recently has this characteristic been associated with virulence and infectivity. *Fitzgerald et al.* [8] demonstrated that only *T. pallidum* Nichols strain and none of the 11 cultivable strains of treponemes examined adhered to cells cultured from normal rabbit testes. The *T. pallidum* seems to have no predilection for any tissues or species; 50–60% of the organisms in the suspension attached well to cell cultures of rabbit, human and rat origin. Antibody-containing serum of *T. pallidum*-infected rabbits interfered with the attachment. Heat killed or 'aged' suspensions of *T. pallidum* did not attach to cells.

The mechanism that enables *T. pallidum* to adhere to cells is not known. It is feasible that *T. pallidum* produces enzymes or toxin-like substances helping the organism in attachment and penetration. We [15] have demonstrated quantitative changes in lipid levels in rabbit organs following infection

---

[1] Space limitations do not permit us to quote all the publications we would like. We apologize to those authors for unavoidable omissions.

with *T. pallidum* Nichols strain. A significant increase in the level of cardiolipin took place in the spleen 3 days after intratesticular infection with 2×10^7 organisms. The lipid changes could not be attributed to the number of treponemes infecting the spleen at that time and, therefore, these changes might have been a product or consequence of the microorganism-cell interaction.

Intracellular Location, Phagocytosis and Persistence

Electron microscopic studies of ultra-thin sections of material from human syphilitic lesions [1, 24] and rabbit testes [23] seem to indicate that some *T. pallidum* can be found inside various cells. The authors agree that most microorganisms are located between epithelial cells but some are within the cytoplasm of macrophages, neutrophils, plasma cells, endothelial cells or, in the rabbit, even in spermatocytes. In spite of this information, some doubt has been raised [14] as to whether the treponemes were actually in the cell or superimposed on it. Furthermore, even if one accepts the intracellular location, the question still remains whether the microorganisms, at the time of the tissue fixation, were alive or dead and whether they contained the extracellular layer. These questions are of basic importance in the discussion of phagocytability of *T. pallidum*. *In vitro* phagocytosis of avirulent *T. pallidum* (Nichols) by rabbit macrophages has been demonstrated [18].

Suppression of growth of *Listeria monocytogenes* has been observed in *T. pallidum* infected rabbits [21]. We [32] have also observed the activation of peripheral blood phagocytic cells in *T. pallidum*-infected rabbits using the nitroblue tetrazolium test. However, the course of *T. pallidum* infection has been found unaltered in rabbits previously immunized with *Mycobacterium bovis*

(BCG) [12, 22] or *Propionibacterium acnes* [2], microorganisms known to stimulate phagocytic cells. Therefore, in *T. pallidum* infection there seems to be a 'selective failure' of phagocytosis which must be ascribed to the biologic properties of the microorganism itself, not to the phagocytic cell. Thus, if we accept these conclusions, the virulence of treponemes in phagocytic cells might be in question and the persistence of virulent *T. pallidum* long after natural [37] or experimental [9] infection, easier to explain. The factors helping the organisms to persist in the host are not well known. The extracellular mucopolysaccharide or antibodies covering *T. pallidum* and their location within cells other than phagocytic cells may play a key role in the persistence phenomenon.

If phagocytosis of *T. pallidum* does not take place, how then can one account for humoral and cellular immunity? We are tempted to assume that not all treponemes in the infectious inoculum have the same morphological properties and the concept of a 'two-organism' disease is not inconceiveable. Those treponemes which may have only little, if any, protective extracellular layer would eventually be phagocytized and used for stimulation of antibody production. Those *T. pallidum* covered with the protective layer might not be phagocytized; they would multiply, increase in mass, and be responsible for the lymphocyte suppression observed in the early stage of the disease in rabbits [20, 29]. This might explain why the infective course progresses in spite of the increasing levels of antibodies present in the serum.

Humoral Response

The Wassermann antibodies have for a long time been suspected of being auto-antibodies to cardiolipin of the host's cells [17]. Our [15] information on the changes of lipids in organs of *T. pallidum*-infected rabbits suggests such a possibility. The second cardiolipin autoantibody described by *Wright et al.* [35] is a mitochondrial cardiolipin antibody detected by a fluorescence method. The cardiolipin antibody can be detected in the patient's serum approximately 4 weeks after the appearance of the primary chancre and it disappears within 2–7 weeks after antibiotic treatment.

A number of antibodies to treponemal antigens are produced. Antibodies detected by the *T. pallidum* immobilization test (TPI) are different from those detected by the fluorescent treponema antibody test [34]. Most likely, in the latter test multiple antibodies participate. Which antibody is responsible for the partial protection demonstrated in experimental infection is not known [26]. It is possible that not all antibodies produced in the course of *T. pallidum* infection have been detected. For example, antibodies to the mucoid material of *T. pallidum* might be present in low titer; however, detection of such antibodies would require special treponemal preparations.

In spite of the autoimmune mechanism prevailing in syphilis, patients with this disease do not show an increased prevalence of the tissue antibodies found in autoimmune disorders [5]. In experimental syphilis, we [3] have found transient autoantibodies to rabbit heart tissue. These antibodies are organ-specific with cross-reactivity to skeletal muscle but they do not have species specificity. We [33] have also occasionally found autoantibodies reacting with rabbit smooth muscle. It is possible that rabbit infected with a larger number of treponemes (ca 10^7) may experience more intense changes.

Cellular Response

With the introduction of newer *in vitro* methods, correlating with the *in vivo* delayed hypersensitivity the cell-mediated immune mechanism in *T. pallidum*-infected man and rabbits has been explored by several research groups. The results [20, 29] suggest that, in experimentally infected rabbits, transitional suppression of cellular response to mitogens and treponemal antigens, as determined by *in vitro* lymphocyte transformation, takes place. We [30] have found that sera of infected rabbits inhibit the cell response to mitogens and antigens, and that the supernatant from cultured lymph node lymphocytes decreased blastogenic activity of antigen-stimulated lymphocytes [31].

Less clear-cut results were obtained in naturally acquired syphilis in man. Lymphocyte transformation in syphilitic patients has been examined since 1965 by various researchers who reported conflicting findings. However, in most cases the results correlated with the appearance of treponemal antibodies. More recently, *Musher et al.* [19], examining lymphocytes of patients with primary and secondary syphilis, observed suppressed response to streptolysin 0 but not to other mitogens or *T. refringens*. *Friedmann and Turk* [10, 11] found differences in lymphocyte reactivity to *T. pallidum* between Ethiopians and Englishmen suffering from syphilis. The lack of agreement in the results of syphilis in man might be explained by the variety of antigens and techniques used.

Immunopathology in Syphilis

In the pathology of syphilis not too much new information has been gained. The depletion of lymphocytes with an increase of histiocytes in lymphatic tissues seems to be the hallmark of syphilis [6, 16, 28]. Characteristically, plasma cells seem to accompany *T. pallidum* throughout the course of the disease. It is feasible that the cells are attracted by the treponemes and may be responsible for local production of specific antibodies which may, later on, interfere with the *T. pallidum*-cell attachment and, in part, be responsible for cessation of the lesions. The treponemal antibodies we [36] have demonstrated in infected rabbit testes seem to be locally produced since they were detected in the testes extract several days earlier than in the serum.

Lesions appearing in the late active stage might be a consequence of the cell-mediated immune mechanisms against the host's own tissue. Since virulent *T. pallidum* have been found [37] in a variety of tissues such as heart, brain, eye, etc., it may be that the late syphilitic lesions are the effect of reactivated *T. pallidum*. The late active lesions, in most cases, represent similar cell infiltration as the lesions of early syphilis and, with some exceptions, the clinical symptoms respond to antibiotic therapy. However, a cell-mediated mechanism against the host's own tissue cannot be excluded since some symptoms, e.g. interstitial keratitis in congenital syphilis respond to steroids but not to antibiotic therapy. The transitional cellular response to heart and skin extracts observed in experimental syphilis [28] gives support to the concept that although the persistence and reactivation of *T. pallidum* may account for many of the immunopathological phenomena observed in late active syphilis, sensitization during and most likely as consequence of infection, to the host's own tissue components cannot be disregarded. In some cases, this may be the sole triggering mechanism of autoaggression.

The mechanism of immunopathology of syphilis is now clearer than it was a decade ago; however, some key information is not yet available.

References

1 Azar, H. A.; Pham, T. D., and Kurban, A. K.: An electron microscopic study of a syphilitic chancre: Engulfment of *T. pallidum* by plasma cells. Archs. Path. *90:* 143–150 (1970).

2 Baughn, R. E.; Musher, D. M., and Knox, J. M.: Effect of sensitization with *Propionibacterium acnes* on the growth of Listeria monocytogenes and *T. pallidum* in rabbits. J. Immun. *118:* 109–113 (1977).

3 Casavant, C. H.; Wicher, V., and Wicher, K.: Host response to *T. pallidum* infection. III. Demonstration of autoantibodies to heart in sera from infected rabbit. Int. Archs Allergy appl. Immun. *56:* 171–178 (1978).

4 Christiansen, S.: Protective layer covering pathogenic treponemata. Lancet *i:* 423–425 (1963).

5 Doniach, D.: Autoantibodies in syphilis and in chronic biological false positive reactors; in Catterall and Nichol, Sexually transmitted diseases, pp. 210–218 (Academic Press, New York 1976).

6 Festenstein, H.; Abrahams, C., and Bokkenheuser, V.: Runting syndrome in neonatal rabbits infected with *T. pallidum*. Clin. exp. Immunol. *2:* 311–320 (1967).

7 Fitzgerald, T. J.: Syphilis: an experimental model. Proc. Int. Symp. on Sexually Transmitted Diseases, Montreal 1977 (in press, 1978).

8 Fitzgerald, T. J.; Johnson, R. C.; Miller, J. N., and Sykes, J. A.: Characterization of the attachment of *T. pallidum* (Nichols strain) to cultured mammalian cells and the potential relationship of attachment to pathogenicity. Infec. Immun. *18:* 467–478 (1977).

9 Frazier, C. S.; Bensel, A., and Keuper, C. S.: Further observations on the duration of spirochetemia in rabbits with asymptomatic syphilis. Am. J. Syph. *36:* 167–173 (1952).

10 Friedmann, P. S. and Turk, J. L.: A spectrum of lymphocyte responsiveness in human syphilis. Clin. exp. Immunol. *21:* 59–64 (1975).

11 Friedmann, P. S. and Turk, J. L.: The role of cell-mediated immune mechanism in syphilis in Ethiopia. Clin. exp. Immunol. *31:* 59–65 (1978).

12 Graves, S. R. and Johnson, R. C.: Effect of pretreatment with *Mycobacterium bovis* (strain BCG) and immune syphilitic serum on rabbit resistance to *T. pallidum*. Infec. Immun. *12:* 1029–1036 (1975).

13 Holt, S. C.: Anatomy and chemistry of spirochetes. Microbiol. Rev. *42:* 114–160 (1978).

14 Knox, J. M.: in Catterall and Nichol Sexually transmitted diseases, p. 232 (Academic Press, New York 1976).

15 Kumar, V.; Klingman, J. D., and Wicher, K.: Host response to *T. pallidum* infection. I. Quantitative changes of lipids in rabbit organs. Int. Archs Allergy appl. Immun. *55:* 476–480 (1977).

16 Levene, G. M.; Wright, D. J. M., and Turk, J. L.: Cell-mediated immunity and lymphocyte transfor-

mation in syphilis. Proc. R. Soc. Med. *64:* 14–16 (1971).

17 Milgrom, F. and Witebsky, E.: Autoantibodies and autoimmune disease. J. Am. med. Ass. *181:* 706–716 (1962).

18 Musher, D. M.; Izzat, N. N.; Min, K. W., and Györkey, F.: *In vitro* phagocytosis of avirulent *T. pallidum* by rabbit macrophages. Acta derm. vener., Stockh. *52:* 349–352 (1972).

19 Musher, D. M.; Schell, R. F., and Knox, J. M.: *In vitro* lymphocyte response to *T. refringens* in human syphilis. Infec. Immun. *9:* 654–657 (1974).

20 Pavia, C. S.; Folds, J. D., and Baseman, J. B.: Depression of lymphocyte response to concanavalin A in rabbits infected with *T. pallidum.* Infec. Immun. *14:* 320–322 (1976).

21 Schell, R. F. and Musher, D. M.: Detection of nonspecific resistance to Listeria monocytogenes in rabbits infected with *T. pallidum.* Infec. Immun. *9:* 658–662 (1974).

22 Schell, R. F.; Musher, D. M.; Jacobson, K.; Schwethelm, P., and Simmons, C.: Effect of macrophage activation on infection with *T. pallidum.* Infec. Immun. *12:* 505–511 (1975).

23 Sykes, J. A. and Miller, J. N.: Intracellular location of *T. pallidum* (Nichols strain) in the rabbit testes. Infec. Immun. *4:* 307–314 (1971).

24 Sykes, J. A.; Miller, J. N., and Kalan, A. J.: *Treponema pallidum* within cells of primary chancre from a human female. Br. J. vener. Dis. *50:* 40–44 (1974).

25 Turner, T. B. and Hollander, D. H.: Biology of the Treponematoses, Wld. Hlth. Org. Ser. No. 35, pp. 35–87 (WHO, Genève 1957).

26 Turner, T. B.; Hardy, P. H.; Newman, B., and Nell, E. E.: Effect of passive immunization on experimental syphilis in the rabbit. Johns Hopkins med. J. *133:* 241–251 (1973).

27 Turner, D. R. and Wright, D. J. M.: Lymphadenopathy in early syphilis. J. Path. *110:* 305–308 (1973).

28 Wicher, V. and Wicher, K.: Host response to *T. pallidum* infection. II. Rabbit leukocyte migration inhibition in the presence of homologous organ extracts. Int. Archs Allergy appl. Immun. *55:* 481–486 (1977).

29 Wicher, V. and Wicher, K.: *In vitro* cell response of *T. pallidum*-infected rabbits. I. Lymphocyte transformation. Clin. exp. Immunol. *29:* 480–486 (1977).

30 Wicher, V. and Wicher, K.: *In vitro* cell response of *T. pallidum*-infected rabbit. II. Inhibition of lymphocyte response to phytohaemagglutination by serum of *T. pallidum*-infected rabbits. Clin. exp. Immunol. *29:* 387–495 (1977).

31 Wicher, V. and Wicher, K.: *In vitro* cell response of *T. pallidum*-infected rabbit. III. Impairment in production of lymphocyte mitogenic factor. Clin. exp. Immunol. *29:* 496–500 (1977).

32 Wicher, V.; Blakowski, S., and Wicher, K.: Nitroblue tetrazolium test in experimental syphilis. Br. J. vener. Dis. *53:* 292–294 (1977).

33 Wicher, K. and Mlodozeniec, P.: Unpublished observation (1978).

34 Wilkinson, A. E.: Fluorescent treponemal antibody inhibition test. Br. J. vener. Dis. *43:* 186–190 (1967).

35 Wright, D. J. M.; Lessof, M. G.; Grimble, A. S.; Doniach, D.; Turk, J. L., and Catterall R. D.: New antibody in early syphilis. Lancet *i:* 740–743 (1970).

36 Yeagle, N.; Kalinka, C.; Nakeeb, S.; Wicher, V., and Wicher, K.: Immunopathology of rabbit testes infected with *T. pallidum.* Abstr. Annu. Meet. Am. Soc. Microbiology, B20, Las Vegas 1978.

37 Yogeswari, L. and Chacko, C. W.: Persistency of *T. pallidum* and its significance in penicillin-treated seropositive late syphilis. Br. J. vener. Dis. *47:* 339–347 (1971).

38 Zeigler, J. A.; Jones, A. M.; Jones, R. H., and Kubica, K. M.: Demonstration of extracellular material at the surface of pathogenic *T. pallidum* cells. Br. J. vener. Dis. *52:* 1–8 (1976).

Dr. K. Wicher, Department of Microbiology,
School of Medicine, State University of New York
at Buffalo, Buffalo, NY 14214 (USA)

Immunopathology. 6th Int. Convoc. Immunol., Niagara Falls, N.Y., 1978, pp. 262–267 (Karger, Basel 1979)

Immunopathology of Chagas' Disease[1]

C. A. Santos-Buch, D. Schecter, M. Sadigursky[2] *and A. M. Acosta*

Cornell University Medical College, Department of Pathology, New York, N.Y.

Introduction

The etiologic agent of American try-panosomiasis or Chagas' disease is the hemoflagellate protozoan *Trypanosoma cruzi*. Recent studies indicate that immunopathogenic mechanisms contribute to the development of the chronic form of the disease [16]. Most individuals, usually children, who are infected by the vector (*Hemiptera, Reduviidae*) develop an acute illness which is no different from other systemic parasitic infections. 90–95% of these patients survive acute *T. cruzi* parasitemias without difficulty [11]. However, an unknown number of these survivors later develop the chronic form of the disease. The onset of the chronic form of the disease heralds a very bad prognosis because usually the heart is fatally affected [11]. In a smaller group of patients with chronic Chagas' disease, the esophagus or the colon lose the ability to develop peristaltic contractions, and megaesophagus or megacolon are recognized pathologic sequelae of *T. cruzi* infections [9]. The target organs of the immunopathogenic mechanisms involved in chronic Chagas' disease

appear to be the primitive conduction fibers [16]. The heart conduction fibers, principally those of the right bundle of His and the anterior fibers of the left bundle of His, are destroyed in a lymphocytic myocarditis which is followed by fibrous replacement, and these changes may not be related to intracellular parasitosis by *T. cruzi* [1]. Similarly, the parasympathetic nervous system of Auerbach in the esophagus and large intestine is damaged in a lymphocytic infiltrate and the subsequent denervation leads to asynchronous peristalsis or paralysis, with the development of proximal dilatation of the hollow viscera [9, 13].

Antibody Reactions

Autoantibodies are formed following *T. cruzi* infection of humans and other vertebrates. Anti-γ-globulin activity and high heterophile antibody titers have been described in acute Chagas' disease [2]. It has been shown that *T. cruzi* inoculated mice also develop antinuclear antibody activity [20].

Tejada-Valenzuela and Castro [24] showed that the sera from 3 patients with chronic chagasic myocarditis formed precipitin lines with human heart extracts. *Jaffe et al.* [8] and *Kozma and Dräyer* [10] showed a high degree of correlation between precipitin autoantibodies to heart

[1] Supported by a grant from the American Heart Association and by The Rockefeller Foundation.

[2] Research Fellow, The Rockefeller Foundation, Cornell-Bahia Program.

extracts and chronic Chagas' disease. *Cossio et al.* [3] have demonstrated the presence of serum autoantibody activity in 95% of patients with chagasic myocarditis and in 45% of asymptomatic patients infected with *T. cruzi.* Sera from a large number of control patients from nonendemic areas did not show this autoantibody activity. Sera from patients with many other parasitic diseases lack this autologous antibody activity, with the exception of Kala-azar [21], but a cross-reacting antigen has been described between *T. cruzi* and *Leishmania donovani* organisms [15]. Biopsy of the myocardium of patients with positive complement fixation tests for *T. cruzi* shows spotty deposits of autologous IgG in the sarcolemma of myofibers, of skeletal muscle fibers, and of the plasma membrane of endothelial cells [3]. The autologous reactivity can be eliminated by exposure to freeze-dried epimastigotes of *T. cruzi* or to cardiac muscle from murine, bovine, or human sources. Since neither blood group A nor blood group B substances nor the Forssman antigen appear to quench or abolish the autologous reactivity of the EVI (endothelial-vascular-interstitial) antibody, it is reasonable to believe that *T. cruzi* and cardiac muscle possess a common antigenic system capable of eliciting autoreactive antibody activity [4, 6]. The EVI antibody can interact with and produce lesions of isolated rat atrial myofibers [19] and may act as a β-adrenergic agonist at the cell plasma level [19]. Data from *Teixeira et al.*'s [23] studies suggest that the antigen common to both *T. cruzi* and the myocardium, responsible for the elicitation of autologous antibody reactivity, may be present in the soluble intracellular compartment of the parasite, the cytosol.

T Lymphocyte Cytotoxicity Induced by *T. cruzi* Infection

Intracellular antigens of *T. cruzi* that appear to possess a high capacity to induce cell-mediated immunity are found in preparations rich in reticulum, ribosomes, and intracytoplasmic DNA [18]. So far, the specific antigens involved in the elicitation of cell-mediated immunity to *T. cruzi* infections have not been completely identified. Evidence that both chronic chagasic myocarditis and myenteric denervation could result from antigenic substances present in both target organs and *T. cruzi* comes from both laboratory and clinical studies.

T. cruzi-sensitized lymphocytes obtained from chronically infected rabbits and from rabbits immunized with a small particle or membrane fraction derived from homogenates of *T. cruzi* organisms destroyed both parasitized and non-parasitized monolayers of heart cells grown in tissue culture [18]. Destruction of heart cell monolayers by *T. cruzi*-sensitized lymphocytes had a high degree of specificity, since no destruction of allogeneic kidney cells was observed in control experiments. Moreover, the small particle or membrane fraction derived from homogenates of allogeneic hearts produced inhibition of migration of blood mononuclear cells derived from *T. cruzi*-sensitized rabbits [18]. Immune sera from *T. cruzi*-sensitized rabbits conveyed some degree of cytotoxicity to normal, non-sensitized lymphocytes, suggesting that antibody may also participate in the cell-mediated killer phenomenon *in vivo.* *Teixeira et al.* [23] incubated Auerbach's parasympathetic myenteric plexus of the colon of normal rabbits with *T. cruzi*-sensitized lymphocytes in nutrient medium, and increased adherence of mononuclear cells to the interlacing fibers and ganglion cells was noted overnight at 37 °C [16]. Control non-sensitized lymphocytes were not observed to adhere to these structures in similar experiments. Nor were macrophages involved, since *T. cruzi*-sensitized blood lymphocyte suspensions were incubated in plastic flasks prior to these cytotoxic studies to remove adherent cells. Thus, it is likely that the cytotoxic effects are engineered by T lymphocytes. *Santos-Buch and Acosta* [unpublished data] have shown that infection of mice with a sublethal dose of a clone of the Y strain of *T. cruzi* induces splenic T lymphocyte cytotoxicity to red blood cell targets coated with proteins of a lysate of the clone. These experiments suggest that T lymphocytes probably are implicated in the pathogenesis of the cardiopathy observed in chronic Chagas' disease.

There is evidence that lymphocytes derived from *T. cruzi*-infected humans with EVI antibody may be cytotoxic to allogeneic and heterogeneic heart cells [5]. Lymphocytes from 3 of 12 EVI antibody-positive, asymptomatic patients adhered to and strongly interacted with myocardial cells, and this reaction appeared to be organ specific since no reaction occurred with preparations of liver [5]. Antibody-mediated lymphocyte cytotoxicity to homologous ganglion cells of *T. cruzi*-infected mice was reported recently [*Dos Santos*, personal commun.].

Teixeira et al. [23] have shown that multiple injections of the small membrane fractions of *T. cruzi* in complete Freund's adjuvant result in focal lymphocytic infiltrates and myocytolysis in rabbits. Injections of the particulate antigens of *T. cruzi* in complete Freund's adjuvant also resulted in neuronolysis of Auerbach's plexus [23]. It would appear that these experiments indicate that the small membrane fractions of *T. cruzi* have the capacity to induce lesions of target organs of Chagas' disease and that autoreactive cell-mediated mechanisms engineer this experimental disease [18, 22, 23].

Cross-Reacting Immunogens of Target Organs and *T. cruzi*

Ricardo Dos Santos of Ribeirão Preto University (Brazil), in a provocative series of experiments using *T. cruzi*-infected mice, has provided data that suggest that diffusing antigenic material from nearby intracellular pseudocysts of amastigotes attaches to the surface membrane of the neurons of Auerbach's plexus of the intestine in the early moments of experimental disease.[3] There follows, in sequence, the appearance of lymphocytes, adherence of lymphocytes to ganglion cells, and neuronophagia and lysis. IgG and *T. cruzi* antigen were present on the surfaces of neurons when the cytotoxic lymphocytes made their appearance. Experiments of *Teixeira et al.* [23] have shown lymphocytic adherence to Auerbach's plexus of uninfected allogeneic targets effected by T lymphocytes derived from *T. cruzi*-infected rabbits [16].

The cross species reactivity of antibody and immune competent cells of chagasic patients and mammalian heart is discussed above. The evidence presently at hand appears to suggest that the principal cross-reacting immunogen of cellular reactivity with heart is present in fragments of the membranes of small organelles of *T. cruzi* [18].

Santos-Buch and Acosta [unpublished data] have developed a method of isolating a water-soluble antigen common to both *T. cruzi* and the myocardium of mice.

[3] Communication presented at the March 1977 Meeting of the Brasilian Society of Tropical Medicine, Brasilia, Brazil.

The procedure is based on studies which have determined that the small membrane myocardial fraction obtained by differential centrifugation (30,000 g × 35 min) stimulates lymphocytes to produce a substance which inhibits migration of monocytes derived from rabbits with chronic chagasic myocarditis.

The antigen from *T. cruzi* was derived from the Maria Cristina strain, isolated from a patient with Chagas' disease. The antigen from heart was derived from the myocardium of outbred, white, Swiss, HaM/CR-CD mice which were originally obtained from Charles River, Inc., Cambridge, Mass.

T. cruzi or mouse heart ventricles were broken up in Potter homogenizers, and the 30,000 g × 15 min fraction was obtained [18]. This fraction was thoroughly washed in cold phosphate-buffered saline. The pellet was treated with DNAase and RNAase (Sigma, St. Louis, Miss.) in 0.15 M NaCl in 0.05 M acetate buffer pH 4.6 with 2mM Mg^{2+} for 1 h at room temperature to solubilize DNA and RNA contaminants in the preparation. Following repeated washings in 0.15 M NaCl in 0.01 M phosphate buffer, pH 7.4, the fraction was rapidly suspended in cold distilled water and homogenized (15 sec, 12,000 rpm) in ice. 0.1 % (w/v) Lubrol (Imperial Chemicals, Ltd., Bridgeport, Conn.), a non-ionic detergent, was added to give a final concentration of 0.01 %. About 5 mg of a mixed-bed resin was added as recommended by *Mazia and Ruby* [12]. After 1 h equilibration, the preparation was centrifuged at 100,000 g × 2 h at 4 °C. ^{3}H-leucine-labelled mouse heart preparations indicated that about 40 % of the membrane was solubilized. The solubilized membrane proteins in the supernate were collected and passed through a 2.5 × 50 cm Sephadex G-200 column. Nearly $\frac{3}{4}$ of the proteins were present in the void volume. This preparation yielded a single protein band after 1 % SDS (lauryl sulfate), 8 M urea disc electrophoresis in acrylamide gels [7], and coincidence of migration of single bands for both the *T. cruzi* Maria Cristina strain and HaM/CR-CD murine myocardium was observed (fig. 1) [17]. Bovine serum albumin markers in SDS-urea gels have indicated that this protein has an approximate molecular weight of 67,000. We have obtained larger yields of cross-reacting small membrane immunogens by solubilization of myocardium in hot 1 % SDS in 0.01 M NH$_4$HCO$_3$ [25]. The solubilized, denatured proteins are partitioned into two sequential peaks in Sephadex G-100 and the proteins of the first peak have an approximate molecular weight of 76,000, whereas those in the second peak have an approximate molecular weight of 68,000. Rabbit antisera to two of three preparations (Lubrol soluble, peak I and SDS peak II) bind immunoglobulins to the surface of *T. cruzi* forms detected by indirect immunofluorescence (fig. 2; table I).

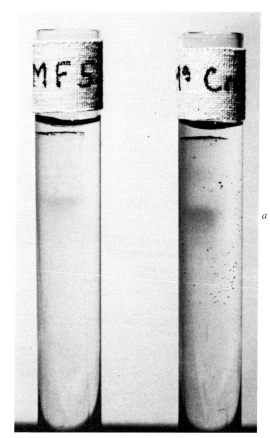

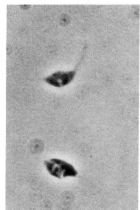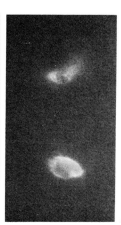

Fig. 2. a Phase contrast photomicrograph of two developing intracellular forms of *T. cruzi.* The upper form is a spheromastigote which has just unfolded the flagellum. The lower form is an amastigote with prominent nucleus and nucleoli and kinetoplast. Both forms were derived from infected rabbit renal cell monolayers in tissue culture. × 750. *b* Indirect immunofluorescence. The two forms were treated with a rabbit antiserum against the Lubrol-soluble antigen of small membranes of mouse heart; after appropriate washings, this was followed by treatment with fluorescein-labeled goat anti-rabbit IgG. × 750.

Fig. 1. 1% SDS-8 *M* urea disc acrylamide electrophoresis, in 2-mercaptoethanol, of solubilized protein obtained from DNAase-RNAase-treated small particles of mouse heart (HaM/CR-CD) after passage through Sephadex G-200. Coincidence of migration of protein band was obtained when compared with electrophoresis from similarly treated small particles of *T. cruzi* (Maria Cristina strain). [17].

Conceivably, *T. cruzi* may have the capacity to synthesize cross-reacting myocardial cell antigen through a process acquired in its intracellular cycle in mammals. If *T. cruzi* does not acquire the capacity to synthesize cross-reacting myocardial cell antigen of mammalians, then it is reasonable to suppose that it might carry the antigen piggyback during its intracellular cycle in the parasitized myocardial cell. This possibility may seem unlikely, since our own observations indicate that many passages of a known strain possessing cross-reacting myocardial cell antigen in NNN (Nicole, Neil and McNichol) [14] medium does not 'dilute' the antigen from amastigotes, as shown by immunofluorescent titers. If these observations are correct, they would seem to indicate that certain strains of *T. cruzi* have the capacity to synthesize cross-reacting mammalian heart antigen.

It is interesting to speculate that *T. cruzi*, in a sense, behaves like a virus which may adaptively incorporate portions of the host's genome during its interiorization of the mammalian cell. Whether the intracellular form of *T. cruzi* is coated in transit by the host's antigens or whether the parasite carries the capacity to synthesize host antigen in its outer coat, it is clear that this phenomenon is of survival advantage because the parasite would be masquerading as self and would not be totally recognized as a foreign intruder

Table I. Cross-reacting immunogens of small membranes of mouse heart and *Trypanosoma cruzi* [1]

Rabbit antibody raised against:	Indirect immunofluorescence (titer) [2]	
	unabsorbed	absorbed [3]
T. cruzi lysates	>1 : 320	1 : 10
Mouse heart SDS peak I	1 : 5	1 : 5
Mouse heart SDS peak II	1 : 40	0
Mouse heart lubrol peak I	1 : 20	0
Normal rabbit serum	0	0

[1] Solubilization of 30,000 $g \times 35$ min pellet of homogenized hearts of HaM/CR-CD mice either with hot SDS or cold lubrol (see text).
[2] Epimastigotes, trypomastigotes and amastigotes $10^3/10$ μl per well were acetone-fixed onto slides and indirect immunofluorescence was done using an optimal dilution of fluorescein-labeled goat anti-rabbit IgG.
[3] Specific immunofluorescence was determined when absorption by acetone-dried *T. cruzi* was seen. *T. cruzi* (Y-strain clone) was derived from infected monolayers of rabbit renal cells.

by the host's immune apparatus. On the other hand, it is theoretically possible that *T. cruzi* coating with host antigen may induce an autoimmune response in the host, thereby giving rise, in genetically selected individuals, to the nosological forms encountered in chronic Chagas' disease. Certainly, this hypothesis is worthy of further study.

References

1 Andrade, Z. A.; Andrade, S. G.; Oliveira, G. B., and Alonso, D. R.: Histopathology of the atrioventricular conduction system in chagasic myocarditis. Am. Heart J. *95:* 316–324 (1978).
2 Cabral, H. R. A.; Paolasso, E. W. De; Iniguez-Montenegro, C.; Soich, A. y Avalos, G.: Valoración clínica de la reacción de Rose-Ragan en la enfermedad Chagas aguda. Pren. Méd. Argent. *54:* 1713–1721 (1967).
3 Cossio, P. M.; Diez, C.; Szarfman, A.; Kreutzer, E.; Candiolo, B., and Arana, R. M.: Chagasic cardiopathy: demonstration of a serum γ-globulin factor which reacts with endocardium and vascular structures. Circulation *49:* 13–21 (1974).
4 Cossio, P. M.; Laguens, R. P.; Diez, C.; Szarfman, A.; Segal, A., and Arana, R. M.: Chagasic cardiopathy: antibodies reacting with plasma membrane of striated muscle and endothelial cells. Circulation *50:* 1252–1259 (1974).
5 Cossio, P. M.; Damilano, G.; Vega, M. T. de la; Laguens, R. P.; Cabeza-Meckert, P.; Diez, C., and Arana, R. M.: In vitro interaction between lymphocytes of chagasic individuals and heart tissue. Medicina, Buenos Aires *36:* 287–293 (1976).
6 Cossio, P. M.; Laguens, R. P.; Kreutzer, E.; Diez, C.; Segal, A., and Arana, R. M.: Chagasic cardiopathy: immunopathogenic and morphologic studies in myocardial biopsies. Am. J. Path. *86:* 533–544
7 Dulaney, T. T. and Touster, O.: The solubilization and gel electrophoresis of membrane enzymes by use of detergents. Biochim. biophys. Acta *196:* 29–34 (1970).
8 Jaffe, R.; Jaffe, W. G. und Kozma, C.: Experimentelle Herzveränderungen durch organspezifische Autoantikörper. Frankfurt Z. Path. *70:* 235–244 (1959).
9 Koberle, F.: Patogenia da molestia de Chagas: estudo dos orgãos musculares ocos. Rev. Goiana Med. *3:* 155–167 (1957).
10 Kozma, C. y Dräyer, B.: Estudios immunopatológicos en diversas cardiopatías. Gac. Med. Caracas *70:* 251–264 (1961).
11 Laranja, F. S.; Diaz, E.; Nobrega, G., and Miranda, A.: Chagas' disease: a clinical, epidemiological and pathologic study. Circulation *14:* 1035–1060 (1956).
12 Mazia, D. and Ruby, A.: Dissolution of erythrocyte membrane in water and comparison of the membrane protein with other structural proteins. Proc. natn. Acad. Sci. USA *61:* 1005–1012 (1968).
13 Mott, K. E. and Hagstrom, J. W. C.: The pathologic lesions of the cardiac autonomic nervous system in chronic Chagas' myocarditis. Circulation *31:* 273–286 (1965).
14 Neva, F. A.; Malone, M. F., and Myers, B. R.: Factors influencing the intracellular growth of *Trypanosoma cruzi in vitro*. Am. J. trop. Med. Hyg. *10:* 140–149 (1961).
15 Pessoa, S. B. and Cardoso, F. A.: Nota sobre a immunidade cruzada na leishmaniose tegumentar e na molestia de Chagas. Hospital *21:* 187–192 (1942).
16 Santos-Buch, C. A.: American trypanosomiasis: Chagas' disease; in Miescher, Immunopathology. 7th Int. Symp., Bad Schachen, 1974, pp. 205–220 (Schwabe, Basel 1977).

17 Santos-Buch, C. A.: Autoimmunity and Chagas' disease: demonstration of a common immunogen of heart and *T. cruzi*; in Miescher, Proc. Int. Symp. on Organ-Specific Autoimmunity, Cremona 1977 (Schwabe, Basel 1978).

18 Santos-Buch, C. A. and Teixeira, A. R. L.: Immunology of experimental Chagas' disease. III. Rejection of allogeneic heart cells *in vitro*. J. exp. Med. *140:* 38–53 (1974).

19 Sterin-Borda, L.; Cossio, P. M.; Gimeno, M. F.; Gimeno, A. L.; Diez, C.; Laguens, R. P.; Meckert, P. C., and Arana, R. M.: Effect of chagasic sera on the rat isolated atrial preparation: immunological, morphological and functional aspects. Cardiovasc. Res. *10:* 613–622 (1976).

20 Szarfman, A.; Cossio, P. M.; Laguens, R. P.; Segal, A.; Vega, M. T. de la; Arana, R. M., and Schmunis, G. A.: Immunological studies in Rockland mice infected with *T. cruzi*. Development of nuclear antibodies. Biomedicine, Paris *22:* 489–495 (1975).

21 Szarfman, A.; Khoury, E. L.; Cossio, P. M.; Arana, R. M., and Kagan, I. G.: Investigation of the EVI antibody in parasitic diseases other than American trypanosomiasis. Am. J. trop. Med. Hyg. *24:* 19–24 (1975).

22 Teixeira, A. R. L. and Santos-Buch, C. A.: Immunology of experimental Chagas' disease. II. Delayed hypersensitivity to *Trypanosoma cruzi* antigens. Immunology *28:* 401–410 (1975).

23 Teixeira, A. R. L.; Teixeira, M. L., and Santos-Buch, C. A.: Immunology of experimental Chagas' disease. IV. Production of lesions in rabbits similar to those of chronic Chagas' disease in man. Am. J. Path. *80:* 163–180 (1975).

24 Tejada-Valenzuela, C. and Castro, F.: Miocarditis crónica en Guatemala. Rev. Col. Med. Guatemala *9:* 124–131 (1958).

25 Weber, K. and Osborne, M.: Proteins and sodium dodecyl sulfate: molecular weight determination on polyacrylamide gels and related procedures; in Neurath and Hill The proteins, 2nd ed.; vol. 1, pp. 180–223 (Academic Press, New York 1975).

Dr. C. A. Santos-Buch, Department of Pathology, Cornell University Medical College, 1300 York Avenue, New York, NY 10021 (USA)

Immunopathology. 6th Int. Convoc. Immunol., Niagara Falls, N.Y., 1978, pp. 268–273 (Karger, Basel 1979)

Immunopathology of Infestation with Animal Parasites

Studies on the Helminthic Infection Schistosomiasis[1]

D. G. Colley and S. G. Kayes

Veterans Administration Hospital and the Department of Microbiology, Vanderbilt University, Nashville, Tenn.

The worldwide magnitude of disease caused by protozoan and metazoan parasites remains staggering. The annual mortality due to malaria is greater than one million persons. Amebiasis, schistosomiasis, filariasis, ancylostomiasis, trichuriasis and ascariasis all affect more than 200 million people, while trypanosomiasis, strongyloidiasis and onchocerciasis affect at least 20 million. Many of these parasitic infections afford extensive opportunities for immunopathologic interactions. All four classifications of hypersensitivity mechanisms described *Coombs and Gell* [11] have been shown to occur in infestations with many of these parasites. .

Immediate hypersensitivity reactions (type I) are elicited by specific antigen interactions with IgE antibodies on the surfaces of mast cells. This induces the release of the distinctive pharmacological mediators which initiate local or systemic anaphylactic reactions. Elevated levels of IgE and peripheral blood and tissue eosinophilia are associated with infestations by parasites that invade tissues or undergo somatic migration. These observations have provided the basis for wide

spread conjecture as to the role of immediate hypersensitivity in such infections.

While it remains attractive to postulate that the augmented IgE responses seen in these helminthic infections play a positive role in protective immunity mechanisms against the parasites, there is still not unequivocal evidence that IgE-mediated mechanisms are responsible for acquired resistance to any of these diseases [4]. It is postulated that immediate hypersensitivity may play an accessory role in protective immunity by altering vascular permeability and allowing the actual protective immune components more ready access to the tissue-dwelling or gut-dwelling parasites.

Reactions characterized as type II hypersensitivities involve antigen-antibody and complement interactions with antigens on the surfaces of cells or tissues, and result in either lesion formation, lysis, enhanced phagocytosis, or intravascular coagulation. The hemolytic anemias of certain protozoal infections (primarily malaria, kala azar, and African trypanosomiasis) are pathologic presentations commonly considered to result from type II mechanisms [4, 18].

Immunopathologic events attributable to immune complex interactions have been described in a wide variety of parasitic infections. In some situations, the complexes have

[1] Supported by the Medical Research Service of the Veterans Administration, and grants from the USPHS, NIH AI 11289, under the auspices of the US-Japan Cooperative Medical Science Program and the Rockefeller Foundation (RF 74084).

been shown to contain antigens derived from the etiologic agents, and in other cases auto-antigens have been described. Substantial data concerning immune complexes and complement interactions have been developed in regard to malaria and schistosomiasis [4, 15, 18, 19].

It is not feasible to deal in depth with all the immunopathologic aspects of the many parasitic diseases cited. Therefore, this presentation will focus on the disease schistosomiasis with an emphasis on the immunopathology of chronic infections and the immunoregulatory controls which may govern the magnitude of such responses.

Schistosomiasis is often considered to be an infection with which immunopathogenic mechanisms provide the basis for disease [16]. Infection is contracted by the mammalian host by contact with fresh water containing the infectious stage of the lifecycle, the cercariae. The cercariae result from asexual replication of schistosomes within the appropriate snail intermediate host. Following penetration through the dermis a cercaria transforms into a schistosomula which migrates to the lungs and the hepatic-portal vasculature. After about 4 weeks, the schistosomulae of *Schistosoma mansoni*, the human schistosome found in Africa, South America and Caribbean, mature into male or female adult worms, begin to produce and fertilize eggs, and may live up to 30 years within the mesenteric venules of the host. The eggs work their way into the lumen of the gut, and are thereby excreted to the environment. In fresh water the embryos within hatch, seek to infect specific host snails, and thus complete the cycle.

Schistosomes are small, intravascular, worms that do not themselves divide in the body, and which are so adept at evading, or subverting, the host's normal defense systems that their presence—even within the portal system—does not appear to contribute

directly to the ill health of the host. In the future, this statement may prove entirely too simplistic, but it does reflect our current knowledge about clinical and experimental infections with the human schistosomes [7]. Studies by *Warren* and his colleagues over the last 15 years have firmly established that hepatosplenomegaly, portal hypertension, and esophageal varices due to *S. mansoni* infection in the mouse are the result of hepatic granulomas formed in response to those schistosome eggs which are not defecated by the host, but rather impact in the presinusoidal capillaries of the liver. The etiology of these granulomas is largely cell-mediated in nature, i.e. they are primarily type IV hypersensitivity reactions against soluble antigens derived from the schistosome eggs (SEA) [16]. Antibodies are also made against SEA [14]. While their participation in the granulomatous process is less than clear, they are not absolutely required for granuloma formation [3], but may play an important role in sequestration of antigenic materials [3, 14] and regulatory processes [9, 10].

Currently, there is considerable interest in the regulation, or suppression, of this egg-focused granulomatous process. *Andrade and Warren* [cited in 17] were the first to observe that during the course of experimental murine infection the actual size of newly formed granulomas decreased as infection became more chronic. Using a system described by *von Lichtenberg* [14] which employs the injection of eggs into the microvasculature of the lungs and measurement of the resulting granulomas, *Domingo and Warren* [cited in 17] studied this phenomenon of smaller new granulomas late in infection. They determined that it was due to a change in the reactivity of the host during chronic infection, and occurred in the presence of continuous antigenic exposure. Peak granulomatous responsiveness was at 8 weeks after infection, remained strong for a few weeks, and declined to a low level throughout chronic infection. This change paralleled the development of a maintenance state of disease, which replaced the more fulminating hepatomegaly present at about 8 weeks of infection. Studies by *Boros et al.* [2] and our laboratory [5]— see also *Phillips and Colley* [15]—have described a variety of alterations in SEA-specific immune responses which occur concomitantly with this diminution of granuloma formation. Concomitant with the observed modulation of granuloma formation there are decreases in lymphokine production, circulating levels of heat-labile reaginic antibody, and to some extent lymph node cell blastogenesis. Both hemagglutinating antibody, and heat-stable, 72-hour skin sensitizing antibody, increase in the sera of chronically infected mice.

While these alterations in immune reactivities yield information as to the occurrences which parallel lesion modulation, they do not determine the mechanisms responsible for the phenomenon. To look more directly at this question, we have performed passive transfer experiments to ask whether an active suppressive process is involved. Lymphoid cell populations, or sera, from chronically infected mice (exhibiting modulated granuloma responses) were injected into syngeneic recipients which had been infected for 6 weeks. Two weeks later, at the usual time of maximum granuloma formation, their hepatic granulomas were measured, and compared with those of parallel control animals which received only saline injections at 6 weeks of infection [6]. The results demonstrated that lymph node or spleen cells from chronically infected mice could suppress the degree of the specific, immunologically mediated granuloma formation in actively infected animals. Subsequent experiments have shown that the cells responsible for this adoptive suppression are sensitive to *in*

vitro pretreatment with anti-Thy 1.2 alloantiserum and complement [16]. It appears that a population of Thy 1.2-bearing lymphocytes in chronically infected mice is essential for active suppression of ongoing granuloma formation. Large, repeated doses of infected sera did not alter the granuloma responses of the infected recipient hosts. Preliminary data by *Pelley and Warren* [personal commun.] using the pulmonary granuloma system rather than actual infection, indicate that both chronic sera and cells can passively suppress granuloma formation.

In studies on human schistosomiasis, we have utilized several *in vitro* methodologies to study immunoregulation of SEA responsiveness during chronic human schistosomiasis. The rationale for such studies is based on the animal model described, and the clinical observation that morbidity due to schistosomiasis is not always strictly related to the intensity of infection. This implies that the degree of host responsiveness expressed may be important to the outcome of infection. During early infection, mononuclear cells of peripheral blood from patients respond moderately well when exposed to SEA in *in vitro* lymphocyte blastogenesis assays [8]. Subsequently, during chronic infection, this ability is not expressed, yet after antischistosomal chemotherapeutic treatment, SEA-induced activity is again strongly expressed [10]. These patterns were obtained when lymphocyte cultures were maintained in medium supplemented with normal human serum (NHS). However, substitution of human sera from patients with chronic schistosome infections (IHS) altered these patterns such that even responsive lymphocytes failed to express their ability to respond to SEA [9]. This serosuppression was only effective in relationship to schistosomal antigen-induced responses, leaving phytohemagglutinin (PHA) and *Candida albicans*-induced responsiveness intact.

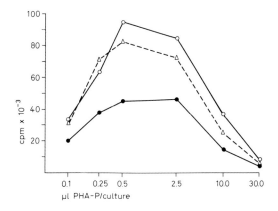

Fig. 1. Tritiated thymidine incorporation by chronic patient cells exposed to PHA and SEA or PHA alone. Triplicate cultures containing 5×10^5 cells/0.2 ml medium supplemented with 5% NHS were maintained for 3 days and exposed to ^{3}H-TdR for last 6 h. o = PHA alone; $\triangle$ = PHA + 5 µg/ml SEA; • = PHA + 50 µg/ml SEA.

Several systems have been tried to allow investigation of potential cellular suppressive mechanisms in the human setting. The data in figure 1 demonstrate the effect of direct addition of SEA to chronic patient cells responding to PHA. This method of demonstrating antigen-induced suppression has been described in experimental suppression models, and was shown to depend on activation of suppressor cell activity [1]. While we do not yet know the basis of our observation, the effect is very similar to that obtained in the animal studies. This antigen-induced suppressive effect was obtained with many, but not all chronic patients tested. It was only infrequently observed with cells from uninfected or recently infected patients.

More direct evidence of schistosome antigen-induced suppressor cell activity was obtained by exposing mononuclear cell preparations of patient's peripheral blood to SEA in culture for 2–4 days, treating these cells with mitomycin-C, washing the cells, and adding them to autologous cells, which were

then tested for their responsiveness to PHA. Controls consisted of PHA-exposed cultures which received parallel mitomycin-C treated cells, except that they were not exposed to SEA in the first culture [10]. Eight of 22 chronic patients tested in this manner developed significant suppressor activity upon exposure to SEA. The mean percent of significant suppression corresponded to a 27% decrease in PHA responsiveness.

In a few preliminary experiments, the generation of suppressor activity by SEA exposure was done in cultures containing sera from chronic patients known to exhibit the previously described serosuppression effect on SEA-induced responsiveness. It was observed that when compared to parallel studies in NHS-supplemented medium more chronic patients developed significant suppression upon antigen exposure in the presence of such suppressive sera. Also, the degree of suppression was often more profound [10]. These manipulations do not induce dependable suppressor activity when the cells from uninfected subjects are tested.

We have also established the serosuppression-suppressor activity systems in the mouse model. The aim is to allow a closer correlation of these parameters with the progression of immunopathology (granuloma formation) and its regulation, and to allow a more detailed analysis of the mechanisms operative in these systems. Since our usual mouse lymphocyte culture system employs NHS (2%) as a medium supplement, we have directly tested the schistosome, antigen-specific serosuppressive effects of sera from patients chronically infected with *S. mansoni*. Some examples of the results of this system on the lymphocyte blastogenic capabilities of optimally SEA-responsive lymphocytes from 8-week infected mice are seen in figure 2. Sera from more than 50 patients have now been tested. As in the completely human system, when compared to NHS-supplement-

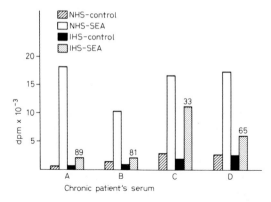

Fig. 2. Suppressive effect of 4 different patient sera on 8-week infected mouse lymphocyte blastogenic response to 4 μg/ml SEA. In 4 separate experiments, 2.5 × 10⁵ CBA/J lymph node cells were cultured in 0.2 ml RPMI-1640 medium supplemented with 5% of either normal human serum (NHS) or infected human serum (IHS) for 5 days. Cultures were exposed to ³H-TdR for last 8 h of culture; incorporation was assayed by liquid scintillation spectroscopy. Numbers over IHS-SEA bars indicate the percent suppression $\left(\dfrac{[\text{NHS/SEA} - \text{IHS/SEA}]}{\text{NHS/SEA}} \times 100\%\right)$.

ed media, media containing chronic patient sera almost always suppressed the specific SEA-induced response, but did not interfere with the PHA-induced blastogenesis.

Initial experiments [*Kayes and Colley*, in progress] testing the efficacy of suppressive sera from chronic patients to promote SEA-induced cellular suppressor activity have indicated that lymphoid cells of chronically sick mice behave similarly to their human counterparts. When spleen cells from 25-week infected mice are cultured in the presence of both SEA and chronic suppressive human serum, they develop increased cellular suppressive activity as measured on syngeneic lymphocyte reactivity to PHA. Spleen cells from 8-week infected mice are not always induced to develop suppressor activity by exposure to SEA in NHS, but do so if this is done in the presence of chronic suppressive

human serum. Spleen cells from uninfected mice are generally unaffected by exposure to SEA, regardless of the source of the human serum in the medium.

Egg-induced granulomas are the most prominent immunopathologic lesions induced in mice by *Schistosoma mansoni.* Mechanistically, they are predominantly dependent upon cell-mediated immune responses, while the immunoregulation of lesion formation and of immune responses induced by egg antigens involves both humoral and cellular suppressive capabilities, and further suggests the existence of interplay among chronic lymphoid cells, chronic sera and specific antigen. Yet there are other pathologic and perhaps immunopathologic events which occur during schistosomiasis. The actual pathogenesis of Symmer's clay-pipestem fibrosis is still debated [15], while lesions as disparate as those of cercarial dermatitis are thought to involve types I, III and IV hypersensitivities. Acute, toxemic schistosomiasis may represent disseminated immune complex lesions [7, 15, 16] and immune complex-mediated nephropathies have been documented in chronic disease [7, 15, 19]. Also, type II autoimmune hemolytic anemia has been proposed to develop during this infection [4].

It should be apparent from this brief discussion of schistosomiasis, and a few examples of other parasite infestations, that the complete spectrum of immunopathology is readily available in the host dealing with these heterogeneous groups of infectious organisms.

References

1 Bash, J. A. and Waksman, B. H.: The suppressive effect of immunization on the proliferative responses of rat T cells *in vitro*. J. Immun. *114:* 782–787 (1975).

2 Boros, D. L.; Pelley, R. P., and Warren, K. S.: Spontaneous modulation of granuloma hypersensitivity in schistosomiasis mansoni. J. Immun. *114:* 1437–1441 (1975).

3 Byram, J. E. and Lichtenberg, F. von: Altered granuloma formation in nude mice. Am. J. trop. Med. Hyg. *26:* 944–956 (1977).

4 Cohen, S. and Sadun, E. H.: Immunology of parasitic infections (Blackwell, Oxford 1976).

5 Colley, D. G.: Immune responses to a soluble schistosomal egg antigen preparation during chronic primary infection with *Schistosoma mansoni.* J. Immun. *115:* 150–156 (1975).

6 Colley, D. G.: Adoptive suppression of granuloma formation. J. exp. Med. *143:* 696–700 (1976).

7 Colley, D. G.: The immunopathology of schistosomiasis. Rec. Adv. Clin. Immunol. *1:* 101–123 (1977).

8 Colley, D. G.; Cook, J. A.; Freeman, G. L., jr.; Bartholomew, R. K., and Jordan, P.: Immune responses during human schistosomiasis mansoni. I. *In vitro* lymphocyte blastogenic responses to heterogeneous antigenic preparations from schistosome eggs, worms and cercariae. Int. Archs Allergy appl. Immun. *53:* 420–433 (1977).

9 Colley, D. G.; Hieny, S. E.; Bartholomew, R. K., and Cook, J. A.: Immune responses during human schistosomiasis mansoni. III. Regulatory effect of patient sera on human lymphocyte blastogenic responses to schistosome antigen preparations. Am. J. trop. Med. Hyg. *26:* 917–925 (1977).

10 Colley, D. G.; Lewis, F. A., and Goodgame, R. W.: Immune responses during human schistosomiasis mansoni. IV. Induction of suppressor cell activity by schistosome antigen preparations and Concanavalin A. J. Immun. *120:* 1225–1232 (1978).

11 Coombs, R. R. A. and Gell, P. G. H.: Clinical aspects of immunology (Davis, Philadelphia 1963).

12 Davis, B. H.; Mahmoud, A. A. F., and Warren, K. S.: Granulomatous hypersensitivity to *Schistosoma mansoni* eggs in thymectomized and bursectomized chickens. J. Immun. *113:* 1064–1067 (1974).

13 Lewis, F. A. and Colley, D. G.: Cellular suppression of granuloma formation (abstr.). Fed. Proc. Fed. Am. Socs exp. Biol. *35:* 860a (1976).

14 Lichtenberg, F. von: Studies on granuloma formation. III. Antigen sequestration and destruction in the schistosome pseudotubercle. Am. J. Path. *45:* 75–93 (1964).

15 Phillips, S. M. and Colley, D. G.: Immunologic aspects of host responses to schistosomiasis: resistance, immunopathology, and eosinophil involvement. Prog. Allergy, vol. 24, pp. 59–182 (Karger, Basel 1978).

16 Warren, K. S.: Worms; in Samter, Immunological diseases, vol. I, pp. 668–686 (Little, Brown, Boston 1971).

17 Warren, K. S.: Modulation of immunopathology in schistosomiasis; in Parasites in the immunized host: mechanisms of survival. Ciba Found. Symp. 25 (new series), pp. 243–252 (Elsevier-Excerpta Medica-North Holland, Amsterdam 1974).

18 WHO: Developments in malaria immunology. Tech. Rep. Ser. 579 (1975).

19 WHO: The role of immune complexes in disease. Tech. Rep. Ser. 606 (1977).

Dr. D. G. Colley, Veterans Administration Hospital, Nashville, TN 37203 (USA)

Immunopathology. 6th Int. Convoc. Immunol., Niagara Falls, N.Y., 1978, pp. 274–279 (Karger, Basel 1979)

Association of Immune Complex Disease with Complement Deficiency

P. J. Lachmann

MRC Group on Mechanisms in Tumour Immunity, The Medical School, Cambridge

Introduction

Where the auto-allergic process is directed against antigenic components other than those represented on cell membranes, the pathogenetic mechanism of auto-allergic diseases involves principally the formation of immune complexes. Immune complexes produce their harmful effects by inducing inflammation and in this process the role of the complement system is known to be of great importance [25]. Thus, the fixation of C3 on immune complexes allows them to interact with the C3b receptors on phagocytic cells which promotes phagocytosis and exocytosis of proteolytic enzymes and of other mediators [7]. The generation of C3a and C5a gives rise to further mediator release also from mast cells and causes the chemotaxis of leukocytes.

The Clinical Association of Complement Deficiency

Armed with this type of information derived from *in vitro* studies and from studies of experimental animals showing that complement depletion reduces the pathogenicity of immune complexes [25], the expectation was that complement deficiency in man would give rise to impaired ability to deal with infection but that it would carry a compensating freedom from diseases of immune complex pathogenesis.

Complement deficiencies with increased liability to infection were indeed discovered [11]. Generalised immune deficiency to bacterial infection has been found among subjects with deficiencies of C3 itself or with disorders which lead to severe C3 deficiency. Recurrent or disseminated neisserial infections (meningococcal or gonococcal, but usually not both) have been found largely with deficiencies of the later-acting complement components.

The second prediction, that of freedom from immune complex disease, however, has been found to be quite false, and an undue prevalence of various immune complex diseases of which systemic lupus erythematosus (SLE) is the commonest, has been recorded in a number of complement deficiencies (table I) [11]. The association is seen particularly with deficiency of the components making up the 'classical pathway C3 convertase': C1, C4 and C2. Of these deficiences

Table I. Clinical associations of complement deficiency

Component	Total number of affected subjects	Healthy	Immune complex disease			Bacterial defects	
			SLE or SLE-like syndrome	glomerulo-nephritis	other	multiple (pyodermal, etc.)	neisserial
C3	5	0	0	0	2	4	0
C3b inactivator	4	1	0	0	0	1	2
C5	4	1	1	0	0	0	2
C6	5	1	0	0	0	0	4
C6 + C7	1	1	0	0	0	0	0
C7	9	2	0	1	2[1]	0	4
C8	9	4	3	0	0	0	2
C1r	3	0	2	1	0	2	0
C4	2	0	2	0	0	0	0
C2	>40	approx. half	approx. 10	approx. 5	6[2]	0	0
C1 inhibitor	many	–	7	11	0	0	0

[1] One Raynaud's; 1 rheumatoid arthritis.
[2] Three Henoch-Schönlein purpura; 1 rheumatoid arthritis; 1 chronic vasculitis; 1 polymyositis.

in man, the deficiency of C2 is the most common. Not all cases of C2 deficiency are now reported, but of the two dozen or so pedigrees recorded in the literature, about half have suffered from SLE or other immune complex disease; the other having been in good health. Deficiencies of C1 and C4 are markedly less common but all have had diseases likely to be immune complex in nature. A further complement deficiency to be included within this group is that of the C1̄ inhibitor. This is relatively common because the heterozygotes suffer from hereditary angio-oedema (HAE) which is caused by the production of a kinin-like mediator from C2 by the combined action of plasmin and C1̄. Although the majority of affected subjects suffer only from angio-oedema, in recent years a number of HAE patients have been shown to have SLE or glomerulonephritis [11]. This is of interest because patients with HAE have a life-long severe deficiency of C2 and C4 which is due to hypercatabolism rather than to hyposynthesis.

Explanations for the Association of Complement Deficiency with Immune Complex Disease

It is pertinent to ask how it should come about that patients with complement deficiency, who appear to lack one of the major pathogenetic pathways of immune complex damage, should nevertheless be unduly prone to immune complex diseases.

The first possibility to be considered is that the association is false and results from ascertainment problems. It is argued that since it is patients with putative immunological diseases that most frequently have their complement levels measured, it is in this group of patients that complement deficiencies will be discovered. The argument has some plausibility and can be countered effectively only by knowing the true incidence of complement deficiencies in normal populations. There must be much more information on this point, now that many clinical laboratories measure complement components, than is as yet pub-

Table II. Incidence of complement deficiency in normal populations

Source	Population	Number studied	Complement deficiency encountered	Nature of deficiency
Hässig et al. [5]	Swiss army recruits	40,000	14	largely C4↓ + C2↓ (no genetic data)
Torisu et al. [21]	Japanese mass medical examination	42,000	3	C4↓ (sera inactivate C4) (no genetic data)
Stratton [19]	Manchester blood transfusion panel	> 10,000	1	C2-deficient (no family data)
Lachmann [10]	Cambridge hospital outpatients	2,000	1	C6 + C7 deficient (inherited)
			1	⌠C1↓ C4↓ C2↓ C1 inhib.↓ C3↓ ⌡HAE with SLE
			2	⌠C1↓ C4↓ C2↓ C1 inhib.↓ I/C + + ⌡Caldwell's syndrome

lished. The data known to the author are shown in table II. The two earlier studies by *Hässig et al.* [5] and by *Torisu et al.* [21] suffer from the fact that it is not clear whether any of the complement deficiencies were genetic. It seems likely from their data that the subjects studied suffered either classical pathway activation (e.g. mixed cryoglobulin disease) or asymptomatic HAE. Even so, they show that any complement deficiency is very uncommon—less than 1/3,000 in the Swiss and less than 1/10,000 in the Japanese. The study by *Stratton* [19] involved a blood transfusion panel and excluded patients with chronic disease. In Cambridge, an outpatient population has been studied which includes a large number of chronic sick and whose age distribution is much slanted towards the elderly. None of these surveys is wholly satisfactory since none used random samples from the population as a whole and the young women who form the majority of patients with systemic lupus erythematosus are markedly under-represented. Nevertheless, if one accepts an incidence for homozygous C2 deficiency within the population of not more than one in 5,000, then it is fairly clear that the incidence of homozygous C2 deficiency among patients with systemic lupus erythe-

matosus must be at least an order of magnitude greater than this. *Glass et al.* [4], for example, found one C2 deficiency subject among 142 lupus patients. It does therefore seem most unlikely that the association of complement deficiency with immune complex disease is entirely an artefact.

The second explanation that has been put forward is that the complement deficiency itself is not responsible for the association with immune complex disease but that it acts as a marker for a true susceptibility gene in close linkage disequilibrium with it. This argument has been adduced particularly for the deficiencies of those complement components that are coded in the HLA region: C2 and C4. (No factor B deficiency is yet known.) C2 deficiency does show strong linkage disequilibrium with a particular HLA haplotype, A10, B18, DW2, BfS both in the US and in Europe [2, 6] and the possibility that there is an immune response gene (for example) predisposing to SLE in linkage disequilibrium with this haplotype cannot be lightly discarded. Since immune response genes are dominant in their effects and the effects of complement deficiency itself would be expected to be recessive (half level of C2 not affecting any of the known complement functions to a significant extent), the study of heterozygotes for C2 deficiency offers an interesting test of the marker-gene hypothesis. Such studies have been performed by *Glass et al.* [4] who have reported a significant association between apparent heterozygous C2 deficiency and SLE and juvenile rheumatoid arthritis. Similarly, *Trouillas and Betuel* [22] have claimed that there is a group of patients with multiple sclerosis that show a high association with low complement levels and B18; and *Turner et al.* [23] have claimed that a similar association exists for the atopic state. Neither of these two latter diseases have been reported in homozygous C2 deficiency. There are, however, difficulties in the ascertainment of heterozygotes except in families where homozygous C2 deficient subjects are found. In a survey of blood donors, *Nerl et al.* [17] have shown that some 63% of HLA, DW2-positive donors have low levels of C2 compatible with a 'heterozygous deficiency state' and 39% had similarly low C4 levels. Since the gene frequency for DW2 is 0.0953 in European caucasoids (figure from the 7th International Histocompatibility Workshop) one can calculate that 0.5% of the whole population should be homozygous for C2 deficiency and 0.4% for C4 deficiency. These figures are much too high and it is therefore clear that the low levels cannot be taken as a marker for a null gene at a single structural locus! An explanation for this conundrum is likely to come from the studies of *O'Neill et al.* [18] who have shown that the C4 locus is likely to be tandemly duplicated so that low levels can result from null alleles at either of the two tandem loci and total deficiency will be rare. If such a gene duplication involved not only the C4 locus but the C2 locus as well, then the high incidence of half normal levels of C2 would have a similar explanation. At any event, if the figures of *Nerl et al.* are at all representative, there is such a high incidence of half normal levels of C2 and C4

in the population that one must regard the associations with caution until more extensive studies have been performed.

In the case of the HLA-linked loci, the hypothesis that the complement deficiency is acting as a marker gene cannot be rejected; but it becomes difficult to accept for the similar association with complement loci which do not show linkage with HLA, for example, deficiencies of C1, C5 and C8, and in patients with hereditary angio-oedema where the complement component deficiency is secondary.

The third explanation is that the deficiency of complement components itself predisposes to immune complex disease and it is then necessary to enquire into the mechanisms that may be involved.

One possible mechanism has been described by *Miller and Nussenzweig* [14, 15]. These workers have pointed out that complement is required for the solubilisation of immune complexes in serum and for their liberation from receptors on cells. In the absence of a fully functioning complement system, complement-containing immune complexes are held more firmly and for a longer time on cell receptors and this may be instrumental in enhancing their phlogistic activity and perhaps in particular in localising them in the kidney where C3b receptors have been described.

A second possibility is that the immune complex disease is associated with antigens from persisting infections with organisms that do not give rise to overt infective disease. On this view, the complement deficiency is producing a subtle form of immunity deficiency allowing the persistence of organisms that are not obviously pathogenic but, by shedding of antigen, can provoke immune complex disease. There is, at least in New Zealand mice, some suggestion that persistent infection with oncornaviruses is a correlate of the lupus-like disease [12] although more recently doubt has been cast on the causal nature of the association [1]. It is, however, of some interest in this connection that *Welsh et al.* [24] have demonstrated that oncornaviruses can be lysed in human serum in the absence of antibody by a mechanism involving the classical pathway of complement activation. Similarly, it has been demonstrated by *Mills and Cooper* [16] that vesicular stomatitis virus can be destroyed in normal human serum by a complement-dependent pathway also involving a low density lipoprotein.

It has further been demonstrated [8] that cells persistently infected with measles virus can be modulated in the presence of antibody but in the absence of complement so that antigens are no longer presented at the cell membrane and the cells become insusceptible to immune attack. The virus in these cells, however, does replicate and can shed virus into the supernatant fluid. Similarly, it has been shown in the author's laboratory that cells transformed by the EB virus develop the capacity to activate the alternative pathway of complement and this is pictured as a mechanism by which such cells may be eliminated *in vivo* [13]. All these complement-dependent mechanisms would serve to control infections which in the absence of an intact complement system might well persist and give rise to immune complex disease.

This type of explanation remains to be proven in any of the human diseases. It has been shown in one case of human C2 deficiency that structures resembling mycoplasma were present in the circulation of a patient with Henoch-Schönlein purpura [20]. Attempts to demonstrate that patients with complement deficiencies show increased antibody levels to oncornaviruses have so far met with little success although the number of subjects studied has been small [9].

The paradox of the title of this talk has certainly not been resolved. However, there seems little doubt that there is a real association of immune complex disease with complement deficiencies and it seems most likely that this association is a direct consequence of the absence of the complement components. This would suggest firstly, that at any rate the classical pathway of complement is not *necessary* for the generation of immune complex damage. Although it was originally suggested that the patients with C2 deficiency and lupus did not have severe renal disease, this is now known not to be always true [3]. It also shows that some complement-mediated function is necessary for the adequate control of immune complexes. It remains to be seen whether this affects primarily their catabolism or whether complement is involved in the control of infectious antigens whose continued presence in the body may be the essential factor in the induction of these diseases.

References

1 Datta, S. K.; Manny, N.; Andrzejewski, C.; Andre-Schwartz, J., and Schwartz, R. S.: Genetic studies of autoimmunity and retrovirus expression in crosses of New Zealand Black mice. I. Xenotropic virus. J. exp. Med. *147:* 854–871 (1978).

2 Fu, S. M.; Stern, R.; Kunkel, H. G.; Dupont, B.; Hansen, J. A.; Day, N. K.; Good, R. A.; Jersild, C., and Fotino, M.: Mixed lymphocyte culture determinants and C2 deficiency: LD-7A associated with C2 deficiency in four families. J. exp. Med. *142:* 495–506 (1975).

3 Gewurz, A.; Lint, T. F.; Roberts, J. L.: Zeitz, H., and Gewurz, H.: Homozygous C2 deficiency with fulminant lupus erythematosus: severe nephritis via the alternative complement pathway. Arthritis Rheum. *21:* 28–36 (1978).

4 Glass, D.; Raum, D.; Gibson, D.; Stillman, J. S., and Schur, P. H.: Inherited deficiency of the second component of complement. Rheumatic disease associations. J. clin. Invest. *58:* 853–861 (1976)

5 Hässig, A.; Borel, J. F.; Amman, P.; Thoni, M. und Butler, R.: Essentielle Hypokomplementaemie. Path. Microbiol. *27:* 542–547 (1964).

6 Hauptmann, G.; Tongio, M. M.; Grosse-Wilde, H., and Mayer, S.: Linkage between C2 deficiency and the HLA-A10, B18, DW2/BfS haplotype in a French family. Immunogenetics 4: 557–565 (1977).
7 Henson, P. M.: The immunologic release of constituents from neutrophil leukocytes. J. Immun. 107: 1535–1546, 1547–1557 (1971).
8 Joseph, B. S.; Cooper, N. R., and Oldstone, M. B. A.: Immunologic injury of cultured cells infected with measles virus. I. Role of IgG antibody and the alternative complement pathway. J. exp. Med. 141: 761–774 (1975).
9 Kurth, R.; Teich, N., and Lachmann, P. J.: Unpublished observations (1978).
10 Lachmann, P. J.: Unpublished observations (1978).
11 Lachmann, P. J. and Rosen, F. S.: Genetic defects of complement in man. Sem. Immunopath. 1: 339–353 (1978).
12 Levy, J. A.: Xenotropic C-type viruses and autoimmune disease. J. Rheumatol. 2: 135–148 (1975).
13 McConnell, I.; Klein, G.; Lint, T. F., and Lachmann, P. J.: Activation of the alternative complement pathway by human B cell lymphoma lines is associated with Epstein Barr Virus transformation of the cells. Eur. J. Immunol. 9: 339–340 (1979).
14 Miller, G. W. and Nussenzweig, V.: Complement as a regulator of interactions between immune complexes and cell membranes. J. Immun. 113: 464–469 (1974).
15 Miller, G. W. and Nussenzweig, V.: A new complement function: solubilisation of antigen-antibody aggregates. Proc. natn. Acad. Sci. USA 72: 418–422 (1975).
16 Mills, B. J. and Cooper, N. R.: Analysis of the mechanism of VSV inactivation by human serum. J. Immun. (in press).

17 Nerl, Ch.; Grosse-Wilde, H., and Valet, G.: Association of low C2 and C4 serum levels with the HLA-DW2 allele in healthy individuals. J. exp. Med. 148: 204–213 (1978).
18 O'Neill, G. J.; Yan, S. Y., and Dupont, B.: Two HLA-linked genes controlling complement C4. Proc. natn. Acad. Sci. USA 75: 5165–5169 (1978).
19 Stratton, F. S.: Personal commun. (1978).
20 Sussman, M.; Jones, J. H.; Almeida, J. D., and Lachmann, P. J.: Deficiency of the second component of complement associated with anaphylactoid purpura and presence of mycoplasma in the serum. Clin. exp. Immunol. 14: 531–539 (1973).
21 Torisu, M.; Sonozaki, H.; Inai, S., and Arata, M.: Deficiency of the fourth component of complement in man. J. Immun. 104: 728–737 (1970).
22 Trouillas, P. and Betuel, H.: Hypocomplementaemic and normocomplementaemic multiple sclerosis. Genetic determinism and association with specific HLA determinants (B18 and B7). J. neurol. Sci. 32: 425–435 (1977).
23 Turner, M. W.; Mowbray, J. F.; Harvey, B. A. M.; Brostoff, J.; Wells, R. S., and Soothill, J. F.: Defective yeast opsonisation and C2 deficiency in atopic patients. Clin. exp. Immunol. 34: 253–259 (1978).
24 Welsh, R. M.; Jensen, F. C.; Cooper, N. R., and Oldstone, M. B. A.: Inactivation and lysis of oncornaviruses by human serum. Virology 74: 432–440 (1976).
25 WHO: The role of immune complexes in disease. Tech. Rep. Ser. Wld Hlth Org. 606 (1977).

Dr. P. J. Lachmann, MRC Group on Mechanisms in Tumour Immunity, The Medical School, Hills Road, Cambridge (England)

Immunopathology. 6th Int. Convoc. Immunol., Niagara Falls, N.Y., 1978, pp. 280–285 (Karger, Basel 1979)

IgE Antibody Response and the Theoretical Basis of Immunotherapy [1]

Kimishige Ishizaka

The Johns Hopkins University, School of Medicine, Baltimore, Md.

Introduction

The crucial role of IgE antibody in reaginic hypersensitivity and atopic diseases suggests strongly that prevention or suppression of IgE antibody formation is beneficial for atopic patients. In order to achieve this goal, however, one has to understand the mechanisms of IgE antibody response. Extensive studies on the antibody response using several different animal models showed that the IgE antibody response is highly dependent on T cells [2]. It became clear also that precursor B cells of IgE-forming cells are different from those for the other immunoglobulin isotypes. In this presentation, therefore, I would like to summarize briefly the involvement of T and B cells in the IgE antibody response and then discuss some approaches to regulate IgE antibody response.

[1] Supported by Research Grants AI-11202 from US Public Health Service and PCM 74–857 from National Science Foundation. Publication No. 310 from O'Neill Laboratories at the Good Samaritan Hospital.

Precursor B Lymphocytes of IgE-Forming Cells

Previous studies on the surface immunoglobulin on B cells in the mouse showed that virgin B cells bear IgM determinants and that the lymphocytes bearing the other heavy chain determinants are derived from the virgin B cells [7]. This principle is effective in the IgE system as well. Ontogenetic development of IgE-bearing B lymphocytes in the rat shows that IgE-bearing B cells appear in the spleen within 24 h after the birth. These cells are detected in the bone marrow as well, and bear both IgE and IgM determinants [4]. Accumulated evidence indicates that the cells with IgE and IgM surface immunoglobulins ('double bearing' cells) are derived directly from IgM-bearing virgin B cells and that neither antigen nor T cells are involved in the differentiation. It has been shown that IgE-bearing lymphocytes increase in all lymphoid tissues except the thymus following infection of rats with the nematode, *Nippostrongylus brasiliensis* (Nb) [6]. This response was observed even in neonatally thymectomized rats, which failed to form antibodies against hapten-protein conjugates [12]. More recently, we have observed that the conversion of IgM-bearing cells to IgE-IgM-'double-bearing' cells can be achieved by a soluble factor which is derived from mesenteric lymph node cells of the parasite infected rats [13]. Addition of cell-free culture supernatants of the mesenteric lymphnode cells to normal bone marrow cell culture induced a significant increase of IgE-bearing cells. The increase in IgE-bearing cells is not due to passive binding of IgE or its fragments to lymphocytes. The effect of the factor is specific; the factor does not increase the number of either IgM-bearing cells or IgG-bearing cells in the bone marrow culture. It was also found that essentially all IgE-bearing cells appeared in the culture were IgE-IgM 'double bearing' cells [11]. Separate experiments showed that this factor is derived from B cells rather than T cells [14]. It is apparent that IgM-bearing virgin B cells can differentiate into IgM-IgE 'double bearing' cells by a B cell factor without participation of T cells.

Evidence was obtained that IgE-IgM 'double bearing' cells are actually precursors of IgE-forming cells. If one cultures normal mesenteric lymphnode cells with pokeweed mitogen (PWM), both IgM- and IgE-forming

plasma cells developed in the culture within 5 days. Removal of IgE-bearing cells before stimulation with PWM diminished the number of IgE-forming cells, without affecting the development of IgM-forming cells (table I). Since a large proportion of IgE-bearing cells is actually IgE-IgM 'double bearing' cells, removal of IgM-bearing cells was accompanied by a marked decrease of IgE-bearing cells, and diminished both IgM-forming cells and IgE-forming cells developed in the culture (cf. table I). The results indicate that IgE-IgM 'double bearing' cells are already committed to IgE synthesis. Similar experiments were carried out using mesenteric lymphnode cells from Nb-infected animals, and the cell suspensions were cultured with parasite (Nb) antigen to observe the secondary response. The results confirmed that antigen-specific B memory cells for IgE bear surface IgE.

Requirement for T Helper Cells

The differentiation of IgE-bearing cells into IgE-forming cells requires T cells. If one cultures B cell-rich fractions from Nb-infected rats with T cells from either infected or normal rats in the presence of the Nb antigen, IgE-forming cells develop only in the presence of T cells from infected animals. It is apparent that antigen-primed T cells are required for the development of IgE-forming cells from B memory cells. The same principle applies to the polyclonal response of IgE-bearing B cells to PWM. B cells from normal mesenteric lymphnode cells stimulated with PWM do not differentiate to IgE-forming cells in the absence of T cells.

Accumulated evidence in adoptive transfer experiments using high responder mice and *in vitro* culture systems indicate that helper T cells are involved in at least two stages in B cell differentiation. One is the last stage of

Table I. Effect of depletion of IgE-B cells or IgM-B cells on the development of Ig-forming cells

Fractionation[1]	Ig-bearing cells		Ig-forming cells[2]	
	IgE, %	IgM, %	IgE	IgM
Unfractionated	3.5	14.3	50	190
IgE-B cell depletion	0.9	9.7	12	150
IgM-B cell depletion	1.0	1.4	20	60

[1] A mesenteric lymphnode cell suspension was treated with either rabbit anti-IgE or anti-IgM antibody and cell suspensions were placed on tissue culture dishes coated with anti-rabbit IgG. Non-adherent cells were cultured in microplates (2×10^5 cells per well).

[2] The number of Ig-forming cells per 10 wells in which 2×10^6 nucleated cells were cultured.

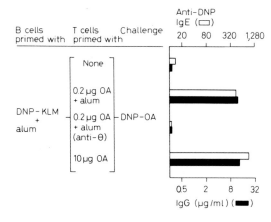

Fig. 1. Adoptive secondary IgE antibody response in irradiated mice. Spleen cells from mice primed with alum-absorbed DNP-KLH were transferred into irradiated syngeneic mice together with spleen cells from either unprimed mice (none) or those primed with ovalbumin, and the recipients were challenged with 10 μg of DNP-OA. Both IgE and IgG anti-hapten antibody responses in the recipients are shown. A portion of spleen cells from mice primed with 0.2 μg alum-absorbed OA were treated with anti-θ antiserum plus C to remove T cells to prove that helper activity of OA-primed cells is associated with T cells.

differentiation in which B memory cells differentiate into IgE-forming cells for secondary IgE antibody response. A representative result of adoptive transfer experiments is shown in figure 1 [1]. Thus, anti-hapten antibody response was not obtained by transfer of spleen cells from DNP-KLH primed mice into irradiated syngeneic mice followed by challenge with DNP-heterologous carrier such as DNP-OA. If one co-transfers OA-primed cells together with DNP-KLH primed B cells, and the recipients are challenged with DNP-OA, a marked IgE anti-DNP antibody response is obtained. As expected, OA-specific helper cells in this system are sensitive to anti-θ-antiserum and complement, indicating that T cells are responsible for helper function.

Another role of helper T cells in the IgE antibody response is their participation in the development of B memory cells committed for IgE. In the experiment shown in table II, two groups of BDF1 mice were immunized with alum-precipitated, urea-denatured antigen, or with the same antigen with-

Table II. Effect of T cells on the development of B memory cells

Carrier priming	Secondary challenge	Anti-DNP response[1]		B memory cells[2]	
		IgE	IgG, μg/ml	IgE	IgG, μg/ml
0.2 μg UD-OA + alum	10 μg DNP-OA	160	12.5	160	10
10 μg UD-OA	10 μg DNP-OA	< 5	0.3	< 5	3.0
None	10 μg DNP-OA	< 5	0	< 5	2.0

[1] IgE antibody titer at 2 weeks, and IgG antibody concentration at 4 weeks after challenge with DNP-OA.
[2] B memory cells in the spleen were determined by adoptive transfer technique. B cell fraction of DNP-OA-immunized mice were obtained at 4 weeks, transferred to irradiated mice together with KLH-primed T cells and the recipients were challenged with DNP-KLH. Numerals represent IgE antibody titer at day 10, and IgG antibody concentration at day 14 in the serum of recipients.

out adjuvant. The reason for using urea-denatured ovalbumin (UD-OA) in this experiment was that the modified antigen can prime T cells specific for native OA but does not prime B cells specific for the major antigenic determinants in the native OA molecules. The primed mice as well as control mice were then immunized with DNP-OA without adjuvant. Under this condition, control mice failed to produce IgE antibody, but the mice primed with alum-absorbed UD-OA formed anti-hapten antibodies. After 4 weeks, these mice were sacrificed and hapten-specific B memory cells in their spleen were assessed by adoptive transfer technique. The results showed that hapten-specific B memory cells for IgE antibody developed in the mice primed with alum-absorbed UD-OA but not in the other two groups. It appears that priming with alum-precipitated carrier enhanced the development of B memory cells committed for IgE. Indeed, the transfer of splenic T cells from the carrier-primed mice also enhanced the development of IgE-B memory cells.

Regulation of IgE Antibody Response by Suppressor T Cells

Both the development of IgE-B memory cells and the differentiation of B memory cells into IgE-forming cells are regulated by antigen-specific suppressor T cells. In previous studies on IgG and IgM antibody responses, most of the antigen-specific suppressor T cells were raised in low responder mice. These cells, however, can be generated even in high responder strains. For example, $B_6D_2F_1$ mice are among the highest responders to OA and produce a high and persistent IgE antibody response when they are immunized with alum-absorbed OA. However, repeated intravenous injections of OA or UD-OA into OA-primed mice induce

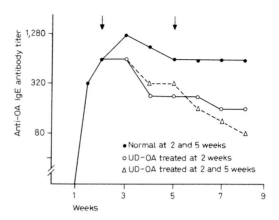

Fig. 2. Depression of ongoing IgE antibody formation by suppressor T cells. All animals were immunized with alum-adsorbed ovalbumin. At 2 weeks, 2×10^7 splenic T cells from normal mice (●) or UD-OA-treated mice (○, △) were transferred. Transfer of either normal (●) or suppressor T cells (△) was repeated at week 5.

the generation of OA-specific suppressor T cells. The splenic T cells from mice treated with urea-denatured antigen suppress primary IgE antibody response of the recipient to alum-absorbed DNP-OA [8]. Suppression of IgE antibody response is specific for carrier; splenic T cells from the UD-OA-treated mice fail to suppress anti-DNP antibody response to DNP-KLH.

Antigen-specific suppressor T cells depress ongoing IgE antibody formation as well [9]. In the experiment shown in figure 2, BDF1 mice were immunized with a minute dose of OA included in alum. After IgE antibody titer reached a maximum, 20 million splenic T cells of UD-OA-treated mice were transferred to the animals. Control mice received normal T cells. IgE antibody titer declined after the transfer of suppressor T cells. Repeated transfer of suppressor T cells further diminished IgE antibody titer. The effect of suppressor T cells on the ongoing IgE formation suggests an important role for suppressor T cells on the regulation of IgE antibody response.

It is well known that IgE-antibody titers in the sera of ragweed-sensitivie patients are persistent, and that the antibody titer increases after the pollen season. It is also known that the major immunological effects of immunotherapy are: (1) an increase of IgG antibody level; (2) gradual decline of IgE antibody level, and (3) suppression of secondary IgE antibody response after pollen seasons [3]. Animal models of the treatment actually reproduced the effect of the treatment. If one gives weekly injections of urea-denatured antigen E or α-polypeptide chain to antigen E-primed mice [5], IgE antibody titer diminished and the treated animals did not show secondary IgE-antibody response to native antigen E [4]. Determination of T helper cells and B memory cells in the treated and untreated mice showed that the treatment depressed helper activity of T cells and prevented the development of B memory cells [10]. When the antigen E-primed mice were treated by weekly injections of native antigen E, B memory cell activity in the treated mice became higher than those in untreated mice. However, helper activity of T cells diminished by the treatment. Thus, the primary effect of repeated injections of antigen is depression of helper activity which account for suppression of secondary IgE antibody response. As already discussed, antigen-specific suppressor T cells are induced by repeated injections of antigen. It appears, therefore, that depression of helper activity by repeated injections of antigen is due to generation of suppressor T cells. If this is actually the mechanism, modification of allergen to tolerogen and the generation of suppressor T cells by changing the schedule of antigen administration would be reasonable approaches to improve the effect of immunotherapy.

References

1 Hamaoka, T.; Katz, D. H., and Benacerraf, B.: Hapten-specific IgE antibody response in mice II. Cooperative interactions between adoptively transferred T and B lymphocytes in the development of IgE responses. J. exp. Med. *138:* 538–556 (1973).

2 Ishizaka, K.: Cellular events in the IgE antibody response. Adv. Immunol. *23:* 1–75 (1976).

3 Ishizaka, K. and Ishizaka, T.: Role of IgE and IgG antibodies in reaginic hypersensitivity in the respiratory tract; in Austen and Lichtenstein, Asthma, physiology, immunopharmacology and treatment, pp. 55–70 (Academic Press, New York 1973).

4 Ishizaka, K.; Ishizaka, T.; Okudaira, H., and Bazin, H.: Ontogeny of IgE-bearing lymphocytes in the rat. J. Immun. *120:* 655–660 (1978).

5 Ishizaka, K.; Okudaira, H., and King, T. P.: Immunogenic properties of modified antigen E. II. Ability of urea-denatured antigen and α-poly-peptide chain to prime T cells specific for antigen E. J. Immun. *114:* 110–115 (1975).

6 Ishizaka, T.; Urban, J. F., jr., and Ishizaka, K.: IgE formation in the rat following infection with *Nippostrongylus brasiliensis*. I. Proliferation and differentiation of IgE-bearing cells. Cell. Immunol. *22:* 248–261 (1976).

7 Lawton, A. R.; Kincade, P. W., and Cooper, M. D.: Sequential expression of germ line genes in development of immunoglobulin class diversity. Fed. Proc. Fed. Am. Socs exp. Biol. *34:* 33–39 (1975).

8 Takatsu, K. and Ishizaka, K.: Reaginic antibody formation in the mouse. VII. Induction of suppressor T cells for IgE and IgG antibody responses. J. Immun. *116:* 1257–1264 (1976).

9 Takatsu, K. and Ishizaka, K.: Reaginic antibody formation in the mouse. VIII. Depression of the ongoing IgE antibody formation by suppressor T cells. J. Immun. *117:* 1211–1218 (1976).

10 Takatsu, K.; Ishizaka, K., and King, T. P.: Immunogenic properties of modified antigen E. III. Effect of repeated injections of modified antigen on immunocompetent cells specific for native antigen. J. Immun. *115:* 1469–1476 (1975).

11 Urban, J. F., jr. and Ishizaka, K.: IgE-B cell generating factor from lymphnode cells of rats infected with *Nippostrongylus brasiliensis*. II. Effector mechanisms of IgE-B cell generating factor. J. Immun. *121:* 199–203 (1978).

12 Urban, J. F., jr.; Ishizaka, T., and Ishizaka, K.: IgE formation in the rat following infection with *Nippostrongylus brasiliensis*. II. Proliferation of IgE-bearing cells in neonatally thymectomized animals. J. Immun. *118:* 1982–1986 (1977).

13 Urban, J. R., jr.; Ishizaka, T., and Ishizaka, K.: IgE formation in the rat following infection with *Nippostrongylus brasiliensis*. III. Soluble factor for the generation of IgE-bearing lymphocytes. J. Immun. *119:* 583–590 (1977).

14 Urban, J. F., jr.; Ishizaka, T., and Ishizaka, K.: IgE-B cell generating factor from lymphnode cells of rats infected with *Nippostrongylus brasiliensis*. I. Source of IgE-B cell generating factor. J. Immun. *121:* 192–198 (1978).

Dr. K. Ishizaka, The Johns Hopkins University, School of Medicine, Baltimore, MD 21239 (USA)

Immunopathology. 6th Int. Convoc. Immunol., Niagara Falls, N.Y., 1978, pp. 286–290 (Karger, Basel 1979)

The Role of IgE Receptors in the Triggering Mechanism of Reaginic Hypersensitivity

Teruko Ishizaka, Kimishige Ishizaka, Daniel H. Conrad and Arnold Froese[1]

The Johns Hopkins University, School of Medicine, Baltimore, Md., and University of Manitoba, Winnipeg

Studies on immunoglobulin E in the past 10 years revealed the mechanisms of reaginic hypersensitivity reactions [6]. It was established that IgE binds to specific receptors on mast cells and basophil granulocytes with a high affinity and the reaction of cell-bound IgE with multivalent antigen induces the release of a variety of chemical mediators [1, 6]. Much evidence supported the idea that bridging of cell-bound IgE molecules or possible interaction of the Fc portion of cell-bound IgE may induce signals for activation of membrane-associated enzymes which initiates mediator release [6]. Recent progress in the studies on cell-bound IgE and receptors for IgE, however, raised another possibility. Since IgE molecules are firmly bound to receptors, bridging of cell-bound IgE molecules probably brings receptor molecules into close proximity. It is conceivable that such local changes in membrane structure or possible interaction between adjacent receptor molecules may induce activation of membrane-associated enzymes. In order to examine this hypothesis, we prepared antibodies against

IgE receptors and studied whether the antibodies could induce mediator release without participation of IgE.

Availability of monoclonal rat IgE [2] and of rat basophilic leukemia (RBL) cells [10] facilitated the preparation of antibodies against IgE receptors [9]. RBL cells were saturated with rat E myeloma protein and their cell membrane was solubilized with 0.5 % Nonidet P-40. The IgE-receptor complexes were precipitated by monospecific rabbit anti-IgE [3], and a rabbit was immunized by repeated injections of the specific precipitates included in complete Freund's adjuvant. Antibodies against RBL cell membrane were specifically purified by using a modification of the method of *Goldschneider and McGregor* [5]. The antiserum was incubated with RBL cells and antibodies bound to the cells were disassociated at acid pH. Purified antibody preparation was then absorbed with mast cell-depleted peritoneal exudate cells. The final preparation (anti-RBL) did not contain a detectable amount of anti-IgE but contained antibodies specific for mast cells. If one treats normal rat peritoneal cells with anti-RBL, followed by fluoresceinated anti-rabbit γ-globulin (anti-RGG), mast cells were selectively stained [9]. Anti-RBL inhibited the binding of ^{125}I-IgE to RBL cells, normal mast cells and solubilized receptors, indicating that anti-RBL contained anti-receptor antibodies [9].

Evidence was obtained that the major antibody in anti-RBL was actually anti-receptor [4]. In the experiment shown in figure 1, surface-labeled RBL cells were solubilized with NP-40 and the solubilized material was incubated with anti-RBL. Analysis of anti-

[1] Supported by Research Grants No. AI-10060 from the US Public Health Service and in part by a grant from Lillia Babbit Hyde Foundation and by the Medical Research Council of Canada. Publication No. 311 from O'Neill Laboratories at the Good Samaritan Hospital.

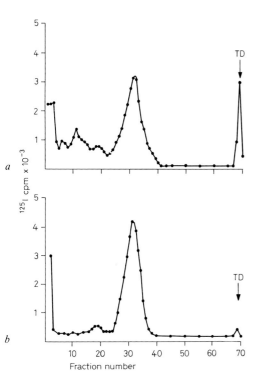

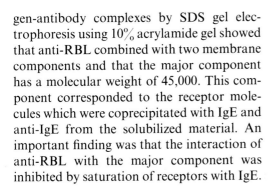

Fig. 1. Comparison of ^{125}I-labeled RBL cell surface components bound by anti-RBL (a) with receptors for IgE (b). *a* An NP-40 extract of surface-labeled RBL cells was incubated with anti-RBL and the antigen-antibody complexes were analyzed by SDS-polyacrylamide gel electrophoresis using 10% polyacrylamide gel (SDA-PAGE). *b* Receptors in the same extract were coprecipitated with IgE and anti-IgE and the complexes were analyzed.

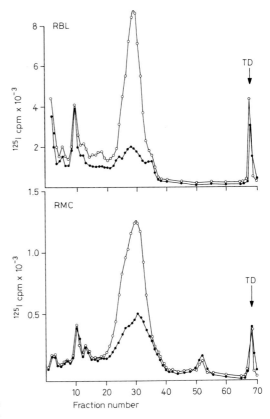

Fig. 2. SDS polyacrylamide gel electrophoresis of RBL cell and purified mast cell (RMC) bound by anti-RBL in the absence and presence of IgE. The NP-40 extract from surface-labeled cells (o) and an extract from those saturated with IgE (•) were incubated with anti-RBL, and the antigen antibody complexes were analyzed by SDS PAGE

gen-antibody complexes by SDS gel electrophoresis using 10% acrylamide gel showed that anti-RBL combined with two membrane components and that the major component has a molecular weight of 45,000. This component corresponded to the receptor molecules which were coprecipitated with IgE and anti-IgE from the solubilized material. An important finding was that the interaction of anti-RBL with the major component was inhibited by saturation of receptors with IgE.

In the experiment shown in figure 2, surface labeled RBL was divided into two parts and one was saturated with IgE. Both preparations were solubilized and each extract was incubated with anti-RBL. Analysis of the antigen-antibody complexes showed that the interaction of anti-RBL with the major component was markedly inhibited by saturation of receptors with IgE. The binding of a minor component with anti-RBL was not affected. Similar results were obtained using normal rat mast cells (fig. 2). The results indicated that the major component is the receptor for IgE, and therefore that the major antibody in our anti-RBL preparation was actually anti-receptor antibody.

In view of these results, we studied the ability of anti-RBL to induce histamine release from normal mast cells. It was found that anti-RBL induced non-cytotoxic histamine release from peritoneal cells as well as purified mast cells of inbred Hooded Lister rats [9]. Furthermore, the histamine release by anti-RBL was inhibited when mast cells were saturated with IgE prior to exposure to anti-RBL. It is apparent that anti-receptor antibodies can induce non-cytotoxic histamine release from normal mast cells without participation of IgE.

As expected, anti-RBL induced immediate skin reactions in normal rats. A 3,200-fold dilution of anti-RBL and a 1,600-fold dilution of anti-IgE gave positive skin reactions [9]. Evidence was obtained that anti-receptor antibody is responsible for the skin reactions by anti-RBL. As reported previously, mast cells in rats infected with *Nippostrongylus brasiliensis* (Nb) are saturated with IgE [8]. Therefore, we tested the skin reactivity of infected rats to anti-IgE and anti-RBL. In the infected rats, a 12,800-fold dilution of anti-IgE gave a positive reaction, whereas a 100- to 200-fold dilution of anti-RBL failed to induce the reaction [9]. In other words, saturation of receptors with IgE increased the sensitivity of the skin to anti-IgE but abolished the reactivity to anti-RBL.

The next question to be asked is whether the bridging of IgE receptors by divalent anti-receptor antibody is essential for the initiation of histamine release. In order to answer this question, anti-RBL was digested by pepsin to obtain $F(ab')_2$ fragments, and a portion of $F(ab')_2$ was reduced and alkylated to prepare Fab′ monomer. The presence of anti-receptor activity in the $F(ab')_2$ and Fab′

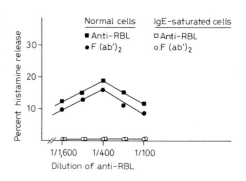

Fig. 3. Histamine release from peritoneal mast cells by the IgG fraction of anti-RBL and its fragments. Anti-RBL was mixed with an 8-fold excess of normal RGG, and mixture was passed through a Sephadex G-200 column to obtain 7S (IgG) fraction. The fraction was digested with pepsin to obtain $F(ab')_2$ fragments. Protein concentration of undigested IgG, $F(ab')_2$ and Fab′ fragments were 5.8, 3.9, and 2.5 mg/ml, respectively.

monomer preparations was confirmed by immunofluorescence and by blocking of IgE-binding to RBL cells and normal mast cells [7]. The $F(ab')_2$ fragments of anti-RBL released a significant amount of histamine from peritoneal mast cells of inbred Hooded Lister rats, whereas Fab′ monomer failed to do so [10]. Representative results of histamine release experiments are illustrated in figure 3. Histamine release by the $F(ab')_2$ and undigested anti-RBL was prevented if peritoneal cells had been saturated with IgE prior to exposure to the antibody.

The $F(ab')_2$ fragments as well as the undigested IgG fraction of anti-RBL induced an immediate skin reaction in normal rats, whereas Fab′ monomer failed to do so [7]. However, the binding of Fab′ monomer to mast cell receptors was demonstrated by the inhibition of the sensitization of normal rat skin with IgE antibodies [10]. In this experiment, Fab′ monomer fragments were injected intracutaneously and the skin sites as well as control sites were sensitized with anti-Nb IgE antibodies 2 h later. The animals were

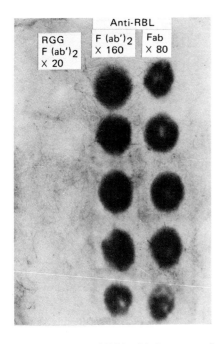

Fig. 4. Reversed PCA with fragments of anti-RBL. Serial dilutions of the F(ab')₂ and Fab' fragments were injected intracutaneously and the animals were challenged by an intravenous injection of goat anti-RGG together with Evans blue 2 h after the sensitization.

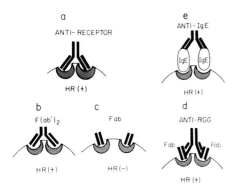

Fig. 5. Schematic models of triggering mechanisms of histamine release by anti-RBL and anti-IgE.

then challenged by Nb antigen 24 h after the sensitization. Skin sites pretreated with the Fab' monomer gave no passive cutaneous anaphylaxis (PCA) reaction, whereas control sites showed clear positive reactions. It appears that the Fab' monomer of anti-RBL bound to receptors on mast cells and blocked the passive sensitization with IgE antibodies.

If the Fab' monomer actually binds to receptors on skin mast cells, one can expect that bridging of cell-bound Fab' monomer by anti-RGG may induce skin reactions. Thus, serial dilutions of the Fab' monomer were injected into normal skin and the animals were challenged with an intravenous injection of anti-RGG 2 h after the sensitization. As shown in figure 4, skin sites receiving Fab' monomer gave positive skin reactions and the sensitizing activity of Fab' monomer was comparable to that of F(ab')₂. Similar experiments were reproduced *in vitro.* If one incubates normal rat peritoneal cells with the Fab' monomer, the sensitized cells released histamine upon exposure to anti-RGG.

These results are summarized schematically in figure 5. Bridging of receptor molecules by divalent anti-receptor or F(ab')₂ induced histamine release without participation of IgE, while the binding of Fab' monomer fragment with the receptor was not sufficient for histamine release. However, if one bridges receptor bound Fab' monomer with divalent anti-RGG, mast cells are triggered. This situation is similar to histamine release induced by anti-IgE in which receptor-bound IgE molecules are bridged by antibody to IgE. One can now visualize that bridging of receptor molecules rather than polymerization of IgE molecules is responsible for triggering mast cells for histamine release.

The new concept of the triggering mechanism does not change the significance of IgE antibodies in reaginic hypersensitivity. In the IgE-mediated reactions, the IgE-receptor serves as an anchor for specific IgE antibody molecules. Thus, receptor-bound IgE molecules permit antigen to bridge adjacent receptor molecules. This, in turn, induces activation of membrane-associated enzymes. Since no immunoglobulins other than IgE will bind with IgE-receptors with high affinity, triggering of histamine release through IgE-receptors will be mediated only by IgE antibodies under physiological conditions.

References

1 Austen, K. F.; Wasserman, S. I., and Goetzl, E. J.: Mast cell derived mediator; structural and functional diversity and regulation of expression; in Johansson, Strandberg and Uvnäs Molecular and biological aspects of the acute allergic reaction, pp. 293–320 (Plenum Publishing, New York 1976).

2 Bazin, H.; Querinjean, P.; Beckers, A.; Heremans, J. F., and Dessy, F.: Transplantable immunoglobulin-secreting tumors in rats. IV. Sixty-three IgE-secreting immunocytoma. Immunology 26: 713–723 (1974).

3 Conrad, D. H. and Froese, A.: Characterization of the target cell receptors for IgE. II. Polyacrylamide gel analysis of the surface IgE receptor from normal rat mast cells and from rat basophilic leukemia cells. J. Immun. 116: 319–326 (1976).

4 Conrad, D. H.; Froese, A.; Ishizaka, T., and Ishizaka, K.: Evidence for antibody activity against the receptor for IgE in a rabbit antiserum prepared against IgE-receptor complexes. J. Immun. 120: 507–512 (1978).

5 Goldschneider, I. and McGregor, D. D.: Anatomical distribution of T and B lymphocytes in the rat. J. exp. Med. 138: 1443–1465 (1973).

6 Ishizaka, T. and Ishizaka, K.: Biology of immunoglobulin E. Molecular basis of reaginic hypersensitivity. Prog. Allergy, vol. 19; pp. 60–121 (Karger, Basel 1975).

7 Ishizaka, T. and Ishizaka, K.: Triggering of histamine release from rat mast cells by divalent antibodies against IgE-receptors. J. Immun. 120: 800–805 (1978).

8 Ishizaka, T.; König, W.; Kurata, M.; Mauser, L., and Ishizaka, K.: Immunological properties of mast cells from rats infected with Nippostrongylus brasiliensis. J. Immun. 115: 1078–1083 (1975).

9 Ishizaka, T.; Chang, T. H.; Taggart, M., and Ishizaka, K.: Histamine release from mast cells by antibodies against rat basophilic leukemia cell membrane. J. Immun. 119: 1589–1596 (1977).

10 Kulczycki, A., jr.; Isersky, C., and Metzger, H.: The interaction of IgE with rat basophilic leukemia cells. I. Evidence for specific binding of IgE. J. exp. Med. 139: 600–616 (1974).

Dr. T. Ishizaka, The Johns Hopkins University, School of Medicine, Baltimore, MD 21239 (USA)

Immunopathology. 6th Int. Convoc. Immunol., Niagara Falls, N.Y., 1978, pp. 291–296 (Karger, Basel 1979)

Inflammation, a Role of the Hageman Factor System

C. G. Cochrane, S. D. Revak, J. H. Griffin and R. Wiggins

Department of Immunopathology, Scripps Clinic and Research Foundation, La Jolla, Calif.

The inflammatory response induced by immunologic reactants is mediated by cellular and humoral factors. One of the humoral systems that is currently being studied is the Hageman factor system. The activated products of this system can lead to a significant number of inflammatory changes as will be shown below. We wish to present the information that is now available on the molecular assembly of the initial components of the system. It is our feeling that the understanding provided by these studies will yield valuable insight into the mechanisms by which these components act *in vivo*.

The initial components of the systems are shown in figure 1. The sequence of protein interactions is the same for components of both human and rabbit plasma. As shown, activation is initiated by the assembly of Hageman factor (HF, clotting factor XII), prekallikrein and high MW kininogen on a negatively charged surface. The reaction is called, therefore, the contact phase in the development of activity of the kinin-forming, intrinsic clotting and fibrinolytic pathway. Activation of the components involves limited proteolytic cleavage which is associated with formation of active proteases with a serine residue in the active site.

The inflammatory activities generated by components of the system include increased vascular permeability (bradykinin, a histidine-rich peptide of high MW kininogen and plasma-cleaved peptides of fibrinogen), smooth muscle contraction and hypotension (bradykinin), chemotaxis of leukocytes (plasmin-generated fragments of fibrinogen and possibly kallikrein), and activation of complement (plasmin). Without doubt, many more links will be found between activated components of the system and the inflammatory response.

The Activation of Hageman Factor

Central to our knowledge of the activation of the system is the mechanism by which HF becomes activated. Work over the past several years has revealed that this activation requires two other molecules acting in concert with HF and that a negatively charged surface augments greatly the reaction. The role of the two additional molecules, prekallikrein and high MW kininogen, will be discussed below. In the presence of a negatively charged surface, HF binds firmly, probably by virtue of positively charged amino acid residues on the heavy chain [16] although these have not yet been identified. It was thought originally that upon binding, the HF molecule underwent a conformational change so as to reveal

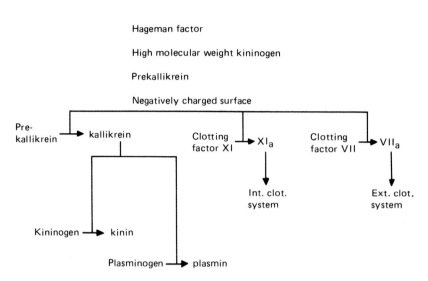

Fig. 1. Protein components of the contact phase of the Hageman factor system.

an enzymatic site. Further studies, however, suggested that this may not be true. The binding of HF to a negatively charged surface does not increase the rate of uptake of [³H] diisopropylphosphofluoridate (DFP) [1, 5, 6]. And in the absence of prekallikrein, HF on the surface and in the presence of other plasma constituents is not readily activated. Nevertheless, the negatively charged surface plays an important role by forming a focus upon which the activating molecules assemble themselves (see below) and also in inducing changes in the HF molecule that make it more sensitive to attack by several activating enzymes [7].

A Role of Kallikrein and High MW Kininogen in the Activation of HF

In the presence of prekallikrein or kallikrein, HF becomes activated [2, 3], a reaction greatly augmented when the HF is bound to a negatively charged surface [7]. A reaction of reciprocal activation is established between prekallikrein and HF on the surface, leading to proteolytic cleavage and activation of both molecules. The initiating event may be provided by the presence of a small amount of either or both HF and prekallikrein in an active form, or by another, as yet unidentified enzyme which contributes the initial cleavage. In any event, the HF and prekallikrein are rapidly cleaved and activated. While it has been shown that kallikrein is markedly active in cleaving HF, it was through the use of prekallikrein-deficient plasma that the requirement of prekallikrein was recognized in the normal, rapid activation of HF [25]. Upon contact with an activating surface, HF in the prekallikrein-deficient plasma activated extremely slowly [9]. Even though it became bound to the surface at a normal rate [17], cleavage of HF in prekallikrein-deficient plasma was much slower than in normal plasma, but was restored to normal upon addition of purified prekallikrein [17].

Prekallikrein activation of surface-bound

HF is greatly augmented by the presence of a cofactor, high MW kininogen. The high MW kininogen serves to stimulate cleavage and activation of HF by kallikrein, and of prekallikrein by activated HF [8, 12]. The high MW kininogen binds prekallikrein [11] and clotting factor XI [21] in plasma so that the molecules circulate in complex form. Upon exposure to a negatively charged surface, prekallikrein and factor XI bind to the surface far more readily in the presence of high MW kininogen [23], suggesting that it is the high MW kininogen that brings the prekallikrein and factor XI to the surface. When binding of the high MW kininogen-prekallikrein complex occurs adjacent to a molecule of HF, proteolytic cleavage and activation of each occurs. The fact that a small, but consistently greater amount of HF becomes bound to the surface in the presence of high MW kininogen may suggest an affinity of the two molecules on the surface [23]. The earliest evidence for a cofactor was obtained by *Shiffman and Lee* [20], and again, the discovery of plasmas deficient in high MW kininogen [4, 19, 25] provided the means by which this molecule was recognized as the important cofactor in the reaction between prekallikrein and HF.

Biologic Importance of the Cleavage of HF at Two Sites by Kallikrein

Cleavage of HF by kallikrein was found to occur predominantly at two positions, immediately adjacent to each other in the polypeptide chain. In each case, a heavy and light chain results, although in 1 case, the molecule remains intact by virtue of a disulfide bridge existing around the cleavage site (fig. 2, site 1). The molecule, when cleaved at site 1, remains bound to the surface, since the light chain is linked to the heavy chain which contains the residues

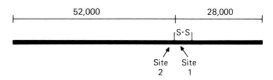

Initial cleavage sites of human Hageman factor during contact activation of plasma

Fig. 2. The structure of Hageman factor. Cleavage sites on the polypeptide chain are noted by arrows. From *Revak et al.* [17].

responsible for binding the molecule to the surface [16]. Cleavage of HF by kallikrein outside of the disulfide loop (fig. 2, site 2) results in release of the active fragment from the surface [16, 17].

Biologic importance has been given to this observation. The fragment released when cleavage occurs at site 2 was found to activate prekallikrein in solution readily, but to activate factor XI poorly or not at all whether the XI was in solution or on a surface [18]. By contrast, the surface-bound HF, cleaved only at site 1, activated both prekallikrein and factor XI readily on the surface. Of interest, kallikrein is rapidly dissociated from the surface while factor XI_a remains surface-bound [18, 23].

Thus, by virtue of dissociation of kallikrein and the 26,000 MW active fragment of HF from the activating surface, a tendency exists for the dissemination of the kinin-generating and fibrinolytic activities of the system. By contrast, activity of the intrinsic clotting system is localized on the surface by virtue of the nearly exclusive activation of factor XI by surface-bound HF_a, and by the slow dissociation of factor XI_a from the surface. The molecular assembly as described above is shown in figure 3.

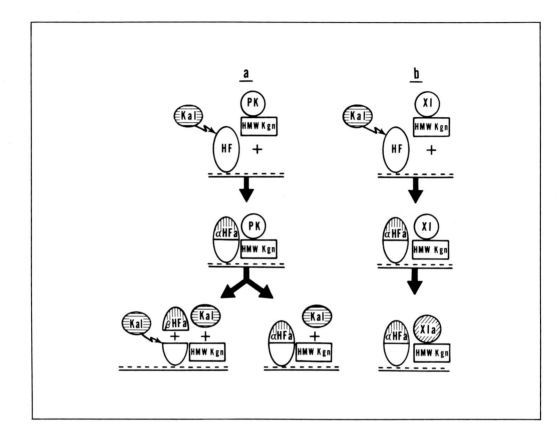

Fig. 3. Molecular model of contact activation of the Hageman factor system. The assembly of molecules is shown in two schemes (a and b), representing alternatives that are observed during activation of the contact system. The surface, bearing negative charges, is shown in each diagram at the bottom. The molecules are labelled as follows: HF = Hageman factor; HF_a = activated Hageman factor; PK = prekallikrein; kal = kallikrein; XI = coagulation factor XI; XI_a = activated XI; HMW Kgn = high MW kininogen. Shaded areas = the activated molecule or light chain of the activated molecule. *a* (top) HF has become bound to the negatively charged surface. The complex of PK and HMW Kgn in solution approaches the negatively charged surface. HF on the surface is susceptible to enzymatic cleavage and activation on the surface as noted by the broken arrow. Kallikrein is the enzyme most often involved in the cleavage of HF in plasma and is therefore designated as the cleaving enzyme. However, other enzymes may also be involved. Although not designated, the kallikrein

acts far more readily when HMW Kgn is bound adjacent to the HF. In the middle and bottom diagrams, HF activated PK to Kal. In the bottom diagrams in *a*, in the first alternative, HF is cleaved at site 2 (fig. 2) to form βHF_a, the 28,000 MW active fragment, which is released into the supernatant. Kal, with low affinity for HMW Kgn, also may be released into the supernatant as shown. In the second alternative at the bottom of *a*, HF is cleaved at site 1 only, i.e. within the disulfide loop (fig. 2), and therefore forms αHF_a which remains bound to the surface. *b* (top) Again HF becomes bound to the surface and is activated by an enzyme, most commonly kallikrein. HMW Kgn with XI bound to it binds to the surface adjacent to HF. In the middle and bottom diagrams, the HF_a in the form of αHF_a cleaved at site 1, then cleaves and activates coagulation factor XI that has been brought to the surface adjacent to the HF by HMW Kgn. Both αHF_a and XI_a remain largely surface-bound.

Activation of the Contact Activation System by Cellular Enzymes

Since proteolytic enzymes are released from cells during immunologic injury, it is of interest to determine if such enzymes could activate components of the HF system. We have recently begun studies of the potential activation of components of the HF system by products of circulating cells and pulmonary cells stimulated by an anaphylactic reaction. The studies were prompted by the observation that rabbits undergoing an IgE-anaphylactic reaction develop abnormalities in their coagulation system [15] and that allergic human beings upon challenge show a fall in high MW kininogen levels [10]. Together with Drs. *Harold Newball* and *Lawrence Lichtenstein*, we have examined the capacity of an enzyme obtained from peripheral leukocytes to cleave and activate HF [14]. The enzyme is obtained from leukocytes of allergic donors after challenge with anti-IgE or sonication, and is isolated by molecular exclusion and ion-exchange chromatography [13]. The enzyme cleaves the HF molecule at site 2 far more rapidly than does plasma kallikrein, yielding fragments of approximately 52,000 and 26,000 MW. A similar although less well studied enzyme has been obtained from washed fragments of human lung after challenge with anti-IgE. Thus, an activator of the HF system is generated during anaphylactic reactions involving human cells and tissues.

Endothelial cells have also been shown to contain an enzyme capable of clearing and activating HF [24]. The importance of this enzyme, which would activate the HF system along a blood vessel wall, may be great.

The importance of such an activation of HF by an anaphylactic reaction will require additional study. But these data offer promise that important relationships may exist between inflammatory cells and this system of plasma proteins.

References

1 Claeys, H. and Collen, D.: Purification and characterization of bovine factor XII. Eur. J. Biochem. *87:* 69–74 (1978).

2 Cochrane, C. G.; Revak, S. D., and Wuepper, K. D.: Activation of Hageman factor in solid and fluid phases. A critical role of kallikrein. J. exp. Med. *138:* 1564–1583 (1973).

3 Cochrane, C. G.; Revak, S. D.; Aikin, B. S., and Wuepper, K. D.: The structural characteristics and activation of Hageman factor, Inflammation: mechanisms and control, pp. 119–138 (Academic Press, New York 1972).

4 Colman, R. W.; Bagdasarian, A.; Talamo, R. C.; Scott, C. F.; Seavey, M.; Guimaraes, J. A.; Pierce, J. V.; Kaplan, A. P., and Weinstein, L.: Williams trait. Human kininogen deficiency with diminished levels of plasminogen proactivator and prekallikrein associated with abnormalities of the Hageman factor-dependent pathways. J. clin. Invest. *56:* 1650–1662 (1975).

5 Fujikawa, K.; Kurachi, K., and Davie, E. W.: Characterization of bovine factor XII$_a$ (activated Hageman factor). Biochem. *16:* 4182–4188 (1977).

6 Griffin, J. H.: Molecular mechanism of surface-dependent activation of Hageman factor (coagulation factor XII) (abstr.). Fed. Proc. Fed. Am. Socs exp. Biol. *36:* 329 (1977).

7 Griffin, J. H.: The role of surface in the surface-dependent activation of Hageman factor (factor XII). Proc. natn. Acad. Sci. USA *75:* 1998–2002 (1978).

8 Griffin, J. H. and Cochrane, C. G.: Mechanisms of involvement of high molecular weight kininogen in surface-dependent reactions of Hageman factor (coagulation factor XII). Proc. natn. Acad. Sci. USA *73:* 2554–2558 (1976).

9 Hathaway, W. E.; Belhasen, L. P., and Hathaway, H. S.: Evidence for a new plasma thromboplastin factor. I. Case report, coagulation studies and physicochemical properties. Blood *26:* 521–532 (1965).

10 Lichtenstein, L. and Kaplan, A.: Personal commun.

11 Mandle, R. J.; Colman, R. W., and Kaplan, A. P.: Identification of prekallikrein and high molecular weight kininogen as a complex in human plasma. Proc. natn. Acad. Sci. USA *73:* 4179–4183 (1976).

12 Meier, H. L.; Pierce, J. V.; Colman, R. W., and Kaplan, A. P.: Activation and function of human Hageman factor. The role of high molecular weight kininogen and prekallikrein. J. clin. Invest. 60: 18–31 (1977).

13 Newball, H.; Talamo, R., and Lichtenstein, L.: Release of leukocyte kallikrein mediated by IgE. Nature, Lond. 254: 635–636 (1975).

14 Newball, H. H.; Revak, S. D.; Cochrane, C. G.; Griffin, J. H., and Lichtenstein, L. M.: Cleavage of Hageman factor (HF) by a basophil kallikrein of anaphylaxis (BK-A) (abstr.). Clin. Res. 26: 519A (1978).

15 Pinckard, R. N.; Tanigawa, C., and Halonen, M.: IgE-induced blood coagulation alterations in the rabbit: consumption of coagulation factors XII, XI, and IX in vivo. J. Immun. 115: 525–532 (1975).

16 Revak, S. D. and Cochrane, C. G.: The relationship of structure and function in human Hageman factor. The association of enzymatic binding activities with separate regions of the molecule. J. clin. Invest. 57: 852–860 (1976).

17 Revak, S. D.; Cochrane, C. G., and Griffin, J. H.: The binding and cleavage characteristics of human Hageman factor during contact activation. A comparison of normal plasma with plasmas deficient in factor XI, prekallikrein, or high molecular weight kininogen. J. clin. Invest. 59: 1167–1175 (1977).

18 Revak, S. D.; Cochrane, C. G.; Bouma, B. N., and Griffin, J. H.: Surface and fluid phase activities of two forms of activated Hageman factor produced during contact activation of plasma. J. exp. Med. 147: 719–729 (1978).

19 Saito, H.; Ratnoff, O. D.; Waldmann, R., and Abraham, J. P.: Fitzgerald trait. Deficiency of a hitherto unrecognized agent, Fitzgerald factor, participating in surface-mediated reactions of clotting, fibrinolysis, generation of kinins, and the property of diluted plasma enhancing vascular permeability (PF/dil). J. clin. Invest. 55: 1082–1089 (1975).

20 Schiffman, S. and Lee, P.: Preparation, characterization and activation of a highly purified factor XI: evidence that a hitherto unrecognized plasma activity participates in the interaction of factors XI and XII. Br. J. Haematol. 27: 101–114 (1974).

21 Thompson, R.; Mandle, R., jr., and Kaplan, A. P.: Association of factor XI and high molecular weight kininogen in human plasma. J. clin. Invest. 60: 1376–1380 (1977)

22 Thompson, R. E.; Mandle, R., jr., and Kaplan, A. P.: Characterization of human HMW-kininogen: procoagulant activity associated with the light chain of kinin-free HMW-kininogen. J. exp. Med. 147: 488–499 (1978).

23 Wiggins, R. C.; Bouma, B. N.; Cochrane, C. G., and Griffin, J. H.: Role of high molecular weight kininogen in surface-binding and activation of coagulation factor XI and prekallikrein. Proc. natn. Acad. Sci. USA 74: 4636–4640 (1977).

24 Wiggins, R. C.; Loskutoff, D. J.; Cochrane, C. G.; Griffin, J. H., and Edgington, R. S.: Activation of Hageman factor by endothelial cells. J. exp. Med. (in press, 1979).

25 Wuepper, K. D.: Prekallikrein deficiency in man. J. exp. Med. 138: 1345–1355 (1973).

26 Wuepper, K. D.; Miller, D. R., and Lacombe, M. J.: Flaujeac trait deficiency of human plasma kininogen. J. clin. Invest. 56: 1663–1672 (1975).

Dr. C. G. Cochrane, Department of Immunology, Scripps Clinic and Research Foundation, 10666 North Torrey Pines Road, La Jolla, CA 92037 (USA)

Immunopathology. 6th Int. Convoc. Immunol., Niagara Falls, N.Y., 1978, pp. 297–301 (Karger, Basel 1979)

Tissue Injury Caused by Cell-Mediated Immunity

J. L. Turk, P. Badenoch-Jones and Marian Ridley

Department of Pathology, Royal College of Surgeons of England, London

Introduction

Many allergic manifestations may be considered as resulting from a spill-over or overproduction of pharmacological mediators produced as part of the mechanism of rejection of foreign antigens. This is particularly so when the antigen is part of an invading microorganism or a proliferating and infiltrating tumour. The release of these mediators in the case of cell-mediated immune processes results in a number of phenomena that together bring about a series of tissue lesions. The reaction in the skin that is characteristically associated with cell-mediated immunity is the delayed hypersensitivity reaction. This is classically an erythematous indurative reaction which may be associated at maximum intensity with tissue necrosis. It is of maximum intensity between 24 and 48 h after intradermal injection of the antigen, or application of a chemical sensitizer to the skin. However, there are many other ways in which cell-mediated immunity can result in damage to tissues as well as the skin. These include rejection of tissue and organ grafts, control of tumours and autoallergic conditions such as experimental allergic thyroiditis and encephalomyelitis in which there is direct damage to the body's own tissues. In addition, cell-mediated immunity can produce local tissue damage by means of the more chronic process of granuloma formation. A granuloma may be considered as an accumulation of cells of the mononuclear phagocyte system (MPS), with or without the addition of other inflammatory cells. In the more acute forms of cell-mediated hypersensitivity reaction, tissue damage is the direct result of changes produced in the vascular system. Thus, there is erythema and oedema which may be both extracellular and intracellular. Tissue necrosis such as that which occurs in the skin graft rejection is also a vascular phenomenon. These tissue changes are probably the result of the release of lymphokines with skin reactive activity (SRF) which could have an effect on vascular permeability and vascular flow either directly or indirectly [3]. It is well known that macrophages accumulate in simple delayed hypersensitivity reactions. However, cell-mediated immunity also is known to contribute to the development of the granulomas of chronic infections such as tuberculoid leprosy and schistosomiasis as well as being involved in the production of fibrosis in chronic inflammatory diseases of the joints such as rheumatoid arthritis.

It is likely that lymphokines are also important in granuloma development. Lymphokines are chemotactic for macrophages which are attracted into the area of inflammation and are inhibited from migrating outwards. They also activate macrophages, increasing their phagocytosis and capacity to kill intracellular organisms. The cells may also take on an appearance resembling that of epithelioid cells. These morphological changes are associated with increased activity in the cells of the hexose monophosphate shunt and of the Krebs cycle. Epithelioid cell transformation of cells of the MPS is a particular feature of chronic inflammatory states produced by cell-mediated immune reactions, associated with a state of delayed hypersensitivity.

Macrophage Activation and Epithelioid Cell Formation

Tissue damage produced by cell-mediated immunity in many cases takes the form of a localised granuloma. In these lesions, cells of the MPS are in many cases transformed into epithelioid cells and multinucleate giant cells. Epithelioid cell granulomas associated with a cell-mediated immune reaction to defined antigens are particularly associated with chronic infections such as tuberculosis, leprosy and schistosomiasis. Similar granulomas can be produced in the skin by exposure to zirconium lactate, a constituent of certain antiperspirant preparations. This has allowed the development of an experimental model of an allergic granuloma in the guinea pig to a skin test with sodium zirconium lactate after a prolonged period of immunization [10]. Animals first develop a typical delayed hypersensitivity lesion which persists for 48 h. Instead of resolving after this time, there is a further increase in skin thickness which reaches its maximum at about 1 week after skin testing. Histologically, the lesions at their peak contain cells of the MPS

resembling epithelioid cells and also multinucleate giant cells. Ultrastructural [11] examination of the lesions shows that the epithelioid-like cells have characteristics similar to those described in zirconium granulomas in man. The association of epithelioid cells and multinucleate giant cells with granulomas that develop on top of established delayed hypersensitivity lesions suggests that these cells may be related to macrophages that have been activated by pharmacological agents of the lymphokine class (fig. 1). In vitro activation of macrophages with lymphokine induces an appearance that under the light microscope gives the impression of movement some way towards epithelioid cell transformation. When macrophages in culture are treated with lymphokine, the immediate effect is for them to round up. This is associated with an inhibition of their ability to migrate out of capillary tubes. After 18–48 h, there is a return to normal morphology. Between 2 and 5 days after the addition of lymphokine, the cells take on what we have called an 'activated' morphology. The cells become larger and contain more cytoplasm and many show long cytoplasmic extensions [4].

During the early stage after contact with lymphokine, there is a decrease in cell wall permeability that parallels the decrease in macrophage mobility. This is associated with a decrease in the surface electrostatic charge. Both the decrease in cell wall permeability and in electrostatic charge can be reversed with agents such as histamine, K^+ and insulin [2]. Activation of macrophages is associated with an increased activity of respiratory enzymes. This especially applies to NADPH oxidase [7, 8]. This enzyme pathway can produce hydrogen peroxide and is related to the peroxide halide bactericidal mechanism that has been demonstrated in polymorphonuclear leucocytes and more recently postulated to reside in exudate macrophages.

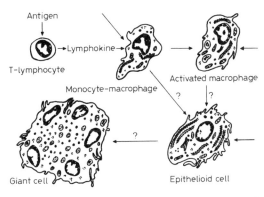

Fig. 1. Diagram showing the possible involvement of lymphokines in the transformation of macrophages to mature epithelioid cells.

The microbiocidal activity of macrophages can also be enhanced by lymphocyte products and it has been postulated that the prime function of lymphokine is to increase the microbiocidal potential of the infected host.

It has been suggested that lymphokines act on the cell membrane via a specific receptor containing α-L-fucose. Lymphokine may then cause an increase in Ca^{++} influx and activation of guanylate cyclase and an increase in cyclic GMP. At the same time, there is a decrease in cyclic AMP. This then leads to tubulin polymerisation and contraction of tubules [6]. An additional finding is that there is a change in the proportion of sulphydryl and disulphide bonds in macrophages after lymphokine activation. Treatment with lymphokine produces a marked increase in disulphide bonds [7].

Macrophage Activation and Fibrosis

Macrophages appear to be part of the body's response to foreign material. They are present in all inflammatory reactions and form the major group of non-specific inflammatory cells in cell-mediated immune reactions, including homograft rejection and reaction to tumours as well as in chronic inflammatory diseases such as tuberculosis and leprosy. As macrophages form the major cell type in granulomas induced by metals and toxic substances such as silica, the question has to be asked as to what is the role of this cell in the final event in such lesions, which may be fibrosis. The first observation is that there is frequently very little fibroblast activation and fibrosis in lesions in which the dominating cell type is the undifferentiated macrophage. Two examples of this are the skin lesion in lepromatous leprosy in man and the lesion induced by the intradermal injection of $Al(OH)_3$ in guinea pigs. In both these conditions, there may be very little evidence of severe scarring despite the presence of visible nodular lesions. Scarring in lepromatous leprosy is either associated with traumatic or infective lesions or with immunological reactions such as erythema nodosum leprosum.

There is little doubt that epithelioid cell transformation can occur in the absence of an immune response, e.g. following a cellophane implant in mice that have been rendered immunologically incompetent by thymectomy and whole body irradiation [5]. One type of non-immunological granuloma associated with an intense fibrogenic effect is that which occurs following the injection of silica. Silica can induce macrophages in a diffusion chamber to produce agents that can stimulate fibroblasts to make collagen [1]. A similar effect on macrophages can also be produced by the soluble products released by specifically sensitized lymphocytes reacting with antigen in a cell-mediated immune reaction. The common factor between silica granulomas and immunological granulomas is the presence of epithelioid cells among other cells of the MPS. A similar granuloma of non-immunological origin is that produced by beryllium. This granuloma also contains epithelioid cells and is associated with intense fibrosis.

Membrane Receptors on Cells of the Mononuclear Phagocyte Series in Relation to Cell-Mediated Immunity

Examination of tissue sections from patients with leprosy and other granulomatous disease has revealed differences in distribution of Fc and C3 receptors on different cell types of the MPS [9]. The technique used was to look for the sticking of EA and EAC to unfixed cryostat sections of the lesions. A sharp distinction could be drawn between undifferentiated macrophages which showed both EA and EAC receptors, while epithelioid cells showed EAC only (table I). In leprosy, EAC was heaviest at the tuberculoid end of the spectrum where cell-mediated immunity is highest, with a gradual diminution towards the lepromatous end of the spectrum where there is a specific failure of cell-mediated immunity. In sarcoidosis, there was also marked EAC adherence but no EA adherence to epithelioid cells, as in the reactional form of borderline tuberculoid leprosy. Macrophages of patients with lepromatous leprosy that had phagocytosed large numbers of bacilli were found to have completely lost their ability to bind EAC.

The reason why epithelioid cells lack EA receptors that are present on other cells of the MPS is not so far understood. Experiments are at the present time in progress to see whether these changes might also be induced in macrophages *in vitro*. Knowledge of the mechanism of loss of Fc receptors under these conditions could give more insight into the basis of tissue reactions in cell-mediated immune reactions. The loss of EAC receptors in undifferentiated macrophages packed with bacilli at the lepromatous end of the leprosy spectrum could be due to the C3 receptors being modified as a result of an intracellular activation of C3 by mycobacterial antigen through either the classical or the alternative pathway.

Table I. Membrane receptors on mononuclear phagocytes in tissue sections across the spectrum in leprosy

Test system	Leprosy spectrum				
	TT	BT	BB	BL	LL
EA	−	±	+ +	+ + +	+ +
EAC	+ + +	+ + +	+ +	+ +	±

Summary

The role of cells of the mononuclear phagocyte system in tissue injury at the sites of cell-mediated immunity is discussed. The effects of locally generated lymphokines on the activation of macrophages and their possible transformation to epithelioid cells is emphasised, together with the involvement of macrophages in fibrosis. Recent work, in this department, on membrane receptors of macrophages and epithelioid cells both *in vivo* and *in vitro* is described.

References

1 Allison, A. C.; Clark, I. A., and Davies, P.: Cellular interactions in fibrogenesis. Ann. rheum. Dis. *36:* 8–13 (1977).
2 Diengdoh, J. V. and Turk, J. L.: Cytochemical studies on the effect of antigen on peritoneal exudate cells from guinea pigs with delayed hypersensitivity. Int. Archs Allergy appl. Immun. *31:* 261–273 (1967).
3 Maillard, J. L.; Pick, E., and Turk, J. L.: Interaction between sensitised lymphocytes and antigen *in vitro*. V. Vascular permeability induced by skin-reactive factor. Int. Archs Allergy appl. Immun. *42:* 50–67 (1972).
4 Nath, I.; Poulter, L. W., and Turk, J. L.: Effects of lymphocyte mediators on macrophages *in vitro*. Clin. exp. Immunol. *13:* 455–466 (1973).
5 Papadimitriou, I. M. and Spector, W. G.: The origin, properties and fate of epithelioid cells. J. Path. *105:* 187–203 (1971).
6 Pick, E.: Lymphokines: physiologic control and pharmacological modulation of their production and action; in Hadden, Coffey and Spreafico, Immunopharmacology, pp. 164–202 (Plenum Publishing, New York 1977).

7 Poulter, L. W. and Turk, J. L.: Studies on the effect of soluble lymphocyte products (lymphokines) on macrophage physiology. I. Early changes in enzyme activity and permeability. Cell. Immunol. *20:* 12–24 (1975).

8 Poulter, L. W. and Turk, J. L.: Studies on the effect of soluble lymphocyte products on macrophage physiology. II. Cytochemical changes associated with activation. Cell. Immunol. *20:* 25–32 (1975).

9 Ridley, M. J.; Ridley, D. S., and Turk, J. L.: Surface markers on lymphocytes and cells of the mononuclear phagocyte series in skin sections in leprosy. J. Path. *125:* 91–98 (1978).

10 Turk, J. L. and Parker, D.: Sensitization with Cr, Ni and Zr salts and allergic type granuloma formation in the guinea pig. J. invest. Derm. *63:* 341–345 (1977).

11 Turk, J. L.; Badenoch-Jones, P., and Parker, D.: Ultrastructural observations on epithelioid cell granulomas induced by Zr in the guinea pig. J. Path. *124:* 45–49 (1978).

Dr. J. L. Turk, Department of Pathology, Royal College of Surgeons of England, Lincoln's Inn Fields, London WC2A 3PN (England)

Immunopathology. 6th Int. Convoc. Immunol., Niagara Falls, N.Y., 1978, pp. 302–307 (Karger, Basel 1979)

Biochemical Studies of Guinea Pig Lymphotoxin

Manfred M. Mayer, Maurice K. Gately and Mitsuhiro Okamoto

Department of Microbiology, The Johns Hopkins University, School of Medicine, Baltimore, Md., Department of Pathology, Harvard Medical School, Boston, Mass., and Department of Biochemistry II, Toyama Medical and Pharmaceutical University, Medical School, Sugitana, Toyama

Interest in the role of lymphokines as mediators of cellular immunity is currently in a phase of rapid growth. We have been especially interested in one of these mediators, lymphotoxin (LT), which may participate in cell-mediated cytotoxicity. At the beginning of our work, about 10 years ago, LT was known only as a cytotoxic activity that is released by immune lymphocytes when treated with specific antigen. It was not known whether this cytotoxic activity is attributable to a single substance or whether several factors are involved. Nor was it known whether LT is a cooperative cytotoxic system like complement. Also unknown was its mechanism of action and its role, if any, in cellular immunity and allergy.

The present article is an excerpted account of our physicochemical studies and subsequent biological investigations which we undertook to answer these questions. A full review has been presented by *Gately and Mayer* [10].

Development of a Biological Assay

Before initiating physicochemical and biological studies, it was necessary to develop a convenient, efficient, precise and reliable method of assay and to characterize the dose-response relationship accurately. We have used a Coulter Counter Microassay to quantitate LT activity against L cells. All samples were assayed at least in triplicate, and the standard deviation for replicate wells was routinely within 15% of the mean. A unit of LT activity is defined on the basis of the amount of LT present in a standard LT preparation. One unit of activity usually produces approximately a 50% reduction in cell count under conditions of our microassay. In each experiment, several dilutions of the standard LT preparation were assayed, and the results were used to construct a dose-response curve. The shape of this curve is entirely concave to the abscissa. The number of units of LT activity in each experimental sample at the dilution tested was then interpolated from this curve [8].

Physical and Chemical Properties

With the aid of the quantitative assay, the sedimentation rate, diffusion rate and buoyant density were measured precisely: from these data, the molecular dimensions were calculated. These measurements serve to identify the LT activity as a substance in terms of its physical properties.

The apparent $S_{20,w}$ of guinea pig LT was

estimated to be 4.2 ± 0.1 S by sucrose density gradient ultracentrifugation. The $D_{20,w}$ was estimated by gel filtration on Sephadex G-100 to be $(8.0 \pm 0.2) \times 10^{-7}$ cm^2/sec. The buoyant density was determined to be 1.302 ± 0.002 g/ml by CsCl isopycnic ultracentrifugation. From these values, the molecular weight of guinea pig LT was calculated to be 45,000, and the frictional ratio was calculated to be 1.1. No evidence was found to indicate that more than a single factor was involved in producing the cytotoxic effect attributed to LT [8].

Purification

Fractionation experiments had to be designed in such a way that a high resolution analysis could be made of the distribution of the active principle in chromatographic or electrophoretic patterns. Careful quantitative accounting of the recovery of lymphotoxin was an important part of the experimental design because in the event of serious loss during the process of purification, the possibility had to be considered that the biological activity in question is mediated cooperatively by two or more factors, as is the case in the complement system. For the same reason, the dose-response curve had to be reassessed as purification proceeded.

The initial objective of this work was the preparation of LT in a state of 'functional' purity, which means freedom from contamination by the other lymphokines in the crude starting material. Isolation in a chemically pure state had to be deferred for lack of the required large quantities of starting material. It was thought that 'functionally' purified preparations would be suitable for initial studies of the mode of action of lymphotoxin and of its role in cell-mediated cytotoxicity.

The functionally purified LT used in our work was made by sequential use of Pevikon block electrophoresis, DEAE-cellulose ion exchange chromatography, and polyacrylamide disc gel electrophoresis [7].

Neutralization by Specific Antibody

Specific immune inhibition offers a valuable tool for characterization by defining the immunodeterminants of LT as a substance. The choice of neutralization tests was based on the assumption that LT would not soon become available in chemically pure form, which is a requirement for most other immunologic tests, such as immunoelectrophoresis.

We have used antigen-induced guinea pig LT which had been partially purified as indicated above to produce an anti-LT serum in rabbits. Anti-LT activity was assayed on the basis of its ability to neutralize the cytotoxic activity of LT. The anti-LT serum was capable of neutralizing all of the cytotoxic activity present in the unfractionated fluids from cultures of antigen-stimulated immune lymph node cells. In addition, it neutralized Con A-induced guinea pig LT [7] and mitogenic factor-induced guinea pig LT [6] with essentially equal efficiency as antigen-induced LT. This indicated these three lymphotoxins to be antigencially similar, and perhaps identical. In contrast, the anti-LT serum did not neutralize guinea pig mitogenic factor or guinea pig MIF [7], suggesting that these two factors are antigenically distinct from guinea pig LT.

Using a radioactive double labelling technique, Sorg and Geczy [18] demonstrated that the anti-guinea pig lymphokine serum of Geczy et al. [11], which is known to contain anti-MIF antibody, reacted primarily with three newly synthesized products of activated lymphocytes. One of the molecules possessed the same molecular weight and pI as had previously been demonstrated for MIF [17]. In similar studies in which they examined the specificity of our anti-LT serum, *Sorg et al.* [19] found that the anti-LT serum reacted with only a single newly synthesized lymphocyte activation product, and this molecule was different from any of the three molecules recognized by the anti-lymphokine serum of *Geczy*. These results support the conclusion that our anti-LT serum does not react with MIF and, in addition, indicate the anti-LT to be highly specific.

Role of Lymphotoxin in Cell-Mediated Cytotoxicity

It has been proposed that lymphotoxin is the mediator of direct T cell-dependent cytolysis [4]. In collaboration with Dr. *Christopher Henney*, we tested this hypothesis by examining the effect of our anti-LT serum on lymphotocyte-mediated cytolysis [9]. In these experiments, the anti-LT serum, which contained neither detectable anti-lymphoċyte nor detectable anti-ovalbumin antibodies, inhibited the lysis of strain 2 guinea pig hepatoma cells incubated with ovalbumin-immune guinea pig spleen cells plus soluble ovalbumin. Likewise, it inhibited the lysis observed when ovalbumin-immune spleen cells were incubated with hepatoma cells to which ovalbumin had been covalently coupled. In contrast, in a system analogous to murine systems in which the effector cell has been identified as a T cell [2], the anti-LT did not inhibit lysis of strain 2 hepatoma cells by alloimmune Hartley or strain 13 guinea pig spleen cells. It cannot be completely excluded that lack of inhibition of cytolysis in the allogeneic system was due to failure of the anti-LT to gain access to the site of lymphocyte-target cell contact at which LT was released locally and, possibly trans-

ferred directly to the target cell. However, the observation that anti-LT did inhibit lysis of ovalbumin-coupled hepatoma cells by ovalbumin-immune spleen cells makes this possibility less likely. These observations are presented graphically in figure 1. Thus, our

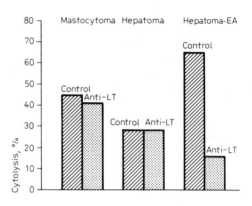

Fig. 1. Effect of anti-lymphotoxin serum on cell-mediated cytolysis. The experiment marked 'mastocytoma' refers to cytolysis of mouse mastocytoma cells by mastocytoma-immune guinea pig spleen cells. Hartley guinea pigs were immunized i.p. with 10^8 P815 mouse mastocytoma cells and spleen cells harvested 10 days later. The ratio of spleen cells to target cells was 100 : 1. ^{51}Cr release was measured after incubation for 4 h. ^{51}Cr release in the presence of normal Hartley spleen cells was 2.7%/h. Hypotonic release was 80%. The experiment marked 'hepatoma' refers to cytolysis of guinea pig hepatoma cells by hepatoma-immune spleen cells. Guinea pigs were immunized i.p. with 3×10^7 hepatoma cells and effector cells harvested 10 days later. The ratio of spleen cells to target cells was 100 : 1 and the incubation time was 4 h. Percentage of ^{51}Cr release in the presence of normal spleen cells varied between 8.7 and 10.0%. Hypotonic lysis released $80.4 \pm 8\%$ of total cell-associated ^{51}Cr. The experiment labeled 'hepatoma-EA' refers to cytolysis of ovalbumin-coupled guinea pig hepatoma cells by ovalbumin immune spleen cells. Hartley spleen cells were obtained 10 days after immunization with 500 µg of ovalbumin in complete Freund's adjuvant into the rear foot pads. The ratio of spleen cells to target cells in the assays was 100 : 1. ^{51}Cr release was assayed after incubation of the spleen cells with ovalbumin-coupled hepatoma cells for 20 h. Percentage of ^{51}Cr release in the presence of normal spleen cells without added rabbit serum was 35.4%. Hypotonic lysis yielded 81% of total cell-associated ^{51}Cr.

experiments provided no evidence that the mechanism of direct T cell-mediated cytolysis involves LT. Rather, the results suggested that there are at least two distinct pathways by which immune lymphocytes can destroy target cells *in vitro*—one which involves secretion of a nonspecific soluble factor, i.e. lymphotoxin, and another which probably requires intimate contact between the plasma membranes of the target and killer cells. As discussed by one of us in a recent review [13], this latter type of mechanism may involve formation of trans-membrane channels in the target cell by insertion of lymphocyte-derived peptides. Further investigation is required to determine under what circumstances and to what extent the LT and the 'intimate membrane contact' mechanisms are operative *in vivo*.

Mechanism of Action of Lymphotoxin

We have studied the effect of various pharmacologic agents on lysis of L cells by guinea pig lymphotoxin in the hope that analyses of the effects of such compounds would provide insight into the biochemical mechanism of cell destruction [14]. Among the many drugs tested, only those that affect plasma membrane functions were found to interfere with the cytolytic action of LT. Dimethyl sulfoxide or lidocaine potentiated L cell resistance against lysis. Stronger protection was provided by ouabain. Addition of ouabain to cells previously injured by LT was also effective in reducing cell death.

In contrast to reports that human lymphotoxin affects RNA [16] and DNA [20] synthesis, we were unable to detect metabolic disturbances in cells before lysis by guinea pig lymphotoxin. The biosynthetic rate of DNA, RNA or protein and the total cellular content of ATP were not significantly changed in guinea pig LT-treated cells [14].

These results suggested that guinea pig LT primarily attacks and disturbs some plasma membrane functions of the target cell, perhaps ionic transport systems, and consequently induces ionic imbalances between the intra- and extracellular milieu which eventually cause cell death.

The nature of these imbalances was explored in a subsequent study [15]. It was found that exogenous addition of $CaCl_2$, but not KCl or NaCl, inhibited the cytotoxic action of LT. Cellular uptake rates of $^{45}Ca^{++}$, but not $^{86}Rb^+$, increased in guinea pig LT-damaged L cells. We were able to show that the factor responsible for increasing the $^{45}Ca^{++}$ uptake rate cochromatographs on a hydroxyapatite column with the cytotoxic activity of LT. Furthermore, we found that ouabain prevented the guinea pig LT-mediated lysis and concomitantly, depressed the guinea pig LT-induced increase of the $^{45}Ca^{++}$ uptake rate.

In control experiments, it was found that addition of guinea pig LT to an LT-resistant L cell mutant affected neither the $^{45}Ca^{++}$ uptake rate nor the viability. This observation further links the cytotoxic activity of LT with its effect on Ca^{++} transport.

On the basis of these observations, two hypotheses were proposed for the mechanism of LT action. According to the first hypothesis, the observed increase of the $^{45}Ca^{++}$ uptake rate during LT action could indicate a failure of the Ca^{++} extruding mechanism. The second hypothesis postulates that LT affects the influx of Ca^{++}, which is ordinarily considered to be a passive process depending on the chemical gradient between the outside and the inside of the cell.

Calcium ion is involved in a wide variety of important processes including cell-cell interactions, membrane transport and cellular proliferation [1, 3, 5]. Hence in a healthy cell, optimal concentrations of calcium are required for a number of intracellular metabolic pathways, and there is little doubt that the cell would be destroyed if the regulatory system of intracellular calcium were sufficiently damaged. From these considerations, the accumulation of calcium resulting from an increase of $^{45}Ca^{++}$ uptake rate observed in our studies might be enough to cause the eventual L cell destruction. Indeed, calcium accumulation in a cell has been proposed to contribute significantly to glucocorticoid-induced lymphocytolysis [12].

While the control experiments with LT-resistant L cells indicate an intimate relationship between the cytotoxic action of LT and its capacity to increase the $^{45}Ca^{++}$ uptake rate, it is not known yet whether this represents a primary or a secondary phenomenon. The primary action of LT on L cells may be a not yet understood biochemical event which would secondarily cause the disturbance of calcium equilibrium. Since we have not observed a significant increase of $^{45}Ca^{++}$ uptake rate during the lag phase of LT action, it is possible that the effect on Ca^{++} transport is secondary. Furthermore, it has to be recalled that the LT preparations used in our studies were not purified to homogeneity. Therefore, there remains a possibility that the increase of $^{45}Ca^{++}$ uptake rate in L cells might be induced by some contaminant.

References

1 Balk, S. D.: Calcium as a regulator of the proliferation of normal but not of transformed, chicken fibroblasts in a plasma-containing medium. Proc. natl. Acad. Sci. USA 68: 271–275 (1971).

2 Cerottini, J. C.; Nordin, A. A., and Brunner, K. T.: Specific in vitro cytotoxicity of thymus-derived lymphocytes sensitized to alloantigens. Nature, Lond. 228: 1308–1309 (1970).

3 Clausen, T.; Elbrink, J., and Dahl-Hansen, A. B.: The relationship between the transport of glucose and cations across cell membranes in isolated tissues.

IX. The role of cellular calcium in the activation of the glucose transport system in rat soleus muscle. Biochim. biophys. Acta 375: 292–308 (1975).

4 Daynes, R. A. and Granger, G. A.: The regulation of lymphotoxin release from stimulated human lymphocyte cultures: the requirement for continual mitogen stimulation. Cell. Immunol. 12: 252–262 (1974).

5 Gail, M. H.; Boone, C. W., and Thompson, C. S.: A calcium requirement for fibroblast motility and proliferation. Expl Cell Res. 79: 386–390 (1973).

6 Gately, C. L.; Gately, M. K., and Mayer, M. M.: Separation of lymphocyte mitogen from lymphotoxin and experiments on the production of lymphotoxin by lymphoid cells stimulated with the partially purified mitogen; a possible amplification mechanism of cellular immunity and allergy. J. Immun. 116: 669–675 (1976).

7 Gately, M. K.; Gately, C. L.; Henney, C. S., and Mayer, M. M.: Studies on lymphokines: the production of antibody to guinea pig lymphotoxin and its use to distinguish lymphotoxin from migration inhibitory factor and mitogenic factor. J. Immun. 115: 817–826 (1975).

8 Gately, M. K. and Mayer, M. M.: The molecular dimensions of guinea pig lymphotoxin. J. Immun. 112: 168–177 (1974).

9 Gately, M. K.; Mayer, M. M., and Henney, C. S.: Effect of anti-lymphotoxin on cell-mediated cytotoxicity. Evidence for two pathways, one involving lymphotoxin and the other requiring intimate contact between the plasma membranes of killer and target cells. Cell. Immunol. 27: 82–93 (1976).

10 Gately, M. K. and Mayer, M. M.: Purification and characterization of lymphokines: an approach to the study of molecular mechanisms of cell-mediated immunity. Prog. Allergy, vol. 25, pp. 106–162 (Karger, Basel 1978).

11 Geczy, C. L.; Friedrich, W., and Weck, A. L. de: Production and in vivo effect of antibodies against guinea pig lymphotoxin. Cell. Immunol. 19: 65–77 (1975).

12 Kaiser, N. and Edelman, I. S.: Calcium dependence of glucocorticoid-induced lymphocytolysis. Proc. natn. Acad. Sci. USA 74: 638–642 (1977).

13 Mayer, M. M.: Mechanism of cytolysis by lymphocytes: a comparison with complement. J. Immun. 119: 1195–1203 (1977).

14 Okamoto, M. and Mayer, M. M.: Studies on the mechanism of action of guinea pig lymphotoxin. I. Membrane-acfive substances prevent target cell lysis by lymphotoxin. J. Immun. 120: 272–278 (1978).

15 Okamoto, M. and Mayer, M. M.: Studies on the mechanism of action of guinea pig lymphotoxin. II.

Increase of calcium uptake rate in LT-damaged target cells. J. Immun. *120:* 279–285 (1978).

16 Rosenau, W.; Goldberg, M. L., and Burke, G. C.: Early biochemical alterations induced by lymphotoxin in target cells. J. Immun. *111:* 1128–1135 (1973).

17 Sorg, C. and Bloom, B. R.: Products of activated lymphocytes. I. The use of radiolabeling techniques in the characterization and partial purification of the migration inhibitory factor of the guinea pig. J. exp. Med. *137:* 148–170 (1973).

18 Sorg, C. and Geczy, C. L.: Antibodies to guinea pig lymphokines. III. Reactions with radiolabeled lymphocyte activation products. Eur. J. Immunol. *6:* 688–693 (1976).

19 Sorg, C.; Geczy, C. L.; Geczy, A. F.; Hämmerling, G. J., and Gately, M.: Evidence that Ia-antigens are not secreted by antigen or mitogen-stimulated mouse or guinea pig lymphocytes (submitted for publication).

20 Williams, T. W. and Granger, G. A.: Lymphocyte *in vitro* cytotoxicity: mechanism of human lymphotoxin-induced target cell destruction. Cell. Immunol. *6:* 171–185 (1973).

Dr. M. M. Mayer, Department of Microbiology,
The Johns Hopkins University, School of Medicine,
Baltimore, MD 21205 (USA)

Immunopathology. 6th Int. Convoc. Immunol., Niagara Falls, N.Y., 1978, pp. 308–310 (Karger, Basel 1979)

Redistribution of Surface Immunoglobulin of Lymphocytes
Mechanisms and Function

Emil R. Unanue

Department of Pathology, Harvard Medical School, Boston, Mass.

The first event that takes place in B cells is the redistribution of surface Ig-ligand complexes [7]. Capping involves the selected segregation of the complexes to one area of the cell surface. It takes place extremely fast, within the first 5–10 min after ligand binding [2, 5]. Capping requires a cross-linking ligand and is energy dependent. Two major questions have been addressed by those studying this phenomenon. What is the mechanism of Ig capping? What is its function? The mechanisms of capping are of great interest to establish since it is a phenomenon in which the surface complexes interact directly or indirectly with the cytoplasm and in which both cytoplasm and membrane reciprocally influence each other. Capping of surface Ig is an expression of the activation of the cell's contractile proteins [6]. This becomes evident when the reaction is closely examined. Capping of Ig complexes takes place within a few minutes after the ligand (antigen or anti-Ig) binds to the membrane. The small microclusters of complexes rapidly flow in a highly coordinated process to one pole of the cell. The rate of Ig complexes during capping is extremely fast and has been estimated to be about 10^{-8} cm^2 sec^{-1}, which is comparable to the rate of flow of lipids and somewhat faster than that estimated for proteins that are not cross-linked by a ligand

[5]. At the time that Ig complexes are redistributing, cytoplasmic actin and myosin also become concentrated to the area of the cap [6]. The coordination between the capping of Ig and the redistribution of cytoplasmic myosin is impressive. Seconds after the cap has formed, an area of constriction develops around it; and at the same time, small ruffles appear on the membrane, always opposite the cap. The small ruffles also contain contractile proteins. This is the stage of translatory motion in which the lymphocyte, if attached to a substratum, now moves at random. The point to emphasize is that ligand-surface Ig interaction stimulates translatory motion in B cells [8]. Indeed, we have found that B lymphocytes can move chemotactically to a gradient of molecules of anti-Ig antibodies [9].

How do the membrane-bound complexes of ligand-surface Ig interact with contractile proteins? The answers are not available. We have hypothesized that the interaction between both may be through some physical linkage perhaps involving a transmembrane protein [2, 6]. So far, the only structure on the membrane which is known to interact with surface Ig is the Fc receptor. This association was found during capping of Ig where the Fc receptor cocaps with it [1, 4]. The reverse is not true, however: capping of

Fc receptors does not cocap surface Ig. Whether the Fc receptor is the transmembrane protein remains speculative.

Experiments using drugs have given clues on how the Ig-contractile protein association may take place. Two drugs that we have used are the Ca^{2+} ionophore A23187 and the local anesthetics. Ca^{2+} ionophores interact with the membrane and induce a flow of extracellular Ca^{2+} into the cell. The local anesthetics are lipophilic chemicals that bind to acidic phospholipids and can displace membrane-bound Ca^{2+}. Both drugs stop formation of Ig caps. Most interestingly, their addition to B cells after caps have formed results in the breaking of the cap. The complexes then disperse as small clusters over the entire surface. At the time the complexes disperse, myosin no longer remains concentrated under the area of the cap. Other observations suggest that the mode of action of both drugs may be different. The dissolution of the cap by the ionophore can be stopped by drugs that affect energy metabolism; these same drugs have no effect on the cap disruption produced by the anesthetic. We have speculated that the Ca^{2+} ionophore, by increasing intracellular Ca^{2+}, results in a systemic activation of the contractile proteins that interfere with the discrete segmental activation during formation and maintenance of the cap. Indeed, cells treated with ionophore show myosin in large, irregular patches. In contrast, our speculation is that the anesthetics may sever the association between surface complexes and the actin-myosin network, which then allows the surface complexes to freely diffuse throughout the membrane [5].

Recent studies by *Braun et al.* [2, 3] have compared capping of various macromolecules in lymphocytes. Our conclusion is that, although all molecules redistribute, there are marked differences among them insofar as kinetics, number of ligands required to induce the reaction, and changes in translatory motion. Ig is the typical example of the molecule that caps fast, while H-2 antigens are molecules that cap slowly and which require two ligands (an antibody to H-2 plus an antibody to the anti-H-2 antibody). The fast capping of some molecules like Ig results, in our view, from the direct or indirect association of the surface complexes with the cell's contractile protein, which will contribute to the reorganization of the surface complexes. The slow capping of other molecules results from the progressive coalescence with time of complexes of increasing size. These complexes are not associated with the cytoplasm. In fact, translatory motion is not triggered by this set of ligands (like H 2); and the ionophores or the anesthetics do not affect their capping. Hence, these drugs clearly separate the two sets of fast and slow capping molecules. Table I compares capping of Ig and H-2 antigens.

In summary, in our view, interaction of surface Ig with a ligand triggers the activation of the contractile elements which serve to organize the membrane and give polarization and orientation to the cell. This step of increased motility in B cells may be crucial in the cellular reorganization taking place in a lymphoid structure at the time of antigen stimulation.

Table I. Comparison of capping of Ig and H-2

	Ig	H-2
Kinetics	fast	slow
Need for two ligands	no	yes
Co-segregation of myosin	yes	no
Stimulation of motility	yes	no
Effect of anesthetics	inhibit capping, break caps	do not inhibit or break caps

References

1 Abbas, A. K. and Unanue, E. R.: Interrelationship of surface immunoglobulin and Fc receptors on mouse B lymphocytes. J. Immun. *115:* 1665–1670 (1975).

2 Braun, J.; Fujiwara, K.; Pollard, T. D., and Unanue, E. R.: Two distinct mechanisms for redistribution of lymphocyte surface macromolecules—contrasting effects of local anesthetics and a calcium ionophore. J. Cell Biol. *79:* 409–418 (1978).

3 Braun, J.; Fujiwara, K.; Pollard, T. D., and Unanue, E. R.: Two distinct mechanisms for redistribution of lymphocyte surface macromolecules—relationship to cytoplasmic myosin. J. Cell Biol. *79:* 419–426 (1978).

4 Forni, L. and Pernis, B.: Interactions between Fc receptors and membrane immunoglobulins on B lymphocytes; in Seligmann, Membrane receptors of lymphocytes, pp. 193–196 (North-Holland, Amsterdam 1975).

5 Schreiner, G. F. and Unanue, E. R.: Capping of the lymphocyte: models for membrane reorganization. J. Immun. *119:* 1549–1551 (1977).

6 Schreiner, G. F.; Fujiwara, K.; Pollard, T. D., and Unanue, E. R.: Redistribution of myosin accompanying capping of surface Ig. J. exp. Med. *145:* 1393–1398 (1977).

7 Taylor, R. B.; Duffus, P. H.; Raff, M. C., and DePetris, S.: Redistribution and pinocytosis of lymphocyte surface immunoglobulin molecules induced by anti-immunoglobulin antibody. Nature new Biol. *233:* 225–238 (1971).

8 Unanue, E. R.; Ault, K. A., and Karnovsky, M. J.: Ligand-induced movement of lymphocyte membrane macromolecules. IV. Stimulation of cell movement by anti-Ig and lack of relationship to capping. J. exp. Med. *139:* 295–312 (1974).

9 Ward, P. A.; Unanue, E. R.; Goralnick, S., and Schreiner, G. F.: Chemotaxis of rat lymphocytes. J. Immun. *119:* 416–421 (1977).

Dr. E. R. Unanue, Department of Pathology, Harvard Medical School, Boston, MA 02115 (USA)

Immunopathology. 6th Int. Convoc. Immunol., Niagara Falls, N.Y., 1978, pp. 311–315 (Karger, Basel 1979)

Physicochemical Aspects of Phagocytosis and of Some Phagocytic Disorders[1]

C. J. van Oss, J. M. Bernstein, B. H. Park, L. J. Cianciola and R. J. Genco

Departments of Microbiology, Pediatrics, and Oral Biology, State University of New York at Buffalo, Buffalo, N.Y.

Introduction

The physical surface properties of phagocytic cells that one can discern to be of importance in cellular attraction (or repulsion), in cellular locomotion, in adhesion and in ingestion, are: cellular surface potential, interfacial free energy, cell shape, and surface viscosity. At present, the first three of these four physical properties are open to measurement. Changes in any of these four properties may result in changes in some aspect of phagocytic activity, and thus give rise to altered resistance to infectious agents *in vivo*.

Physical Surface Properties of Phagocytes

Cellular Surface Potential. The strength of the negative electrical surface potential (ζ-potential) of either bacteria or phagocytic cells is not directly linked with the greater or lesser propensity for bacteria to become adsorbed and/or ingested [8]. Virtually all cells, bacteria and other biological particles normally have a high enough ζ-potential to prevent their mutual approach to a smaller separation distance than $\approx$ 50–80 Å [11,

[1] Supported in part by PHS Grant DE 04898 of the National Institute of Dental Research.

12], and it is only when cellular protrusions attain with radii of curvature < 500 Å that molecular contact becomes a possibility [8, 10–12]. Thus, for allowing intercellular contact, cell shape (see below) is more crucial than cell charge. Disorders involving ζ-potential abnormalities of phagocytic cells are not at present known, nor would they be likely to have a strong influence on phagocytic ingestion.

Interfacial Free Energy. The difference in interfacial free energy between bacteria (and other particles) and phagocytic cells is the major factor in the decision between engulfment and non-engulfment. Bacteria (or other particles) that are more hydrophobic than phagocytes become readily engulfed, and generally are of low virulence; bacteria that are more hydrophilic than phagocytes tend to escape engulfment and are pathogenic [8, 11]. Hydrophilic bacteria are made more hydrophobic by specific antibodies (thermo-stable opsonins), and complement ($C\overline{1423}$) (thermo-labile opsonins) further enhances this hydrophobicity [8, 11, 14–17]. Especially for the most hydrophilic of phagocytic cells, the polymorphonuclear granulocytes (PMNs), their surface hydrophilicity for purely thermodynamic reasons can entirely account for their engulfment of complexes exhibiting Fc tails of several IgG molecules and/or C3b entities, so that at least for these cells, receptor hypotheses are superfluous [8, 11, 14–17]. The pronounced hydrophilicity of PMNs clearly is a strong advantage in the continuing curtailment of the growth of many varieties of bacteria that are only marginally hydrophobic. A decrease in hydrophilicity of peripheral PMNs would therefore tend to lead to a diminished resistance to certain bacterial infections.

In a number of categories of intractable idiopathic bacterial infections in children and young adults, such a decrease in hydrophilicity of PMNs coupled with their diminished *in vitro* phagocytic activity has been encountered and is discussed below.

Cell Shape. As discussed above, the negative ζ-potential of all cells suspended in watery media normally suffices to prevent close intercellular approach, unless at least one of the cell types involved is endowed with protrusions with rather small radii of curvature (< 500 Å) [8, 10–12]. Elevated blood glucose levels, which are known to cause a decrease in phagocytic activity and in leukocyte adhesiveness *in vitro* [7], do not cause a change in either the ζ-potential [8] or the hydrophilicity of phagocytes [8, 10, 12]. But hyperglycemia does induce phagocytes to adopt a more spherical shape and to lose their propensity to form pseudopodia [12]. Thus, under the influence of glucose, hydrophobic-hydrophilic cell interactions are much diminished due to the uniform electrostatic cell repulsion, no longer overcome by the cellular protrusions of small radii of curvature that normally bridge the electrical double layer. The increased incidence of bacterial infections among imperfectly controlled diabetes is surely to an important extent due to this effect of high glucose levels [7, 8, 10, 12], but even intermittent contact with glucose (e.g. during a few seconds, every 2 min, for a few hours) has the same effect [9]. The latter fact may well be connected with the increased suscep-

tibility to bacterial infections among patients with trauma and following surgery [1, 2] who are subjected to frequent and sustained glucose infusions.

Surface Viscosity. In contrast to the three other physical cell surface properties discussed above, there does not as yet appear to exist a reliable method for the measurement of the surface viscosity of cells. The discussion of this parameter, however great its possible importance, must therefore of necessity be brief. The elasticity, the deformability and the mobility of the cell membrane must be linked to the degree of surface viscosity, and these properties are in their turn connected to cell deformability and cell shape (see above) as well as to the cells' general mobility and their response to chemotactic stimuli. The locomotive activity is found to be impaired in certain phagocytic disorders, in conjunction with disorders of surface hydrophilicity of phagocytic cells (see below).

Disorders of Surface Hydrophilicity of PMNs

The most convenient method for the quantitative measurement of the degree of hydrophilicity of living cells is the determination of the contact angle sessile drops of saline water make with flat layers of them. With human PMNs that angle is remarkably constant, it normally is close to $18°$ [7, 8, 11].

Children with Chronic Upper Respiratory Infections. A number of children (with no obvious immunologic disorders) with intractable chronic upper respiratory infections have been studied. It was found that the contact angle of their peripheral PMNs was significantly increased (i.e. PMNs had become less hydrophilic) and that their *in vitro* phagocytic activity was markedly diminished [3, 6, 13]. The contact angle and phagocytic activity data of 1 of these cases [15] are

Table I. The influence of various factors on the contact angle and on the phagocytic activity of the granulocytes of patients and of normal granulocytes

Granulocytes	Pretreatment[1]	Contact angle degrees $\pm$ SE	Phagocytic activity[2] in % of normal $\pm$ SE
A. Pediatric patient B			
Patient's	pat. serum	*19.0 $\pm$ 0.45*[3]	*69.7 $\pm$ 4.1*[4]
Patient's	pat. serum + alb.	17.6 $\pm$ 0.1	104.1 $\pm$ 6.2
Patient's	cont. serum	*17.8 $\pm$ 0.15*[3]	*97.9 $\pm$ 5.5*[4]
Control	pat. serum	*18.3 $\pm$ 0.2*[5]	*77.8 $\pm$ 4.9*[6]
Control	cont. serum + alb.	17.6 $\pm$ 0.25	101.2 $\pm$ 4.9
Control	cont. serum	*17.5 $\pm$ 0.2*[5]	*100.0 $\pm$ 5.6*[6]
B. IJP patient K			
Patient's	pat. serum	*19.2 $\pm$ 0.5*[7]	*64.3 $\pm$ 6.4*[8]
Patient's	pat. serum + alb.	17.7 $\pm$ 0.1	94.9 $\pm$ 7.1
Patient's	cont. serum	*17.7 $\pm$ 0.3*[7]	*97.3 $\pm$ 10.3*[8]
Control	pat. serum	17.6 $\pm$ 0.2	99.1 $\pm$ 4.6
Control	cont. serum + alb.	17.5 $\pm$ 0.2	89.4 $\pm$ 6.1
Control	cont. serum	17.6 $\pm$ 0.2	100.0 $\pm$ 7.1

[1] Granulocytes were incubated alone for 30 min in these media, followed with two washings with Hanks' balanced salt solution, and contact angle and phagocytosis determinations.
[2] Mean number of *Staphylococcus aureus* particles (pre-opsonized with 1 % human IgG) ingested per granulocyte; expressed in percent of activity of control cells.
Significance of difference between values in italics: [3] $p < 0.04$; [4] $p < 0.001$; [5] $p < 0.007$; [6] $p < 0.003$; [7] $p < 0.005$; [8] $p < 0.0002$.

grouped in table I.A. This child's PMNs only had a high contact angle and a decreased phagocytic activity when the cells had been previously incubated in the child's own serum. After incubation of the child's PMNs in normal serum, or in the child's own serum after addition of serum albumin (raising its albumin concentration from 4.5 to 5.1%), the phagocytic activity and the contact angle of his PMNs reverted to normal values. Conversely, PMNs from a normal subject, previously incubated in the child's serum, had an increased contact angle and diminished phagocytic activity. Also in this case, addition of serum albumin to the child's serum restored the contact angle and the phagocytic activity of the control cells to

normal levels. Increases in the serum albumin content of normal sera had *no* effect on the properties of granulocytes incubated in them (table I). There appears to be a factor in this child's (and in some other children's) serum that causes a decrease in the hydrophilicity and in the phagocytic activity of PMNs. That factor does not seem to be serum albumin. An increase in serum albumin level does, however, counteract its effects *in vitro*, and *in vivo* administration of serum albumin to another child (whose PMNs showed very similar properties *in vitro*) brought about a remarkable, if temporary, clinical improvement. The latter child's PMNs in addition showed an impaired chemotactic response *in vitro*, but with normal intracellular metabolism and lysosomal enzymes [3]. It should be noted that our monolayer method for the *in vitro* measurement of phagocytic ingestion [7, 8, 11] is not directly affected by the chemotactic properties of the phagocytes.

Patients with Idiopathic Juvenile Periodontitis. The PMNs of 10 young people with localized idiopathic juvenile periodontitis (IJP) were studied [4]. It was found that in all cases their peripheral PMNs had significantly (p < 0.05) higher contact angles (19.5° average) than matched normal subjects (17.9° average). Also, the IJP patients' PMNs *in vitro* phagocytic activity was significantly less (i.e. ≈ 36%) than that of the matched normal subject's PMNs. The locomotive activity of the IJP patient's PMNs was also significantly diminished [4].

Further IJP patients have been studied since, and in the light of the findings with the children with upper respiratory infections, discussed above (table I.A), the influence of the patients' sera on their (and other) PMNs was also studied. Table I.B shows the findings of a typical IJP case. Again, precisely as in the pediatric case depicted in table I.A, this patient's PMNs only had a high contact angle and a decreased phagocytic activity when the cells had been pre-incubated in the patient's own serum. After incubation of the patient's PMNs in normal serum, or in the patient's own serum after addition of 0.5% serum albumin, the phagocytic activity *and* the contact angle of her PMNs reverted to normal values. However, contrary to the pediatric cases exemplified in table I.A, the sera of these dental patients did not have the power to increase the hydrophobicity and depress the phagocytic activity of PMNs from normal subjects. There nevertheless also appears to be a factor in these IJP patients' sera that causes a decrease in hydrophilicity and in the phagocytic activity of their own PMNs, which can be counteracted on *in vitro* by the addition of serum albumin.

Discussion and Conclusions

Various physical surface properties of phagocytic cells can play a role in their ingestive capacities: electrical potential, interfacial free energy, shape (radius of curvature of parts of the cell) and surface viscosity. The electrical surface potential generally prevents intercellular contact by mutual electrostatic repulsions, unless processes with small radii of curvature are present that can overcome the repulsion and establish contact. Elevated blood glucose levels cause a decrease in the formation of such pseudopodia and thus inhibit intercellular contact, resulting in a decrease in phagocytic ingestion. This is probably one of the major factors in the high incidence of bacterial infections among imperfectly controlled diabetes, and a possible contributing cause in the increased susceptibility to bacterial infections among trauma and surgery patients who receive frequent glucose infusions. However, once contact can be made the interfacial free energy differences of cell surfaces play the major role in causing or preventing engulfment: hydrophilic phagocytes tend to engulf hydrophobic bacteria and other cells or particles. Normally, human peripheral PMNs are quite hydrophilic (their contact angle is about 18°), and their phagocytic activity is correspondingly diminished. That leukocyte defect appears linked to a factor present in the sera of these patients. Increasing the serum albumin level of the sera makes the patients' PMNs revert to normal *in vitro*, and has at least in one instance brought about a striking but temporary improvement *in vivo*.

Little is known as yet about possible changes in cellular surface viscosity and their effects. Increases in cell surface viscosity could plausibly result in a decrease in locomotive capacity, and thus in a diminished chemotactic response. The same factors that cause a cell's surface to become more hydrophobic may well also influence its surface viscosity, which in turn can readily affect a cell's propensity to extend pseudopodia and hence its locomotive power.

All four principal physical cell surface properties discussed above thus appear to be linked together in various ways, and as demonstrated above with a number of cases, changes in one or more of these surface properties can have important pathological effects that bear directly upon patients' capacity to resist microbial infections.

References

1 Alexander, J. W. and Good, R. A.: Immunobiology for surgeons, p. 10 (Saunders, Philadelphia 1970).
2 Altemeier, W. A.: The significance of infection in trauma. Bull. Am. Coll. Surg. 1: 7–16 (1972).
3 Bernstein, J. M. and Gillman, C. F.: Phagocytic dysfunction as a cause of recurrent upper respiratory disease (abstr.) Trans. Am. Acad. Ophthal. Otolar. 82: 509 (1976).
4 Cianciola, L. J., Genco, R. J.; Patters, M. R.; McKenna, J., and Oss, C. J. van: Defective polymorphonuclear leukocyte function in a human periodontal disease. Nature, Lond. 265: 445–447 (1977).
5 Cunningham, R. K.; Söderström, T. O.; Gillman, C. F., and Oss, C. J. van: Phagocytosis as a surface phenomenon. V. Contact angles and phagocytosis of tough and smooth strains of Salmonella typhimurium and the influence of specific antiserum. Immunol. Commun. 4: 429–442 (1975).
6 Gillman, C. F.; Bernstein, J. M., and Oss, C. J. van: Decreased phagocytosis associated with increased surface hydrophobicity of neutrophils of children with chronic infections (abstr.). Fed. Proc. Fed. Am. Socs exp. Biol. 35: 227 (1976).
7 Oss, C. J. van: The influence of glucose levels on the in vitro phagocytosis of bacteria by human neutrophils. Infec. Immun. 4: 54–59 (1971).
8 Oss, C. J. van: Phagocytosis as a surface phenomenon. Annu. Rev. Microbiol. 32: 19–39 (1978).

9 Oss, C. J. van and Border, J. R.: Influence of intermittent hyperglycemic glucose levels on the phagocytosis of microorganisms by human granulocytes in vitro. Immunol. Commun. 7: 669–676 (1978).
10 Oss, C. J. van; Gillman, C. F., and Good, R. J.: The influence of the shape of phagocytes on their adhesiveness. Immunol. Commun. 1: 627–636 (1972).
11 Oss, C. J. van; Gillman, C. F., and Neumann, A. W.: Phagocytic engulfment and cell adhesiveness (Dekker, New York 1975).
12 Oss, C. J. van; Good, R. J., and Neumann, A. W.: The connection of interfacial free energies and surface potentials with phagocytosis and cellular adhesiveness. J. electroanal. Chem. 37: 387–391 (1972).
13 Oss, C. J. van; Park, B. H.; Bernstein, J. M., and Gillman, C. F.: Diminished hydrophilicity of granulocytes in children who are prone to bacterial infections. Influence of serum factors. Abstr. 51st Colloid Surf. Sci. Symp., Grand Island, New York 1977 pp. 100–101.
14 Stendahl, O.; Tagesson, C., and Edebo, L.: Influence of hyperimmune immunoglobulin G on the physicochemical properties of the surface of Salmonella typhimurium 395 MS in relation to interaction with phagocytic cells. Infec. Immun. 10: 316–319 (1974).
15 Stendahl, O.; Tagesson, C.; Magnusson, K. E., and Edebo, L.: Physicochemical consequences of opsonization of Salmonella typhimurium with hyperimmune IgG and complement. Immunology 32: 11–18 (1977).
16 Stjernström, I.; Magnusson, K. E.; Stendahl, O., and Tagesson, C.: Liability to hydrophobic and charge interaction of smooth Salmonella typhimurium 395 MS sensitized with anti-MS immunoglobulin G and complement. Infec. Immun. 10: 261–265 (1977).
17 Tagesson, C.; Magnusson, K. E., and Stendahl, O.: Physicochemical consequences of opsonization: perturbation of liposomal membranes by Salmonella typhimurium 395 MS opsonized with IgG antibodies. J. Immun. 119: 609–613 (1977).

Dr. C. J. van Oss, Department of Microbiology, School of Medicine, State University of New York at Buffalo, Buffalo, NY 14214 (USA)

Workshops

Immunopathology. 6th Int. Convoc. Immunol., Niagara Falls, N.Y., 1978, pp. 316–317 (Karger, Basel 1979)

Workshop A

New Trends in Immunohistology

Chairmen: *G. A. Andres*, Departments of Microbiology, Pathology, and Medicine, State University of New York at Buffalo, Buffalo, N.Y., and *G. Wick*, Institute for General and Experimental Pathology, University of Innsbruck, Innsbruck

Contributors: *A. G. Engel*, Department of Neurology, Mayo Medical School, Rochester, Minn.; *N. K. Gonatas*, Department of Pathology, University of Pennsylvania, Philadelphia, Pa.; *S. Shibata*, The Third Department of Internal Medicine, University of Tokyo, Tokyo, and *T. Sugisaki*, Department of Internal Medicine, Showa University, Tokyo

G. Andres opened the Workshop by giving a brief historical review of recent developments in immunohistology. He mentioned the use of new tracers in combination with scanning electron microscopy, the preparation of hybrid antibodies with dual specificity, the application of labeled lectins, and recent progress in immunoautoradiography.

G. Wick then gave a short review on what he considered to be some major areas of present and future immunohistological investigations. The following examples were listed: (1) *Technical developments:* use of laser illumination for immunofluorescence; fluorescent-activated cell sorter (FACS); microfluorometry and pattern recognition; automation of immunohistological procedures. (2) *Methods:* use of enzyme (e.g. pronase)-treated paraffin sections for immunohistological studies; combination of immunofluorescence and cytoadherence techniques. (3) *Reagents:* use of Fab and F(ab')$_2$ conjugates; labeling with new fluorochromes, e.g., the blue-fluorescing SITS (4-acetamide-4'-isothiocyanato-stilbene-2, 2'-disulphonic acid); purification of IgG antibodies and conjugates by affinity chromatography with staphylococcal protein A (SPA); use of reference preparations from WHO; standardization of immunofluorescence and immunoenzymatic methods using the defined antigenic substrate spheres (DASS) system. (4) *Applications:* detection of immune complexes by immunohistological methods; demonstration of hormone receptors on cell surfaces; development of leukemia-specific antibodies; use of cell hybridization for the production of monoclonal, high titered antibodies; diagnostic use of specific antibodies to polymorphic variants of collagen, such as type IV basement membrane collagen.

N. K. Gonatas discussed the use of lectins coupled to horseradish peroxidase (HRP) for the analysis of cell surfaces, especially for the process of adsorptive endocytosis. He used the two-step conjugation method recommended by *Avrameas and Ternynck* and separated the conjugate from free HRP and free ligand by column chromatography on Sephadex G-200. These procedures were exemplified by data obtained with ricin and wheat germ agglutinins. Although the yield of conjugate was low, the final product proved to be highly pure and active. The use of this wheat germ agglutinin conjugate for the analysis of absorptive endocytosis was demonstrated both in suspensions of neuroblastoma cells and on tissue sections of the central nervous system. For development of staining, *N. K. Gonatas* recommended tetramethylbenzidine. The staining pattern on the sections corresponds to that found after silver impregnation. The description of technical details can be found in the following review: *Gonatas, N. K. and Avrameas, S.:* Detection of carbohydrates with lectin-peroxidase conjugates. Methods in cell biology, vol. XV, chap. 23, pp. 387–406; Academic Press, New York 1977.

The next speaker, *A. G. Engel*, presented extensive data on immunohistological investigations on the motoric end plate (MEP) in normal muscle and in muscle from patients with myasthenia gravis (MG). He specifically addressed himself to: (1) the ultrastructural identification of the acetylcholine receptors (ACHR), (2) light and electron microscopical localization of ACHR at the end plate, and (3) the demonstration of complement at the MEP in MG. The immunohistological reagents employed included HRP-bungarotoxin, SPA-HRP for the demonstration of bound IgG, and HRP-labeled rabbit anti-rat C$_3$. The HRP-bungarotoxin was found to bind to the MEP in preparations of fresh, living muscle. Ultrastructurally, the binding sites were identified at the internal extensions of the junctional folds of normal MEP. In MG the abundance of ACHR was significantly reduced. Using morphometric methods, the receptor surface area and the electric potential of the MEP showed a clear-cut correlation. Using the HRP-SPA, conjugate IgG was demonstrated at the MEP of MG patients. C3 could be located at this site too. Ultrastructural analysis revealed that the immune complexes were localized in the synaptic space and in the altered postsynaptic membrane.

T. Sugisaki discussed the question whether the immune response of various strains of rats to homologous brush border antigens might result in antibody formation to different antigens and hence in different renal lesions. The following recipient strains were used: Sprague-Dawley (SD), Fisher, Buffalo, August, Brown Norway (BN), Lewis (L), Wistar and Brown Norway X Lewis hybrids (L/BN). The renal antigen preparation consisted of homogenized kidney from SD rats. Groups of rats were sacrificed 2–8 weeks after the second injection of antigen and the kidneys were studied by immunofluorescence. The following staining patterns were observed: (1) granular deposit of IgG and C3 along the glomerular basement membrane (GBM) in all strains; (2) granular deposits of IgG and C3 along the tubular basement membrane (TBM), particularly prominent in Lewis rats; (3) linear staining of the basement membrane of proximal tubules in BN and L/BN rats; (4) homogenous deposits of IgG in the loops of Henle and distal convoluted tubules in SD, Fisher and August rats; (5) mononuclear cell infiltrates in the peritubular and perivascular areas, without concomitant deposits of IgG, in Lewis and Wistar rats.

The last speaker, *S. Shibata*, presented the results of studies concerning experimental glomerulonephritis induced in rats by injection of a glycopeptide ('nephritogenoside') purified from the GBM. The principle of the preparation of the nephritogenic peptide was outlined by presentation of flowcharts and gel filtration curves. After digestion with trypsin, followed by electrophoresis and gel filtration, a glycoprotein (GP) was obtained that was labile to periodate oxidation. Then, by extensive proteolytic digestion, a small nephritogenic glycopeptide was recovered. Further purification yielded the so-called 'pure nephritogenoside' (NG) which had a molecular weight of about 6,000. The NG contained at least 3 branched glucose residues. The yield was about 10 mg from 1 kg of renal cortex. Both the GP and the NG were found to induce glomerulonephritis when injected into rats. By immunofluorescence, the animals developed granular deposits of IgG along the GBM and in the mesangium. Animals immunized with NG developed mesangial IgG deposits only. Finally, *S. Shibata* showed that the GP can be purified by adsorption to Con A columns. The binding of FITC-Con A to the GBM may then be explained by a possible coating of the GBM with GP.

Immunopathology. 6th Int. Convoc. Immunol., Niagara Falls, N.Y., 1978, pp. 318–319 (Karger, Basel 1979)

Workshop B

Detection of Circulating Immune Complexes

Chairmen: *K. Kano*, Department of Microbiology, State University of New York at Buffalo, Buffalo, N.Y., and *P. H. Lambert*, World Health Organization, Immunology Research and Training Center, Blood Transfusion Center, Cantonal Hospital, Geneva

Contributors: *B. Albini*, Department of Microbiology, State University of New York at Buffalo, Buffalo, N.Y.; *P. Casali*, World Health Organization, Immunology Research and Training Center, Hospital Cantonal, Geneva; *P. Grabar*, Pasteur Institute, Paris; *F. Milgrom*, Department of Microbiology, State University of New York at Buffalo, Buffalo, N.Y.; *T. Nishimaki*, Department of Microbiology, State University of New York at Buffalo, Buffalo, N.Y.; *T. Palosuo*, Central Public Health Laboratory, Helsinki; *E. Penner*, Department of Microbiology, State University of New York at Buffalo, Buffalo, N.Y., and *I. M. Roitt*, Department of Immunology, Middlesex Hospital Medical School, London

This Workshop was devoted to the discussion of recent advances in the methodology of assays for the detection of immune complexes (IC) in sera and tissues. *P. H. Lambert* reviewed various techniques for the detection of circulating IC. As the possible source of false-positive results he identified polyanionic substances (e.g. DNA), aggregated IgG, and various antibodies which may be present in pathologic sera. In a collaborative study performed recently by several laboratories under the auspices of the World Health Organization, 17 different methods based on biological properties of IC were compared (tests based on interaction of IC with Clq; with conglutinin; with rheumatoid factors; with Fc and C3 receptors of cells). All these tests cannot distinguish between IC and aggregated γ-globulins. The sensitivity of each method depends on the reactivity of the various classes and subclasses of immunoglobulin, and on the characteristics of the IC. The methods with the highest sensitivity seem to be tests using Raji cells, followed by the solid-phase rheumatoid factor and solid-phase Clq assays.

P. Casali reported on the use of solid-phase human Clq and bovine conglutinin for the isolation of IC. This procedure involves two steps: (a) the lipid-free serum (lipids are removed by incubation with freon) is precipitated by polyethylene glycol, and (b) the solubilized precipitate is adsorbed on columns of polymethyl methacrylate beads coated with conglutinin or Clq. After washing the column, the IC are eluted with 0.02 M EDTA (in the case of the conglutinin column) or 0.5 M NaCl (in the case of the Clq column). Using these procedures, the following IC prepared *in vitro* were analyzed: (1) IC consisting of bovine serum albumin (BSA) and antibodies to BSA produced in rabbits; (2) tetanus toxoid and its corresponding antibody from human sera,

and (3) HBsAg and the corresponding antibody from patients. In all the final preparations, the antigen, the antibody, Clq, Clr, Cls, and C3 could be demonstrated. In addition, IC formed *in vivo* and present in the sera of patients with disseminated leishmaniasis (Kala Azar) were isolated. It was shown that they contained IgM, IgG, Clq, Clr, Cls, C3c, and C3d. *P. Casali* pointed out that this method seems to be useful in the search for antigens involved and in the analysis of the composition of IC found in the circulation.

F. Milgrom presented the immunological evidence for a molecular transformational change occurring in the antibody molecule after reaction with the specific antigen. In these studies, which were initiated 20 years ago, it was shown that antibody acquired a new antigenic specificity after reaction with the specific antigen. The antibody recognizing this novel antigen on the immunoglobulin molecule was described as 'anti-antibody' (AA); it belongs, in the human system, to the IgM class, and is found with low frequency among normal blood donors. The notion of a molecular transformational change suggested originally on the basis of serological findings found strong support in the physiochemical data obtained by *Robert and Grabar*, and by *Ishizaka and Campbell*.

P. Grabar and *F. Milgrom* discussed the use of electrophoresis (especially electrophoresis at 56°C) for the splitting of IC and for the demonstration of antigen and antibody. This method has been especially useful in the case of IC in systemic lupus erythematosus.

T. Palosuo introduced AA inhibition test and discussed the possible automation of the test. He showed that the AA inhibition test is specific for IC and that its sensitivity is comparable to that of other procedures such as the Raji cell test. The only problem of this test, at present, would be the scarcity of the reagent with AA of high titer. However, *F. Milgrom* assured the audience that his group will soon be able to secure such reagents to distribute them to the interested investigators.

T. Nishimaki utilized the AA inhibition test for the identification of antigens in IC found in rheumatoid arthritis sera. His data clearly demonstrated heterophile Hanganutziu-Deicher antigen or IgG in the IC.

K. Kano presented data on IC in renal transplantation sera and chronically rejected renal grafts. By using the AA absorption test, he was able to detect IC deposition in renal grafts, even in the absence of circulating IC at the time of graft removal.

I. Roitt introduced his procedure of isolation of IC. He employed a sucrose density gradient incorporating PEG followed by SDS-PAGE in a two-dimensional system which allowed for the determination of molecular weights of constituents of IC.

B. Albini discussed a modification of the Raji cell test. In this method, test sera are diluted serially in hemagglutination plates and subsequently are reacted with Raji cells and the appropriate FITC-conjugated antisera. This microtest using immunofluorescent staining procedures renders semiquantitative data expressed as titers. The results show a 'technical' variability of one to two titer steps. Standardization of the methodology is essential; thus, cells have to be harvested 72 h after feeding of the culture, as the ratio of C3 to Fc receptors is optimal at this time; undiluted serum very often gives nonspecific reactions; and the concentration of the anti-serum used has to be kept constant to allow for comparison of tests performed at different times. The use of radiolabelled sera, which allows for expression of the results in 'micrograms of aggregated γ-globulin standard' is more sensitive than the method described here; it seems, however, to have the disadvantage of pretending to be a quantitative test which it clearly is not in view of the variability of the quality of the aggregated γ-globulin used as standard and the probable broad range of differences in the properties of IC tested.

E. Penner presented his studies on IC in various liver diseases employing both AA inhibition test and Raji cell test. Data on alcoholic liver diseases as well as hepatitis B virus (HBV) associated liver diseases obtained by these two tests appeared to be in good agreement. In alcoholic liver disease, IgG-containing immune complexes were detectable only in patients with active disease, as exemplified by acute alcoholic hepatitis and active alcoholic cirrhosis. In addition, IgA-containing immune complexes were demonstrated in the majority of sera positive for IgG complexes. Immune complexes were also quite frequently observed in HBV-associated diseases, with the highest frequency being observed in the prodromal, serum sickness-like stage of acute hepatitis.

In summary, *K. Kano* concluded that the present status of IC technology is quite similar to that of HLA technology 10 years ago and stressed the need of a bench-type workshop for the evaluation of various procedures in the very near future.

Immunopathology. 6th Int. Convoc. Immunol., Niagara Falls, N.Y., 1978, pp. 320–321 (Karger, Basel 1979)

Workshop C

Radioimmunoassays

Chairmen: *K. Ishizaka*, Departments of Medicine and Microbiology, The Johns Hopkins University, Baltimore, Md., and *A. O. Vladutiu*, Immunopathology Laboratory, Buffalo General Hospital, Buffalo, N.Y.

Contributors: *J.-F. Bach*, Nephrology Research Unit, Necker Hospital, Paris; *I. K. Mushawar*, Abbott Laboratories, Chicago, Ill.; *V. Pezzino*, Metabolism Section, Veterans Administration Hospital, San Francisco, Calif.; *D. Pressman*, Roswell Park Memorial Institute, Buffalo, N.Y.; *M. Shimizu*, Allergy Research Laboratory, Buffalo, N.Y., and *C. B. Wilson*, Department of Immunopathology, Scripps Clinic and Research Foundation, La Jolla, Calif.

Procedures for radioimmunoassays (RIA) were first described in the early 1950s. This laboratory technique permits accurate measurement of minute amounts of substances. It revolutionized many fields of medicine, e.g. endocrinology. The RIA owes its exquisite specificity to the use of antibodies and hence immunology was strongly implicated in the development of RIA. Surprisingly, however, RIA is still not used extensively in immunology. Nevertheless, there is little doubt that RIA can help the advancement of immunology in general and also of immunopathology.

It is unanimously accepted that the antibody is the most important constituent of an RIA. The antibody cannot be prepared *in vitro* and we still have to rely on the ability of animals to make antibody. However, it is possible to manipulate the antigenicity of a substance and, by use of various adjuvants and schemes of immunization, it is possible to influence the antibody response. This perhaps is a topic to which the immunologists should pay more attention. If the production of antibody becomes more scientifically controlled, the sensitivity and specificity of RIA will be increased and new RIA will become feasible. Various autoantigens or autoantibodies can be accurately quantitated by RIA and their amount can be related to the degree of tissue damage due to an autoimmune reaction. Mediators of hypersensitivity reaction could be detected by RIA in minute amounts and this can have a diagnostic role in immune diseases. Various cell markers can be measured by RIA. For instance, an RIA for HLA antigens (or other *MHC*-determined antigens) can quantitate their expression on cells. Perhaps one of the important actions of the viruses is to alter the expression of surface antigens on the cell membrane and thus to enhance or decrease the host's T lymphocyte cytotoxicity.

Several specific RIA of importance to immunopathology were discussed at the Workshop. The technical

data and mainly the importance of these RIAs for the investigations of the immune reactions were emphasized. *D. Pressman* pointed out that any test that uses radiolabeled antigens or antibodies should be called radioimmunoassay. He showed that by labelling antibodies to CEA with radioiodine, it is possible to localize the CEA-producing cells. Moreover, if the radiolabeled antibodies are attached to various drugs, these can be made to act only on tumor cells.

A simple, sensitive and reproducible immunoradiometric assay for the detection of the e antigen of hepatitis B virus (HBeAg) and of its corresponding antibody (anti-HBe) was reported by *I. K. Mushawar*. The HBeAg is different from all the other markers of hepatitis B virus and it could be either a part of a host antigen modified by the virus, or a true viral antigen. HBeAg serves as a marker of aggressiveness in chronic active hepatitis and of increased infectivity of HBsAg-positive blood. The RIA for HBeAg is 1,000 times more sensitive than the immunodiffusion and the solid-phase inhibition type of RIA for anti-HBe is 6,000 times more sensitive than the immunodiffusion method. These assays can be used to better understand the pathogenesis of type B viral hepatitis.

An RIA for an organ-specific autoantigen, human thyroglobulin, was described by *V. Pezzino*. Thyroglobulin quantitation is of clinical value for the investigation of various thyroid disorders. The assay is sensitive to 2.5 ng/ml and thyroglobulin is detectable in 84% of euthyroid subjects; elevated values are observed in patients with hyperthyroidism and decreased values in hypothyroidism.

C. Wilson presented RIA for the detection of antibody to glomerular basement membrane (GBM) antigen(s). Chloramine T is used for iodination of this antigen(s). Using this test, antibodies to GBM were detected in many patients with the Goodpasture syndrome. They, however, are transitory in nature. Their role in the follow-up of patients is not yet proven but by use of this assay, the response of patients to plasmapheresis can be monitored. *J. F. Bach* discussed the relationship between the level of circulating anti-GBM antibodies and their fixation in the kidney.

A new solid-phase RIA for measuring IgG to bee venom antigens in allergic patients was reported by *M. Shimizu*. The principle of the test is similar to that of the radioallergosorbent test for IgE antibody. It uses cyanogenbromide-activated paper discs. Various technical points such as addition of Tween 20 in the incubation buffer were discussed.

It became evident from the Workshop that RIA can be used in various animal models of autoimmune diseases as well as in the study of other immunologically mediated diseases in humans. There is quite a large number of RIA techniques. The chloramine T appears to be a commonly used method of iodination of various proteins. Solid-phase assays, which do not require a second antibody, are becoming more common, especially since these assays require less time to be performed. It may be hoped that RIA will be used more often for quantitation of various mediators of hypersensitivity reactions, for lymphokines, and for the detection of idiotypes and anti-idiotypes.

Immunopathology. 6th Int. Convoc. Immunol., Niagara Falls, N.Y., 1978, pp. 322–323 (Karger, Basel 1979)

Workshop D

Diagnostic Relevance of *in vitro* Assays for Cellular Immunity

Chairmen: *T. T. Provost*, Departments of Dermatology and Medicine, State University of New York at Buffalo, Buffalo, N.Y., and *J. L. Turk*, Department of Pathology, Institute of Basic Medical Sciences, Royal College of Surgeons of England, London

Contributors: *B. Arredondo*, The Venezuelian Institute for Sientific Research (IVIC), Caracas; *E. Kondracki*, The Venezuelian Institute for Sientific Research (IVIC), Caracas; *I. B. Malavé*, The Venezuelian Institute for Sientific Research (IVIC), Caracas; *M. Reichlin*, Department of Medicine, State University of New York at Buffalo, Buffalo, N.Y.; *J. S. Smolen*, Second Medical Department, University of Vienna, Vienna, and *V. Untermohlen*, Division of Nutritional Sciences, Cornell University, Ithaca, N.Y.

In opening the discussion, *J. L. Turk* defined four questions to be discussed. (1) Is there a correlation between *in vitro* tests, especially the lymphocyte transformation test (LTT), and effector mechanisms in immunopathologic processes and resistance to infection? (2) Is there a correlation between the delayed hypersensitivity skin test (DHT) and effector mechanisms in immunopathologic processess and resistance to infection? (3) Is there a correlation between DHT with allergic processes rather than with resistance? (4) Are there any new ideas for upgrading the quantitation of tests for cell-mediated immunity (CMI), especially the macrophage migration inhibition test and the leukocyte migration inhibition test (LMIT)?

J. L. Turk illustrated these four questions with examples from the work of his own group. He began with a discussion of the LTT using specific treponemal antigens in syphilis. No reactivity was found in early primary syphilis. Some activity appeared in late primary disease but was lost in secondary syphilis. A high rate of reactivity was found, however, in patients with reinfections. Nonreactive patients with both primary and secondary syphilis became strongly reactive within 1 week of chemotherapy. There was good correlation between the results of the LTT and the 'luo'-DHT described by *Noguchi*. *Noguchi* has already described an increase in DHT reactive in patients with secondary syphilis following the onset of chemotherapy. Neither the LTT nor the DHT could be considered as correlates of resistance to infection in this disease. The highest levels of LTT reactivity were found in patients with reinfections who had manifestly no resistance to the organism. Similar conclusions had been obtained by *Bjune* in leprosy; the highest levels of LTT with specific *M. leprae* were found in borderline tuberculoid leprosy rather than in polar tuberculoid leprosy. In this disease, the test results correlated rather with the allergic po-

tential of the individual to the infection than with resistance to *M. leprae*.

J. L. Turk then presented data on DHT during the development of experimental allergic orchitis in guinea pigs. Female guinea pigs immunized with sperm in complete Freund's adjuvant (CFA) had strong DHT to sperm. Male animals had only weak DHT at the time of strongest cellular infiltration in the testis. Tuberculin reactivity was similarly reduced in males, as compared to females, during the peak of the disease. Thus, skin DHT reactions could be reduced at times of strong immunopathologic reaction, possibly caused by deviation of reactive cells to the sites of strong tissue infiltration. It seems, therefore, that there are situations in autoallergic disease, in which there is no correlation between DHT and tissue damage.

During immunization with dead tularemia vaccine in incomplete Freund's adjuvant, there was strong development of both DHT and LTT despite the poor protective value of the vaccine. Cyclophosphamide (CY), 300 mg/kg given 3 days before vaccination, produced a marked increase in both DHT and LTT.

Finally, *J. L. Turk* reported on a new lymphokine-macrophage assay. Use was made of light scattering to measure *in vitro* lymphokine-induced aggregation of macrophages. The aggregometer produced a permanent, objective, record. The test was 40 times as sensitive as MIF assays. Most of the aggregation activity could be eluted from a Sephadex G-100 column with a MW of 40,000 (similar to MIF). Some material with macrophage aggregation properties seemed to have a MW of 150,000. Whether the latter represented aggregated lymphokine or immunoglobulin is not yet known. More objective and reproducible assays of this type should be developed in the future for use with the autoanalyser.

M. Reichlin described the use of guinea pig peripheral mononuclear cells as a source of lymphocytes in the LTT.

Guinea pigs sensitized with cytochrome c in CFA responded primarily with CMI. Peripheral leukocytes from sensitized animals, isolated by a Ficoll-hypaque gradient and incubated in the presence of cytochrome c produced stimulatory indices of 50–100. This is comparable to the results obtained with peritoneal exudate cells from sensitized animals purified by passage over a nylon column. *V. Untermohlen* discussed further LMIT. She stated that the LMIT was absolutely reproducible in her and in the other investigators' experience. She stressed, however, the importance of meticulous technique for the successful performance of this test. She emphasized the importance to cleanly break the capillary tube at the fluid cell interface; to eliminate air bubbles; to gently pipette; and to avoid cell clumping. In addition, the composition of the mononuclear cells employed in the LMIT assay can be important; e.g., using PPD as the antigen, it was necessary to have a cell mixture composed of roughly 10% mononuclear cells and 90% granulocytes. In contrast, the direct LMIT employing mealses antigen required only mononuclear cells which, however, had to include both macrophages and lymphocytes.

J. S. Smolen presented data on LTT suggesting CMI to denatured human type I collagen in rheumatoid arthritis (RA). LTT performed on 38 patients with RA, 9 patients with Reiters syndrome (RS), and on 32 control individuals, demonstrated that 55% of RA, 11% of RS, and 25% of controls had a positive LTT ($p < 0.05$). The LTT was performed in serum-free RPMI 1640 medium. When heat-treated blood group AB serum was added to the medium of some peripheral blood lymphocytes, some leukocyte preparation of RA patients displayed a marked inhibition of LTT when cultured in the presence of type I collagen. The nature of the inhibitor is unknown. One possibility is that the AB serum contained aggregated IgG and that rheumatoid factor activity occurred in these test sera which were inhibitory to LTT.

I. Malavé presented evidence for significant changes in mitogen-induced LTT in protein-caloric-deficient C57BL/6 mice. The proliferative response to suboptimal doses of PHA and Con A increased with the length of time of deprivation. This was secondary to a failure in the adherent cell-mediated suppressor control.

B. Arredondo presented data on an *in vivo* model for cutaneous leishmaniasis. Balb/c mice infected with *Leishmania mexicana*, which presented with chronic disseminated cutaneous leishmaniasis, developed nonspecific suppressor cells. Splenic lymphocytes from infected Balb/c mice that were cocultured with spleen lymphocytes from uninfected Balb/c mice and exposed to PHA, Con A, and lipopolysaccharide, produced a marked suppression of LTT if compared to controls. In addition, the Balb/c mice failed to mount a CMI as well as a specific antibody response against *L. mexicana*.

E. Kondracki described a technique for lymphocyte stimulation in agarose gels, which allows for the investigation of the proliferative response of single lymphocytes to specific and nonspecific mitogens. The antigen or mitogen in tissue culture medium is layered over the agarose gel containing the lymphocytes. The technique can be adapted for either liquid scintillation or autoradiographic techniques.

Author Index

Subject Index